Radio Frequency and Microwave Effects on Biological Tissues

Radio Frequency and Microwave Effects on Biological Tissues

Jitendra Behari

CRC Press
Taylor & Francis Group
Boca Raton London New York

CRC Press is an imprint of the
Taylor & Francis Group, an **informa** business

CRC Press
Taylor & Francis Group
52 Vanderbilt Avenue,
New York, NY 10017

CRC Press is an imprint of Taylor & Francis Group, an Informa business

Printed on acid-free paper

International Standard Book Number-13: 978-0-367-25459-9 (Hardback)

Library of Congress Control Number: 2019949444

Visit the Taylor & Francis Web site at
http://www.taylorandfrancis.com

and the CRC Press Web site at
http://www.crcpress.com

Contents

Preface

Present book is culmination of my teaching experience and particularly researching in the area of bioelectromagnetics, spread over about five decades. Beginning with the exploration of bioelectrical bone behavior leading to the development of the concept of bone fracture healing and osteoporosis treatment has been a long journey. This has been compiled in my earlier book *Biophysical Bone Behavior* (2009) John Wiley Asia (P Ltd.). The research and the one that followed had been supported by various sources of government funding.

The presentation in this book is divided into six chapters. The first chapter introduces the subject to the beginners and outlines the sequence of subject development. The second chapter discusses the basic issues in electromagnetics biointeraction. This chapter connects the basic electrical parameters, for example, the dielectric constant of high and low water content tissues and dielectric variation with frequency starting with MHz to GHz frequency range. Various derived parameters like role of free and bound water and their frequency dependence has been a focus of concern. The third chapter deals with all the important aspects relating to dosimetry. The dose–response relationship in biological media pertaining to nonionizing radiations is truly a complex one, for it depends on a number of environmental parameters as discussed in Chapters 2 and 3. The chapter deals with instrumentation and methods of measurement specific absorption rate (SAR) and the theoretical aspects behind it. While the issue is largely discussed, the microwave-based devices are finding use (microwave ovens and mobile phones, to name a few) by a wide range of population. While data have come up in support of distinct biological effects of microwaves, the contrary results are also reported. Since the mobile phones are right in contact with the body organs they appear to be the biggest bio-hazards and hence a complete chapter (Chapter 5) is devoted to this. Long-term exposure and their effects on central nervous system along with some epidemiological studies are presented here. The last chapter deals with the criteria and magnitude of safe exposure and the measurements of field in an open (unobstructed) environment. This is compared with the field emission from mobile towers and those emitted from mobile phones. Various safety guidelines are also discussed.

Summarily, the book discusses the advancement in the area of bioelectromagnetics vis-a-vis the emission of electromagnetic radiations from mobile phones, and the varying nature of criteria of safe exposure and biohazards presented. It is hoped that this book will serve to fill the need to better the subject and update the knowledge.

The author will consider his efforts rewarded if it serves the purpose.

Jitendra Behari
Ex Professor and Dean
School of Environmental Sciences
Jawaharlal Nehru University
New Delhi India

Acknowledgments

At the very outset, I would like to thank Mr. S. S. Kohli, Scientist G, Department of Science and Technology New Delhi, for initiating the idea of taking up this project and for his constant interest and support, which has led to the completion of the work. Thanks are also due to Amity University Noida, Uttar Pradesh, India for providing infrastructural support for carrying out this work.

The work summarized in the book includes the research carried out by the author in his carrier spanning over four decades in the area of bioelectromagnetics. During this period, the author had an opportunity to work with more than a dozen M.Phil. and doctoral students who significantly contributed in shaping the course of work. During the period various government agencies supported this activity by way of providing financial assistance. This includes Department of Science and Technology, Indian Council of Medical Research, University Grants Commission, Council of Scientific and Industrial Research, Indian National Science Academy, Jawaharlal Nehru University, etc. In the preparation of this book, several individuals have donated their computer skills, without which the work could not have taken the present shape. Profound thanks are due to them.

In the end, financial assistance obtained from Department of Science and Technology in carrying out this project is thankfully acknowledged. The author will consider his efforts rewarded if the present volume triggers more activities to provide links to many unanswered questions.

Author Biography

Jitendra Behari received his Ph.D. in physics from Indian Institute of Technology Delhi in 1971. Thereafter, he joined the Department of Biomedical Engineering, IIT & AIIMS in 1973, and later continued his career in the School of Environmental Sciences, Jawaharlal Nehru University, where he was also the Dean of the school. He retired as professor from JNU in 2012. He was conferred honorary D.Sc. in bioelectromagnetics (Ansted University, UK at Penang, Malaysia, August 2001).

During academic pursuits at JNU he was selected as a Fulbright Fellow and adjunct faculty at Michigan State University; DAAD Fellow; a Fellow of Japanese Association of Cultivation Sciences; and British Council. He has also been a Career Awardee (UGC), Fellow of Institution of Electronics and Telecommunication Engineers, Ultrasonic Society of India and a senior member of IEEE. He was also a member of Commission K of International Union of Radio Sciences (URSI), IEEE Engineering in Medicine and Biology Society and Electromagnetics Academy (USA), Indian Science Congress Association, and had been on executive bodies of Biomedical Engineering Society of India, IEEE, ED, MTT Chapter and Indian Society of Biomechanics. He has been a past chairman of IEEE ED MTT Chapter and member executive of Indian Physics Association and Indian Vacuum Society.

Dr. Behari founded Microwave Applications Society of India and has been serving it as secretary. The society regularly brings out newsletter and organized several workshops/symposia/conferences on an annual basis. His areas of research included microwave soil moisture measurements and modeling, waste water treatment with the use of nanoparticles, has published more than 100 original research publications, written several books and obtained four patents, and have developed several instruments, for example, bone stimulator for fracture heeling, rodent repellar, etc. He has been a referee for various national/international journals and funding agencies.

Summary of All the Chapters

In an attempt to cover all the aspects of RF–microwave field interaction with biological tissues, the book is divided into six chapters. The distribution of the matter over these is divided accordingly.

Biological bodies are complicated structures having spatially varying electrical properties. With water being the major constituent of biological tissues, it gives it a complex dielectric behavior, making data analysis difficult. To make a systematic approach the six chapters are planned sequentially as:

Title of the book: Radiofrequency and Microwave Effects on Biological Tissues

Chapter author: Jitendra Behari

Chapter number and title: Chapter 1: Basics of Bioelectromagnetics

The first chapter starts with introducing the subject of bioelectromagnetics, which deals with the fundamentals of electromagnetic field interaction with the biological systems (EMF biointeraction). It begins with defining the basics of electromagnetics, confines the power and energy specific to microwaves in nonionizing part of the electromagnetic spectrum. It emphasizes the importance of wave shape in relation to the nature of biological effects. The subject has its origin in observation of bioelectricity arisen due to stimulation of tissue by a direct current source and consequently the identification of bioelectric phenomena. The exposure due to time-dependent fields and their wave shape and depth of modulation (besides several others) have been reported to be more bioactive than simple continuous wave fields. Reversible change in behavior pattern is mentioned as the parameter to define the limit of safe exposure. Finally to seek a comparison between theory and experiment, it also introduces the theoretical methods leading to establishing tensor integral theorem to compute field induced inside a biological body leading to the computation of specific absorption ratio.

Key words: EMF biointeraction, specific absorption ratio, tensor integral theorem

Book title: Radiofrequency and Microwave Effects on Biological Tissues

Chapter author: Jitendra Behari

Chapter number and title: Chapter 2: Concepts in EMF Biointeraction

While the existence of low level (extremely low frequency) electromagnetic fields in the environment has been known since antiquity through their biological implications are now confirmed for several decades. As such, dosimetry of such fields and their emissions from various sources of mass utilization, along with those of RF/microwave (over a vast portion of electromagnetic spectrum) has been a subject of constant concern. When RF–microwave energy falls on a biological body the energy is transferred to the biosystem. It considers two basic mechanism of energy transfer: thermal (there is an increase in the temperature of the targeted object) and nonthermal (there is no increase in the temperature). Pertinent to the case of mobile phone frequency exposure to human head, it underlines its interaction and discusses the occurrence of "hot spots" in the brain and its spatial dependence on frequency. Due to the exposure to the E-field parallel to the human body, the resonance absorption in humans standing with and without its contact with the ground is discussed. Whole body rates of energy absorption of models of human and for animals subjected to incident fields of 10 mW/cm^2 show that rates of energy deposition at resonance in the grounded plane or over a reflector are very different. A typical value for the resonance frequency in the grounded human is 70 MHz and in the one insulated from the ground is half of this.

The difference in resonance frequency of absorption in man and child is dependent upon the difference in the head size and that of electrical properties of tissue. An important parameter deciding the amount of energy deposited in the brain is the distance of the head from the mobile antenna.

Coming down to the macroscopic phenomena pertaining to EMF interaction with biosystems is the complex permittivity of tissues. Its variation with frequency gives rise to the three major dispersion regions: alpha, beta, and gamma, with a small dispersion region falling in between beta and gamma, calling it the delta region. Assuming tissue to be a low permittivity, nonconducting sphere in water, the volume fraction solid (p) can be calculated using Maxwell's equation. Water plays a dominant role in controlling dielectric data of tissue. There is no difference between tissue water and bulk water. In brief, the basic tools to understand the interaction processes are outlined. Other processes discussed are: cell signaling, calcium signaling, and ionic diffusion. Role of free radical mechanisms action in biology is emphasized.

Book title: Radiofrequency and Microwave Effects on Biological Tissues

Chapter author: Jitendra Behari

Chapter number and title: Chapter 3: Dosimetry

This chapter deals with the most complicated aspect related to mechanism and methods in dose–response relationship, which is nonlinear. Dosimetry is the most controversial aspect in bioelectromagnetics as it is dependent on number of uncontrollable parameters. Hence to specify the uniqueness of SAR, at a given frequency or in a band of frequencies is beset with difficulties. In this chapter, methods are described, which leads to measurements of SAR describing the inherent controversies. The methods are described for both: in vivo (animal exposure) and in vitro (tissue culture, biological liquids). For in vivo measurements, for total body exposure in a transverse electromagnetic cell (TEM, DC to 500 MHz), specially designed anechoic chambers for higher frequencies up to 10 GHz were used. These chambers (above 500 MHz) can be calibrated using a specially designed probe and may be absolute power measurements are possible for SAR computation. In vitro measurements are usually carried out in a TEM cell, whereby the field is assumed to be uniform over the exposure region. An indigenously developed method for measurement of induced field and other for measurement of increase in temperature of phantom material due to mobile phone frequency exposure is also discussed. For theoretical computation, method of moments and finite-difference time domain (FDTD) are mentioned.

Book title: Radiofrequency and Microwave Effects on Biological Tissues

Chapter author: Jitendra Behari

Chapter number and title: Chapter 4: Biological Correlates of Low Level Microwave Exposure: Stress

Chapter 4 introduces the basis for the effects of nonionizing electromagnetic radiations on biological systems. The systems examined, which may facilitate to form a basis for exemplifying biological results are: immune system, blood brain barrier, nervous system, electrophysiology, electrohypersensitivity, sensory processing, effect on brain and DNA leading to cancer, model of cancer promotion, role of calcium, cell regulatory factors leading to impact on fertility pattern. Amplification process at the membrane site is by far the least understood process and seems to be resulting due to highly cooperative nonequilibrium biomolecular processes and stochastic processes.

The mechanism of signal interaction is also presented and the important role of reactive oxygen species (ROS) is emphasized. The study concludes that a reduction or an increase in antioxidative enzyme activities, protein kinase C, melatonin, caspase 3, and creatine kinase is related to overproduction of ROS in animals due to mobile phone radiation exposure. Testicular function is particularly susceptible to the radiation emitted by mobile phones kept in the waist pocket. Significant decrease in sperm count, increase in the reactive oxygen species causing damage to sperm cells, reduction in seminiferous tubules and testicular weight, and DNA damage were observed following exposure to EMF in male albino rats. The results suggest that mobile phone exposure adversely affects male fertility.

These findings on these biomarkers are clear indications of possible health implications. A chronic exposure of microwave exposure to human constitutes a nonspecific stress, which may have adverse biological effects. All symptoms of a nonspecific stress reaction of EMF exposure are visible on human behavior due to microwave exposure.

Book title: Radiofrequency and Microwave Effects on Biological Tissues

Chapter author: Jitendra Behari

Chapter number and title: Chapter 5: Biological Responses of Mobile Phone Frequency Exposure

In view of the wide ranging perception about adverse biological effects on human health due to the mobile phone frequency use, it seems pertinent to discuss their possible biological effects in particular.

While the existence of low level electromagnetic fields in the environment has been known since antiquity, their biological implications are now noted for several decades. As such, dosimetry of such field parameters and their emissions from various sources of mass utilization has been a subject of concern. Recent advancement in mobile communications has also drawn attention to their biological effects. Handheld phones are used by children and adults alike in various positions with respect to the body. Further, an increasing number of mobile communication base stations has led to wide ranging concern about possible health effects of radiofrequency emissions. There are two distinct possibilities by which health could be affected as a result of radio frequency field exposure. These are thermal effects caused by holding mobile phones close to the body and extended conversations over a long period of time. Secondly, there could be possibly nonthermal effects from both phones and base stations whereby the effects could also be cumulative. Some people may be adversely affected by the environmental impact of mobile phone base stations situated near their homes, schools, or any other place. In addition to mobile phones, appliances like microwave oven, etc., are also increasingly used. Apart from the controversy over the possible health effects due to the nonthermal effect of electromagnetic fields, the electromagnetic interaction of portable radio waves with human head needs to be quantitatively evaluated. Relating to this is the criteria of safe exposure to the population at large. To understand the mechanism by which these effects are precipitated, a number of parameters are considered, which include: blood brain barrier, tumor promotion and the role of melatonin, brain exposure, DNA strand break, and reproduction pattern in male and female. These are central to mobile phones kept in breast or waist pocket. This is followed by reporting of some important epidemiological studies. While a lot of efforts have gone into resolving the issue, a clear picture has yet to emerge. Recent reports indicate effects or no effects. It seems advisable to continue with more such studies with a common protocol to clinch the issue. Radio frequency field exposure, thermal and non thermal effects, Tumor promotion and the role of melatonin, DNA strand break, reproduction pattern, epidemiological study.

Book title: Radiofrequency and Microwave Effects on Biological Tissues

Chapter author: Jitendra Behari

Chapter number and title: Chapter 6: Safety Guidelines for Electromagnetic Field Exposure and Mobile Tower.

Though the data on biological effects on microwave field exposure are huge, yet these are controversial. It is thus suggestive that the criteria for safe exposure need to be redefined, for which some new parameters need to be chosen and standardized. A prerequisite to this is the knowledge of field measurements in free space. Presently, the accepted parameter is the specific absorption ratio (SAR). On the basis of field measurements, several scientific committees (ICNIRP, IEEE, FCC, etc.) have come out with their suggestions on the safe values of SAR for whole body exposure and the part body exposure. A forerunner to this is the knowledge of absolute field values by a standard method, which are internationally accepted. There are two sources of exposure to humans, one the mobile towers and other the mobile phone, the former being continuously applied and the latter is intermittent. The field due to mobile tower is well below the safe level for human exposure.

In the present chapter, methodology has been described and the range and the azimuth of the region, where the field measurements need to be carried out is mentioned. The difference between line of sight and the off sight measurements shows a vast difference.

Key words: specific absorption ratio, IEE, FCC, and ICNIRP guidelines for safe exposure

Abbreviations

ADHD	Attention deficit hyperactivity disorder
AMW	Amplitude modulated wave
ASDs	Autism spectrum disorders
C	Specific
ε^*	Complex permittivity
CT	Computer tomography
CW	Continuous wave
DAMPS	Digital advanced mobile phone systems
DECT	Digital electrical cordless telecommunication
EEG	Electroencephalogram
EHS	Electrohypersensitivity
ELF-EMFs	Extremely low frequency–electromagnetic fields
EMREs	Electromagnetic response elements
EMP	Electromagnetic pulse
FM	Frequency modulation
IDEN	Integrated digital enhanced network
IEEE	Institute of Electrical and Electronics Engineer
FCC	Federal Communication Commission
FDTD	Finite difference time domain
$(FD)^2TD$	Frequency dependent finite difference time domain
GFAP	Glial Fibrillary Acidic Protein
GTEM GHz	Transverse electromagnetic mode
GSM	Global system for mobile communication
HD-FDTD	High definition-finite difference time domain
ICNIRP	International Commission on Non-Ionizing Radiation Protection
IEBCM	Iterative extended boundary condition method
MEG	Magnetoencephalogram
MAPK	Mitogen activated protein kinase
MW	Microwave radiation
ODC	Ornithidine decarboxylase
PKC	Protein kinase C activity
PD	Power density
ROS	Reactive oxygen species
RF-EMWs	Radiofrequency electromagnetic waves
SAA	Saliva-alpha amylase
SAR	Specific absorption ratio/rate
Tanδ	Dissipation factor
TDMA	Time division multiple access

TEM	Transverse electromagnetic cell
TETRA	Terrestrial trunked radio
UHF	Ultra high frequency
σ_{eff}	Effective conductivity

1

Elements of Bioelectromagnetics

1.1 Introduction

Bioelectromagnetics deal with a complexity of biological systems being interrogated by electromagnetic waves, which are emitted by manmade devices or sources. As such the electromagnetic environment consists of natural radiations and manmade EMFs that are produced either by design or as a consequence of the use of electrical devices and systems. Based on this, populations are now blanketed to varying degrees of EMFs, and their levels will continue to increase as technology advances.

Electromagnetic radiations (EMRs) can be characterized by their wavelength, frequency, or energy, which are directly related to each other by the relationship $E = hc/\lambda$, where h is the Planck's constant, c is the velocity of light in vacuum, and λ is the free space wavelength with frequency $\nu = c/\lambda$. The frequency of an EMW is defined as the number of times the electric or magnetic fields change their sign, at a given point, per time unit and it is measured in Hertz (Hz). The wavelength of an EMW is inversely proportional to the frequency of the wave, proportional to the speed of the wave in the medium (usually the medium is considered to be the vacuum, where the speed corresponds to the speed of light $c = 3 \times 10^8$ m/s) (Figure 1.1). As an example, a typical microwave furnace emits a wave of 2.45 GHz, corresponding to a wavelength of about 12 cm. These waves consist of oscillating electric and magnetic fields that influence each other and affect in different ways the biological systems (i.e., cells, plants, animals, and human beings). To better understand this reciprocal influence, it is useful to start with an overall description of the physical properties of electromagnetic waves. Two components of EMWs: (i) an electrical wave creating an electrical field that moves along one plane and (ii) a magnetic wave creating a magnetic field that moves perpendicularly to the electrical ones. The direction of propagation is normal to the plane containing E and B. If there is an electric field, then there is a coupled magnetic field and vice versa. If one is known, the other can be calculated: These are connected together by Maxwell's equation (Stratton 1941).

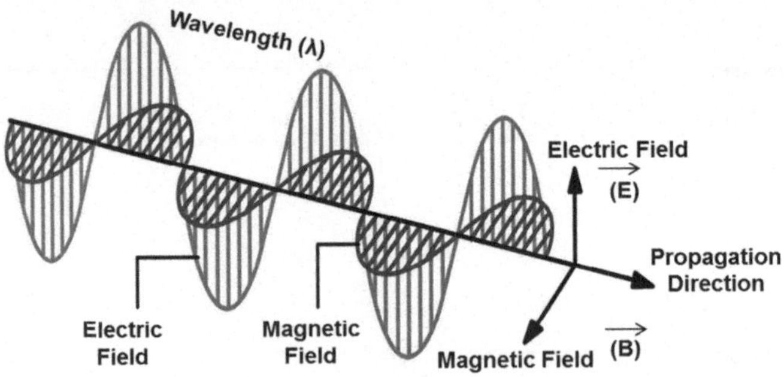

FIGURE 1.1
Propagation of electromagnetic waves.

1.2 Definitions and Basic Concepts

The dielectric permittivity ϵ and conductivity σ of a material are, respectively, the charge and current densities induced in response to an applied electric field of unit amplitude. These definitions are illustrated by examples of an idealized parallel plate capacitor, of plate area A and separation d, which contains the material under investigation. Initially, let the region between the plates be a vacuum. A constant voltage difference V between the plates will induce a charge density D given by

$$D = \varepsilon_0 V/d \tag{1.1}$$

where ϵ_0 is the permittivity of free space (8.85×10^{-12} F/m). The capacitance C is the ratio of the total induced charge on the plates to the applied voltage (ignoring the contribution from the fringing fields outside of the region between the plates)

$$C = \epsilon_0 A/d \tag{1.2}$$

If a material is now introduced between the plates, an additional charge density P_s will be induced on the plates from the polarization of charges within the material. For sufficiently low voltages, this charge density is proportional to E and can be written as follows:

$$D = \epsilon_0 E + P_s = \epsilon_s \epsilon_0 E \tag{1.3}$$

And the capacitance is now

$$C = \epsilon_s \epsilon_0 A/d \tag{1.4}$$

where ϵ_s is the static permittivity of the material. The circuit might also include a conductance G in parallel with the capacitance

$$G = \sigma_s A/d \tag{1.5}$$

where σ_s is the (DC) conductivity of the material. In response to alternating fields, the dielectric properties will vary with frequency if dielectric relaxation processes are present.

The illustration of an ideal parallel plate capacitor is only meaningful at frequencies at which the free space wavelength is much larger than the dimensions of the capacitor. A more general definition of the relative permittivity ϵ and conductivity σ is

$$D = \epsilon \epsilon_0 E \tag{1.6}$$

$$J = \sigma E \tag{1.7}$$

where D and J are, respectively, the displacement and the conduction current densities. Moreover, the measured electrical properties of parallel plate capacitors are quite different from ideally predicted values, because of a variety of parasitic effects that can be modeled as series or shunt impedance elements in the circuit.

Electromagnetic fields are quantified in terms of electric field (Table 1.1) strength **E**, expressed in volt per meter (V m^{-1}) and magnetic field strength **H** expressed as amperes per meter (A m^{-1}). Electric fields are associated only with the presence of electric charge, magnetic fields are the result of the movement of electric charge (electric current). An electric field exerts forces on an electric charge and similarly, magnetic fields can exert physical forces on electric charges, but only when such charges are in motion. A magnetic field can also be specified as magnetic flux density, **B**,

TABLE 1.1

Parameters of SAR Variation over the EM Spectrum

Parameter	
Current Density (J)	Frequency Range upto 10 MHz
Current (I)	Upto 110 MHz
Specific Absorption Rate (W/kg)	100 kHz to 10 GHz
Specific Energy Absorption (SA)	Pulsed Fields (300 MHz to10 GHz)

expressed in tesla (T). The two quantities, **B** and **H**, are related by the following expression:

$$\mathbf{B} = \mu \mathbf{H} \tag{1.8}$$

where μ is the constant of proportionality (the magnetic permeability) in vacuum and in air. In nonmagnetic (including biological) materials, μ has the value $4\,\pi \times 10^{-7}(\text{Hm}^{-1})$.

As a function of the frequency (or wavelength), the EMWs are usually classified into one of the two categories: (i) electromagnetic fields or nonionizing radiations (NIR), that is, low-level radiation which is generally perceived as harmless to humans; and (ii) electromagnetic radiations or ionizing radiation, that is, high-level radiation which has the potential for cellular and DNA damage. The ionizing radiations have a frequency high enough to produce the ionization of molecules and atoms through the breaking of the chemical bonds of the molecules. Examples of these radiations are the X-rays and radiations produced by radioactive sources.

On the other hand, the NIR correspond to those waves of the electromagnetic spectrum whose energy is too low to break the atomic bonds. Among these radiations are the ultraviolet and visible light, the infrared radiation, the radiofrequency and microwave emissions, the extremely low-frequency (ELF) fields, and the static magnetic and electric fields (Figure 1.2). The NIR, even at very high intensity, cannot produce ionization in a biological system. Nevertheless, these radiations have been proven to produce other biological effects, such as heating, alteration of some chemical reactions, or induction of electric currents on tissues and cells (Adey 1993). A single photon of radio frequency (RF) radiation has relatively low energy levels, less than 1.24×10^{-5} eV; therefore, it is not capable of producingionization. A definite amount of photon energy is required to produce ionization by ejection or promotion of orbital electrons from atoms of the material through which an electromagnetic wave propagates. The minimum photon energies capable of producing ionization in water and in atomic carbon, hydrogen, nitrogen, and oxygen are between 10 and 25 eV. Inasmuch as these atoms constitute the basic elements of living organisms, 10 eV may be considered as the lower limit for ionization in biological systems. The deleterious biological effects of such ionizing radiations as gammarays and x-rays that largely result from ionization taking place in biological cells and tissues are not produced by a single photon of RF radiation (Lin 1978). Accordingly, electromagnetic radiation in the RF spectrum is regarded as nonionizing radiation. It is noted that for strong RF fields, simultaneous absorption of 8.06×10^{5} or more low-energy RF photons could potentially produce ionization in biological materials, but the probability of such an occurrence is small. The point is that RF radiation has low-energy photons, and from these considerations this radiation is too weak to affect ionization or cause significant damage to biological molecules such as DNA, which is known for itsongoing repair mechanism.

High-frequency EMFs are part of the electromagnetic spectrum between the low frequency and the optical part of the spectrum. As this part of the spectrum is used for broadcasting and telecommunication, it is termed radio frequency. The RF spectrum is defined in the frequency range between 9 kHz and 300 GHz. Here, the focus is on the effect of frequencies close to 900 MHz. EMFs in this frequency range may have a continuous sinusoidal waveform, but more often they have a complex amplitude distribution over time. For example, for broadcast or telecommunication purposes they are modulated or pulsed. There are many sources of RF that we can encounter during everyday life. Among them, the most common (as a function of their emission frequency) are: (i) TV and PC monitors (3–30 kHz); (ii) amplitude-modulated radio emitters (30 kHz to 3 MHz); (iii) induction heaters for industry (0.3–3 MHz); (iv) thermo-shielding, diathermia systems (3–30 MHz); (v) mobile telephones; (vi) microwave ovens, diathermia devices (0.3–3 GHz); (vii) RADAR, satellite communications systems, microwave communications systems (3–30 GHz); and (viii) solar radiations (30–300 GHz) (Table 1.2, Figure 1.2). In this part of the spectrum covering microwaves, the wavelength stretches between meters

TABLE 1.2

Electromagnetic Wave Spectrum

Frequency	Wavelength	Band
30–300 Hz	10–1 mm	Extremely low frequency
3–300 kHz	10–1 km	Low frequency
3–30 MHz	100–10 m	High frequency
30–300 MHz	10–1 m	Very high frequency
300–3000 MHz	1 m to 10 cm	Ultrahigh frequency
Frequency 890–2250 MHz (mobile phone frequency)		
3–30 GHz	10–1 cm	Super high frequency
30–300 GHz	1 m to 1 mm	Extremely high frequency
300–3000 GHz	1 mm to 100 μm	mm wave frequency
Region of EMF Spectrum	Wavelength range (meters)	Frequency range (Hz)
Ionizing	$<10^{-7}$	$>3 \times 10^{15}$
Nonionizing (visible)	4×10^{-7} to $7 \times <10^{-7}$	4.2×10^{14} to 7.7×10^{14}
Nonionizing nonvisible (shortwave)	10^{-3} to $>10^{5}$	3×10^{11} to $>3 \times 10^{3}$
Nonionizing nonvisible (longwave)	10^{5} to $>10^{8}$	3×10^{3} to $>3 \times 10^{0}$

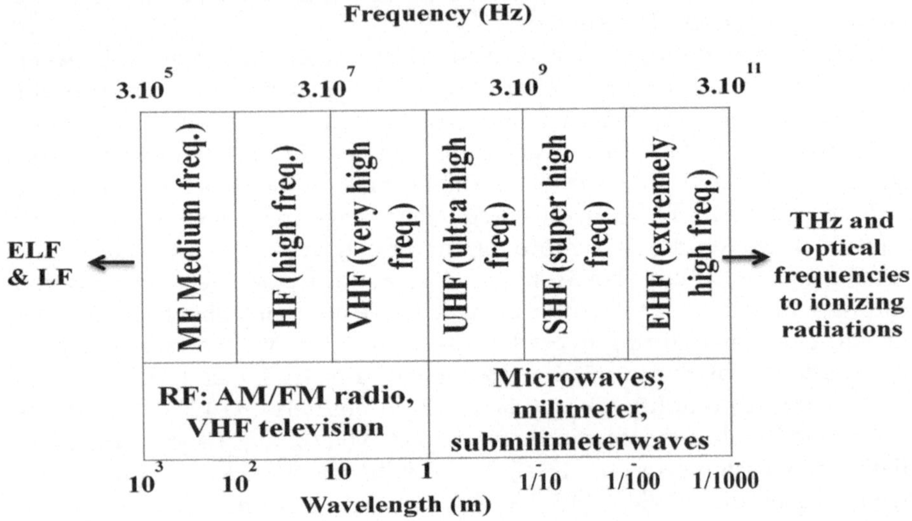

FIGURE 1.2
Electromagnetic frequency spectrum and associated wavelengths (RF/MW frequencies).

to millimeters. This offers a wide range of waveband, where this matches with the dimensions of the living system. Hence, this has remained a matter of investigation, if such wavelength can excite or produce resonance in biological tissues and bodies. An important property of such waves is that they radiate electromagnetic radiations when fed to antennas of manageable dimensions. For example, the wavelength at the power distribution frequencies of 50 and 60 Hz, which are enormous with respect to the objects we use in our day-to-day life. Since electromagnetic waves of all frequency (wavelength) are pervading the environment, their interaction with biological objects is a matter of concern. In this connection, two modes of radiation pattern have to be considered: near field and far field (Figure 1.3). Far-field measurements in connection with dosimetry are easy to perform and are measured most of the time for determining the criteria for safe exposure.

While considering the radiation behavior, when these EMFs fall on various physical objects, one has to operate in time domain (described as function of time), and hence these are real and physically measurable, though, working in frequency domain is correspondingly easy. However, numerical signals, such as for telephony, television, and frequency-modulated (FM) radio, may need time domain analysis and measurements. Radiation is a phenomenon characterizing the RF/microwave range. It is well known that structures radiate poorly when they are small with respect to the wavelength. A basic requirement of a radiating system is

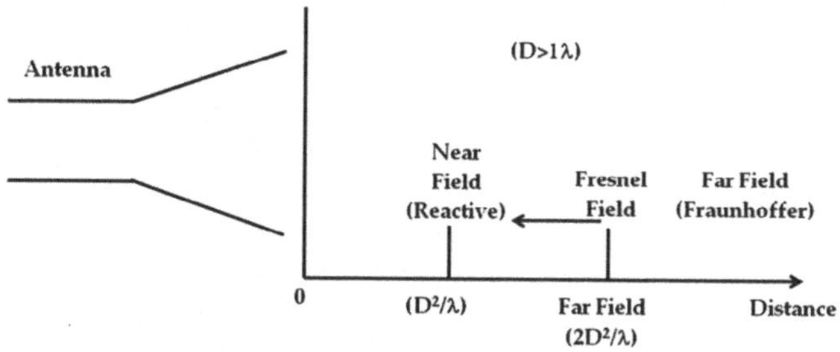

FIGURE 1.3
Field distribution pattern from microwave antenna.

that for it to radiate efficiently the structure has to be large enough with respect to the wavelength λ. The concepts of radiation, antennas, far field, and near field have to be investigated.

With the advent of increasing industrialization and the tendency to increase the power of equipment raised the question of health risks first for personnel, then for the general public has come up. Radiofrequency electromagnetic waves may interact with biological tissues through various processes. Before starting any interpretation of the results obtained, it is necessary to survey the basic phenomena involved in the interaction of RF and microwave radiation with living systems, which falls within the terrain of bioelectromagnetics.

1.3 Bioelectric Phenomena

Electric and magnetic fields are part of all living beings (bioelectricity) and are also found naturally in our environment since time immemorial. Very much like gravitational fields, EM fields are a basic force of nature. Our bodies are bioelectrical in nature; the molecules in our body are held together by electric fields. The messages that flow in our nervous system involve electric and magnetic fields, and the heart is electrically active. The currents in the body can also be induced and influenced by outside magnetic fields. If strong enough, these currents can cause stimulation of nerves and muscles or affect other biological processes. This is accepted and understood in medicine and science as proven fact; however, there is still ongoing debate as to the biological consequences of long-term low-level exposure. Bioelectricity is extremely important in a living body and has long been shown that direct application of an externally generated voltage may have an effect on bone and cartilage repair (Behari 2009). Considerable animal and in vitro experimentation suggests the clinical usefulness of electric currents for soft tissue repair and possibly to enhance repair of nerve fibers that have sustained crush or transaction injury (WHO 1993).

Living cells exhibit bioelectric phenomena. However, a small variety only produces potential changes that reveal their physiological function. There are familiar bioelectric recording. The three most prominent bioelectric effects, those of heart, skeletal muscle, and brain, are recorded by the following: the electrocardiogram (ECG), reflecting the excitation and recovery of the whole heart; the electromyogram (EMG), reflecting the activity of skeletal muscle; and the electroencephalogram (EEG), reflecting the activity of the outer layers of the brain, the cortex. In these cases, the action potentials are used for diagnostic purposes, and extracellular electrodes are used that are both large and distant from the population of cells that become active and recover. The depolarization and repolarization processes send small currents through the conducting environmental tissues and fluids, resulting in a time-varying potential field. Appropriately placed electrodes can record the electrical activity of the bioelectric generators. However, the waveforms of such recordings are vastly different from those of the transmembrane potential (Vander Vorst & Duhamel 1996). Despite the difference in waveform, extracellular recordings can identify the excitation and recovery processes very well (WHO 1993). Furthermore, the eye, ear, sweat glands, and many types of smooth muscles also produce action potentials that are also used for their diagnostic value. There is no doubt that bioelectricity has to be taken into account when investigating possible medical applications of RFs and microwaves as well as when wondering about possible hazards on human beings and animals due to RF or microwave exposure (Rosen et al. 2003; National Institute of Environmental Health Sciences 2004).

Bioelectromagnetics research has laid foundations pointing to a new understanding of living matter, based on physical processes at the atomic level, far beyond the realm of chemical reactions in a biomolecular fabric. Appropriate models describing these bioeffects based on nonequilibrium thermodynamics, with nonlinear electrodynamics at the atomic level as integral features. Tissue heating, modeled in equilibrium thermodynamics, fails to offer suitable models for several spectrums of observed electromagnetic field bioeffects. Indeed, bioelectromagnetic research appears to have gone beyond the immediate goals associated with hazard research.

Laboratory studies have identified cell membranes as the major primary tissue site of interaction with environmental ELF and ELF-modulated RF/microwave fields. They have determined major sequences in the coupling of cell surface signals to a cascade of high-energy enzymatic mechanisms inside cells. Major effects of these fields have been noted in the following: (1) regulation of the immune system; (2) in modulation of brain and central nervous system functions, including regulation of the pineal gland and its hormone melatonin, which regulate the body's 24 h daily rhythm, and are indirectly involved in other hormonal mechanisms, including normal estrogen receptor formation in the breast; (3) in regulation of cell growth, through enzymatic mechanisms mediating DNA synthesis and repair; and (4) in apparently acting at cell membranes with chemical cancer promoters, or with the body's intrinsic hormonal mechanisms as cofactors in tumor formation.

Epidemiological studies have drawn attention to ELF and ELF-modulated RF fields as possible risk factors in leukemia, lymphoma, breast tumors, skin melanoma, and brain tumors. It is clear that these studies are merely pointers to much needed information on an exposure metric for health effects in man. Nevertheless, they emphasize the complexity of tissue effects of nonionizing EM fields. Unlike ionizing radiation, the nonionizing metric must take account of profound tissue effects attributable to intermittency of exposure, and the frequently transient character of the ensuing biological response.

In the present context, we limit ourselves to the RF/microwave range; we may refer to our subject of interaction of electric and magnetic fields with organic matter (as biological effects of nonionizing radiation). Considering a frequency range, we describe the phenomena in what is called the frequency domain, wide or narrow, we need to change the frequency of the source. The general description in the frequency domain implies complex quantities, with a real and an imaginary part, respectively, which are not physical. The frequencydomain description is, however, extremely useful because many sources are monochromatic.

To investigate the actual effect of physical sources, however, one has to operate in what is called the time domain, where the phenomena is described as a function of time and hence it is real and physically measurable. Operating in the time domain may be difficult with respect to the frequency domain. Today numerical signals, such as for telephony, television, andFM radio, may, however, necessitate time-domain analysis and measurements.

There is an interesting feature to note about microwaves. These radiations cover the frequency range where the wavelength is of the order of the size objects of common use, that is, meter, decimeter, centimeter, and millimeter, depending of course on the material in which it is measured. One may, hence, wonder whether such wavelengths can cause resonance in biological tissues and systems.

A field is associated with a physical phenomenon present in a given region of space. As an example, the temperature in a room is sum total of its distribution, over a number of points in the room. Extending this point, one may say the same about the temperature distribution inside a human body. We do not see its spread (field), but it exists, and we can, for instance, visualize constant-temperature or isothermal surfaces. Similar is the phenomena related to the electromagnetic field inside the biological body, dominated by extremely low frequency signals.

There are fields of different nature. First, fields may be either static or time dependent. Considering, for instance, the temperature field just described, the room may indeed be heated or cooled, which makes the temperature field time dependent. The human body may also be submitted to a variety of external sources or internal reasons which affect the temperature distribution inside the body.

Second, the nature of the field may be such that one parameter only, such as its magnitude, is defined as scalar. The temperature field, for instance, inside a room or human body is a scalar field. On the other hand, in a vector field, a vector represents both the magnitude and the direction of the physical quality of points in space, and this vector field may also be static or time dependent. When plotting a static scalar field, that is, one quality, in points of space already requires some visualization effort. On the other hand, plotting a time-dependent vector field, which is described by a set of direction lines, also known as stream lines or flux lines.

1.4 Behavior as an Indicative Property in Bioelectromagnetic Research

From a pathological point of view, it can be hypothesized that a brain with greater indications of oxidative stress along with immune activation and mitochondrial dysfunction might generate different oscillatory activity than a brain without these features. Atrial septal defect (ASD) or neuro developmental and neuropsychiatric conditions would impart it a quantitative support. From this point of view, it can be suggested that compromised whole body health status of at least many patients with ASDs would make it harder for them to maintain the resilience of their brain cells and brain activities in the face of an external environmental challenge. Sleep and consciousness have been considered "emergent properties" (Krueger and Obal 2003; Krueger et al. 2008). Brain oscillatory property is critical for organizing behavior, and it arises from cells and subcellular features that are shaped by the environment and can be differently based on their functional status as well as on account of external sensory or psychosocial activity.

In particular, (a) brain oscillatory activity is intimately connected with cellular, metabolic, and immune status, (b) EMF/RFR is capable of penetrating changes at each of these levels, and (c) problems at each of these levels can add to several others. In particular, EMF/RFR and possibly toxicants can copotentiate damage (Ahlbom et al. 2008; Luukkonen et al. 2009) amplifying allostatic load. From this it is suggestive that the combination of EMF/RFR impact may quite plausibly contribute both to how ASDs happen in individuals and to why there are more reported cases of ASDs than ever before (Hertz-Picciottol & Delwiche 2009; King & Bearman 2009).

There are many complex interactions within and between cells, and these interactions over a wide range of frequency of electromagnetic spectrum play an important role in transmitting and receiving signals through an ion-rich aqueous solutions. However, their mechanism of interaction is not fully understood.

RF fields with frequencies in the range 1 MHz to 10 GHz can penetrate exposed organic tissues and produce heating by absorption of waves. The energy absorbed by the tissues and organs is measured in this case as a specific absorption rate (W/kg), which is the unit of dosimetry (Table 1.3). Since the mode of EMF biointeraction is frequency dependent (Figure 1.4a–c), the magnitude of safe exposure (and hence SAR) is also frequency

TABLE 1.3

Unit Conversations

	Desired unit				
Given unit	**W/m**	**mW/cm²**	**µW/cm²**	**V/m**	**A/m**
W/m	1	0.1	100	√(W/m × 377)	√(W/m/377)
mW/cm²	10	1	1000	√ (mW/cm² × 3770)	√(mW/cm² × 37.7)
µW/cm²	0.01	0.001	1	√ (µW/cm²) × 3.77	√(µW/cm²) × 37700
V/m	(V/m)²/377	(V/m²)/3770	(V/m)²/3.77	1	V/m/377
A/m	(A/m)² × 377	(A/m)² × 37.7	(A/m)² × 37700	A/m × 377	1

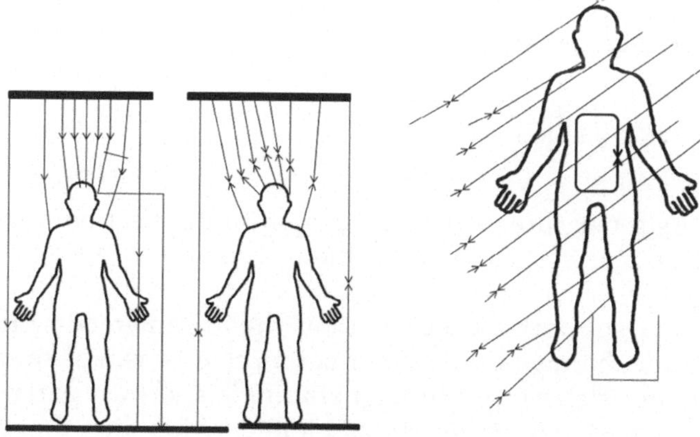

FIGURE 1.4a

Low-frequency signal completely penetrate the biological material.

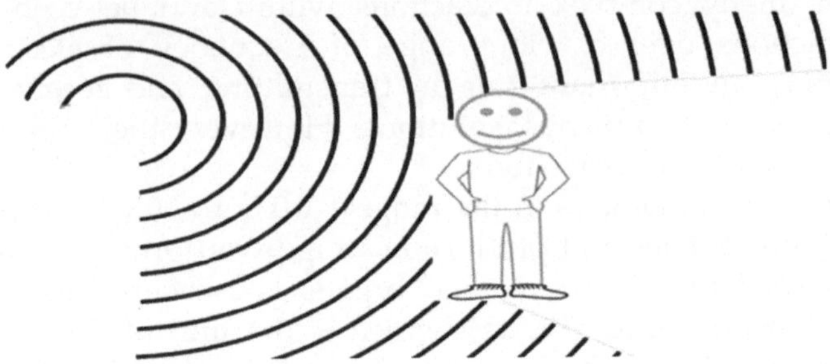

FIGURE 1.4b
Exposure of humans to RFfields.

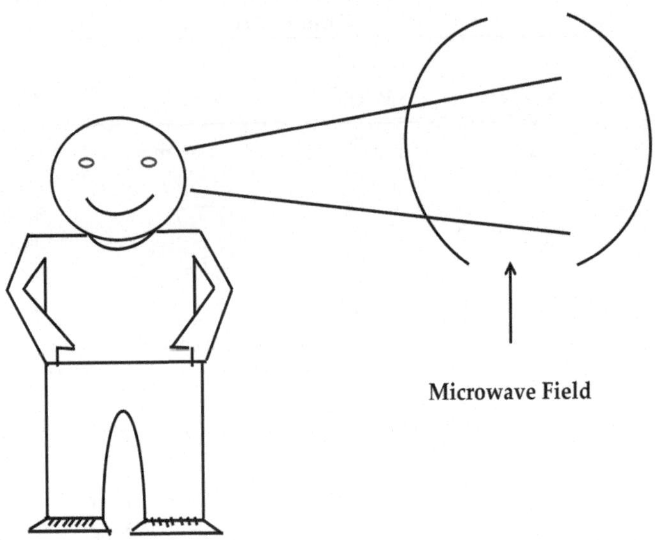

FIGURE 1.4c
Exposure of human to microwave field.

dependent. As a measure of producing a harmful effect on human health (30–300 MHz), a specific absorption coefficient of 4 W/kg is recommended.

Existing data support the observation that biointeraction mechanism applies both for thermal and nonthermal mechanisms. For thermal effect to be visible, measurable rise in temperature is a known parameter to be spatially measured. For nonthermal biointeraction lies the concept of cell-to-cell signaling. If such messages are critical to control, complex biological processes could be disrupted by weak external electromagnetic radiation. One possible impact of nonionizing electromagnetic radiation is DNA damage of brain cells that has been of paramount importance, leading to various patho physiological possibilities, one being the brain cancer. Also manmade radiations in the environment may lead to an adverse impact on reproductive pattern and developmental effects in animals. It may also lead to Alzheimer's disease. EMF affects the biochemical pathways and immunological mechanisms that link the different organ system in our bodies and those for animals. The human body acts as an antenna for RF signals and a small percentage of the population appears to be sensitive to EMF, interfering in their daily life. The complexity of the signal may be important in altering biological responses. Some people feel weak or ill if they are close to electrical, electronic, or wireless devices (electrosensitivity (radiofrequency disease)). Its impact on human includes chronic headaches, digestive disorders, sleep disturbance, memory loss, depression, chronic pain, cold, dizziness, and so on.

Bioelectromagnetics research has laid foundations pointing to a new understanding of living matter, based on physical processes at the atomic level, far beyond the realm of chemical reactions in a biomolecular frame. Appropriate models describing these bioeffects are based on nonequilibrium thermodynamics at the atomic level as integral features. Tissue heating, modeled in equilibrium thermodynamics, fails to offer suitable models for several spectrums of observed EMF bioeffects.

Various set of experiments have identified cell membrane as the primary site of interaction with environmental ELF and ELF-modulated RF/MW fields. They have identified major sequences in the coupling of cell surface signals to a cascade of high-energy enzymatic mechanisms inside cells (Figure 4.6). Major effects of these fields have been noted in (1) regulation of the immune system, (2) modulation of the pineal gland and its hormone melatonin, which regulates body rhythm on 24 h basis, and is also involved in other hormonal-mechanisms, (3) mediating DNA synthesis and repair, and (4) in apparently acting at cell membrane with chemical cancer promoters, or with the body's intrinsic hormonal mechanisms, and cofactors in tumor formation.

Epidemiological studies have drawn attention to ELF and ELF-modulated fields as possible risk factors in leukemia, lymphoma, breast tumors, skin melanoma, and brain tumors. It is clear that these studies are merely pointers to much needed information on an exposure metric for health effects in man. Nevertheless, these interactions emphasize the immense complexity of these effects accountable to intermittency of exposure, and the frequently transient character of the ensuing response.

the only determining factor in evaluating biological effects of RF and microwaves. Other features of the radiation also need to be considered. A radiation diagram typical of a communications antenna is shown in Figure 6.1b. A paraboloid antenna is placed at the coordinate origin. The gain $G_i(\theta, \varnothing)$ of the antenna varies with the direction $(\theta, \varnothing)$. The gain of an antenna is defined as the ratio of the power transmitted by the antenna in a given direction to what which would be transmitted by an isotropic antenna (transmitting the same power in all directions) placed in the same location. It is usually expressed in decibels (dB).

1.6 Influence of the Waveform

Parameters of microwave exposure are an important consideration in the induction of biological effects. One key word is dosimetry, which takes into account the level of exposure as well as its duration. The simplest expression is the product of the level duration. Different durations of acute exposure lead to different biological effects and, consequently, different long-term effects occur after repeated exposure. The waveform of the radiation is also important. Differential effects have indeed been observed after exposure to pulsed-wave with respect to continuous-wave (CW) microwaves. In practice, biological effects have been observed under a variety of exposure types: CW, sinusoidal amplitude-modulated wave (AMW), and pulse-modulated wave (PMW) (Vander Vorst & Duhamel 1996). Hence, there is a difficulty in evaluating the exposure. Thermal effects are of course related to power, so that comparison of biological effects under different types of exposure should be done at constant power. Normally it should be either the CW power or the average power when the excitation is pulse modulated. In this case, however, and especially when the duty cycle is short, as in radar-type waves, the peak power may be much larger than the average power, and possible nonlinearity may induce other effects. In addition to power, other parameters inducing effects are polarization of incident radiation and distance from the emission source.

Natural bioelectric processes are responsible for nerve and muscle function. Externally applied electric currents can excite nerve and muscle cells. The nerve system is concerned with the rapid transfer of information through the body in the form of electrical signals. It is conveniently divided into the central nervous system (CNS) and the peripheral nervous system. The CNS consists of the brain and spinal cord. The peripheral nervous system consists of afferent neurons, which convey information inward to the CNS, and efferent neurons, which convey information from the CNS to the body. The efferent system is subdivided into a somatic nervous system and an autonomic nervous system. The autonomic nervous system consists of neurons that convey impulses to smooth muscle tissue, cardiac muscle tissue, and glands, which are usually considered involuntary, that is, not under conscious control.

Muscles can be stimulated directly or indirectly through the nerves that enervate the muscle. Thresholds of stimulation of nerve are generally well below thresholds for direct stimulation of a muscle. Hence, an understanding of neuroelectric principles is a valuable foundation for investigating both sensory and muscular responses to electrical stimulation.

1.7 Biological Interaction with Matter

EMF effects on biological targets are grossly frequency dependent. Low-frequency waves penetrate all through the biological body and hence signals are all pervading in terms of their wavelength. They penetrate entire organic substances (magnetic field), more and (electric field) less. A specific signal transfer at a particular place in the body is not possible. The signal stimulus is present all over the body. On the other hand, microwave radiation or radiation in the extended light frequency range can aim at and reach a particular part of the body, a particular receptor, but only when the receptor is on or near the surface of the body. This is also possible with the use of microwave applicator. In this case, it is also conceivable that bioinformation could be transmitted on from there, with a corresponding time-lag, into the deeper-lying regions of the body, irrespective of the direction of the incoming radiation. Hence at the millimeter wave region, the point-to-point propagation is more valid (Figure 1.4a–c). Hence, the amount of energy deposition varies and correspondingly the single value of specific absorption rate is not valid.

There are two broad divisions of the mechanism by which biological matter undergo interaction with EM radiations.

(a) Thermal mechanism: Thermal mechanisms are mainly associated with the absorption of the RF energy resulting from the electrical conductivity of most biological tissue. The RF electric field generates an oscillating current and the rapid transfer of the energy of this current into the molecular motion responsible for most of the heat capacity results in an increase in the local temperature. The electrical conductivity is in fact only partly due to the translational motion of charged particles—ions. The other main contribution arises is from the hindered rotation of molecules, principally water. The water molecule has a large permanent dipole moment, which is randomly oriented in the absence of an applied electric field **E**. An electric field partially orients the dipole moments along the direction of the field. Because of the viscosity of the water, the field has to do work to rotate the dipoles resulting in energy transfer into the liquid—heat. This dissipation mechanism is most effective over a fairly broad range of frequencies, close to those given by $\omega\tau = 1$, where $\omega = 2\pi\nu$ and τ is the average time the dipoles take to reorient.

(b) Low-frequency electric fields from demodulation: In view of public concern that pulsed RF signals from mobile phones might interact differently with biological components from continuous wave RF signals, it is surprising that there has been almost no discussion of how this might arise. It is well known that pulsed RF fields can result in acoustic effects (microwave hearing). This is believed to be a thermal effect and is only detectable at much higher peak powers than those of mobile phone signals. So there would need to be another mechanism if, for example, biological effects of pulsing were to occur at the power levels of GSM or TETRA handsets. One possible route would be through demodulation.

The RF fields from the mobile phones used for telecommunications are pulsed at 217 Hz (GSM) and 17.6 Hz (TETRA), so demodulation of these signals would lead to the presence of electric fields at 217 or 17.6 Hz and their harmonics, as well as fields at frequencies relating to the digital stream (tens of kHz). Now, the International Council on Non-Ionizing Radiation Protection (ICNIRP) public exposure guideline for low-frequency electric fields (4–1000 Hz) of 2 mV/m (for tissue of resistivity 1 Ωm) is appreciably less than the corresponding guideline at 1 GHz of around 100 V/m. So even quite weak demodulation of mobile phone signals at these fields might produce low-frequency electric fields above the guidelines.

Demodulation would occur if the electrical conductivity or dielectric constant of a biological component varied significantly with electric field **E**, so that its electrical response was nonlinear. For example, if its conductivity $\sigma = \sigma_0 + \sigma_1\mathbf{E}$, there would be components of current at the modulation frequencies, which would become significant at fields at which $\sigma_1\mathbf{E} \sim \sigma_0$. Symmetry arguments show that these second-order terms should be zero in crystals with inversion symmetry, but there are many other crystals or structures involving interfaces in which second-order terms can be quite significant at high electric fields and these find useful application particularly at optical frequencies.

However, the only known example of a biological component that is detectably nonlinear for average extracellular tissue fields less than 100 V/m is a cell membrane. The neutral lipid bilayer separates regions of opposite polarity, so that the charge distribution is similar to that of a semiconductor junction. The nonlinearity was demonstrated by the observation that membranes rectified RF signals of average field ~1 V/m frequencies below a few kHz. However, the value of the rectified signal fell rapidly at higher frequencies and at 100 kHz was a hundred times less than the low-frequency value (Montaigne & Pickard 1984). At lower frequencies, the field across the membrane is larger than the average field by several thousands; however, this enlargement disappears at higher frequencies. So it seems very unlikely that membranes could produce significant demodulation of the 1 GHz or so RF

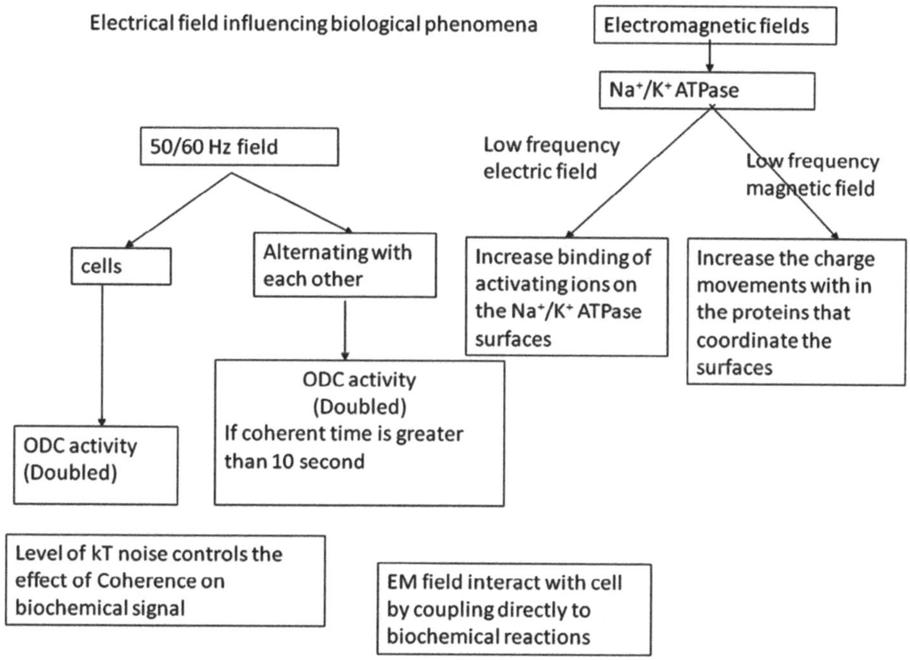

FIGURE 1.5
Electrical field influencing biological phenomena.

signals used in mobile telecommunications. It seems very probable that this is also the case for other biological components. A summary of known effects of fields produced by extremely low frequency EMF fields falling on biological systems is summarized in Figure 1.5, and corresponding RF/microwave field effects will be discussed in Chapters 4 and 5.

1.8 Electrical Properties of the Human Body

Both theoretical and experimental dosimetry require a knowledge of the electrical properties of the object for which this is assessed. In particular, when the object is the human body, its electrical properties must be known to calculate internal fields or to construct phantoms on which measurements can be made. The electrical properties of the human body are usually specified either in terms of relative permittivity and effective conductivity or in terms of complex relative permittivity. In general, the relative permittivity and effective conductivity of body tissues are a strong

wave scattered by the body will be development on its physiological parameters, geometry, frequency, and polarization of the incident electromagnetic field. The electric field induced inside the biological system is the key quantity which determines the induced current and the total power deposition inside it when exposed to electromagnetic radiations. Therefore, our theoretical approach aims to determine this induced electric field.

Consider a biological system as shown in Figure I.6, composed of heterogeneous lossy medium with an irregular shape, being illuminated by incident electric field $\mathbf{E}^{\mathrm{i}}$. The body may further be assumed to be constructed of layers with variable permittivity and conductivity. Therefore, the parameters of the medium constituting the biological system can be expressed as follows:

Permittivity: $\varepsilon = {}^{\varepsilon}(\omega, r)$ dependent on frequency and location

Conductivity: $\sigma = \sigma(\omega, r)$ dependent on frequency and location

Permeability: $\mu = \mu_o$ permeability of free space, since the biological bodies are assumed to be essentially non magnetic in nature.

From the Maxwell's equations, both for the incident and the total electromagnetic field, a tensor integral equation can be derived (Chapter 3). This tensor integral equation provides a link between the known incident electric field $\mathbf{E}^{\mathrm{i}}(\mathbf{r})$ and the unknown total induced field $\mathbf{E}(\mathbf{r})$. Inthe theoretical development, the tensor integral equation involves the unknown total field $\mathbf{E}(\mathbf{r})$ as

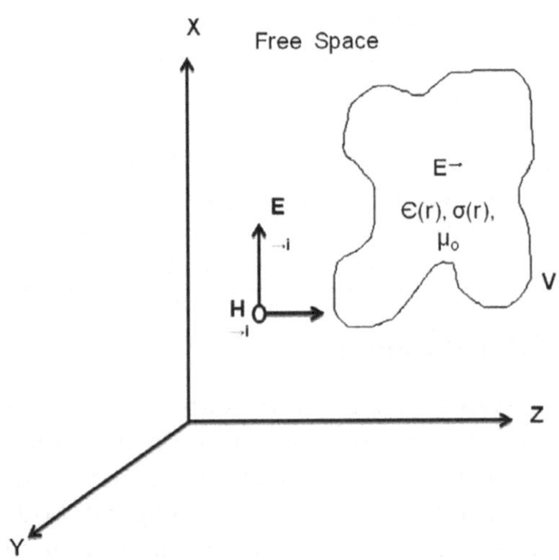

FIGURE 1.6
An arbitrarily shaped biological body in free space, illuminated by an electromagnetic field.

a part of integrand, thereby imposing difficulties in arriving at a direct solution. To circumvent the problem mentioned before, a numerical technique—moment method with pulse function expansion of the unknown electric field **E**(**r**)—is employed to transform the tensor integral equation into a set of simultaneous equations. This set of simultaneous equations can then be solved for the unknown fields at different locations inside the body by known numerical techniques. An exact formulation of the tensor integral equation and its transformation into a set of simultaneous equations have already been reported by Livesay and Chen (1974).

When a biological body is illuminated by the incident electric field **E**(**r**), the total electric field inside and outside the body is the sum of $\mathbf{E}^{i}(\mathbf{r})$ and the scattered electric field $\mathbf{E}^{s}(\mathbf{r})$ maintained by the induced current and charge in the body. Mathematically,

$$\mathbf{E}(\mathbf{r}) = \mathbf{E}^{i}(\mathbf{r}) + \mathbf{E}^{S}(\mathbf{r}) \tag{1.11}$$

and similarly, the total magnetic field **H**(**r**) can be expressed as follows:

$$\mathbf{H}(\mathbf{r}) = \mathbf{H}^{i}(\mathbf{r}) + \mathbf{H}^{S}(\mathbf{r}) \tag{1.12}$$

where $\mathbf{H}^{S}(\mathbf{r})$ is the scattered magnetic field maintained by the induced current and charge in the biological system. Since $\mathbf{E}^{i}(\mathbf{r})$ is known, the problem will be solved if an expression for $\mathbf{E}^{S}(\mathbf{r})$ is obtained. A somewhat detailed formulation of this will be presented in Chapter 3.

References

Adey WR (1993) Biological effects of electromagnetic fields. *J. Cell Biochem.*, 51: 410.

Ahlbom A, Bridges J, de Seze R, Hillert L, Juutilainen J, Mattsson MO, Neubaeur G, Schuz J, Simko M & Bromen K (2008) Possible effects of electromagnetic fields (EMF) on human health—opinion of the scientific committee on emerging and newly identified health risks (SCENIHR). *Toxicology*, 246(2–3): 248.

Behari J (2009) Biological correlates of electromagnetic field exposure. In: *Toxicology General & Applied Toxicology* (Ballantyne B & Syven T, eds., 3rd Edition). John Wiley & Sons Ltd., Chapter 106. p. 1.

Booker HG (1982) *Energy in Electromagnetism*. Stevenage: P. Peregrinus.

Hertz-Picciottol & Delwiche L (2009) The rise in autism and the role of age at diagnosis. *Epidemiology*, 2(1): 84.

King M & Bearman P (2009) Diagnostic change and increased prevalence of autism. *Int. J. Epidemiol.*, 38(5): 1224.

Krueger JM & Obal F Jr (2003) Sleep function. *Front. Biosci.*, 8: 511.

Krueger JM, Rector DM, Roy S, Van Dongen HPA, Belenky G & Panksepp J (2008) Sleep as a fundamental property of neuronal assemblies. *Nat. Rev. Neurosci.*, 9 (12): 910.

Landau LD & Lifschitz EM (1960) *Electrodynamics of Continuous Media*. Oxford: Pergamon.
Lin JC (1978) *Microwave Auditory Effects & Applications*. Springfield, IL: Charles C Thomas Publisher.
Livesay DE & Chen KM (1974) Electromagnetic fields induced inside arbitrarily shaped biological bodies. *IEEE Trans. Micro Theory Tech. (MTT)*, 22: 1273.
Luukkonen J, Hakulinen P, Maki-Paakkanen J, Juutilainen J & Naarala J (2009) Enhancement of chemically induced reactive oxygen species production and DNA damage in human SH-SY5Y neuroblastoma cells by 872 MHz radio-frequency production. *Mutat. Res.*, 662(1–2): 54.
Montaigne K & Pickard WF (1984) Offset of the vacuolar potential of characean cells in response to electromagnetic radiation over the range 250 Hz to 250 kHz. *Bioelectromagnetics*, 5: 31.
National Institute of Environment Health Sciences. Available online: www.niehs.nih.gov (accessed on 25 March 2004).
Ramo S, Whinnery JR & Van Duzer T (1965) *Fields & Waves in Communication Electronics* (3rd Edition). New York: Wiley.
Rosen A, Rosen HD, His RA & Rosen D (2003) Topics in RF/microwave & optics in therapeutic medicine, Part I, opportunities for microwave & photonics in medical diagnostics & therapy. *Proceedings, International Topical Meetings on Microwave Photonics, Hungarian Academy of Science*, Budapest, Hungary.
Stratton JA (1941) *Electromagnetic Theory*. New York: McGraw Hill Book Company.
Tonks L (1938) A new form of the electromagnetic energy when free charged particles are present. *Phys. Rev.*, 54: 863.
Vander Vorst A (1994) *Electromagnetism*. Champs et Circuits. Brussels: De Boeck.
Vander Vorst A & Duhamel F (1996) 1990–1995 Advances in investigating the interaction of microwave fields with the nervous system. *IEEE Trans. Microwave Theory Tech.*, 44: 1898.
WHO (1993) *Environmental Health Criteria 137, Electromagnetic Fields (300 Hz–300 GHz)*. Geneva: World Health Organization, p. 115.

2

Concepts in EMF Biointeraction

2.1 Fundamentals

The effect of RF and microwave radiation interaction with biological tissues has now become a matter of increasing concern. The issue is becoming increasingly complex and the phenomenon is essentially a function of the following three parameters:

a. The frequency and the type of EM waves propagating into the living system.
b. Mode of interaction of the waves with tissues, specific to their electromagnetic properties.
c. Secondary effects induced by the primary interaction.

The word interaction stresses the fact that end results not only depend on the action of the field but also are influenced by the reaction of the living system. Living systems have a large capacity of reprogramming its physiological function in response to the effects induced by external influences. Physiological compensation means that the strain imposed by external factors is fully compensated and the organism is able to perform normally. Extended phenomena, i.e., pathological compensation, means that the imposed strain leads to the appearance of disturbances within the functions of the organism and even structural alterations may result. The borderline between these two types of compensation is obviously not always easy to determine.

The radiation mechanism considered consists of a source that emits EM energy. Part of the incident energy is absorbed and transformed within the biological system. Hence, there is the sequence:

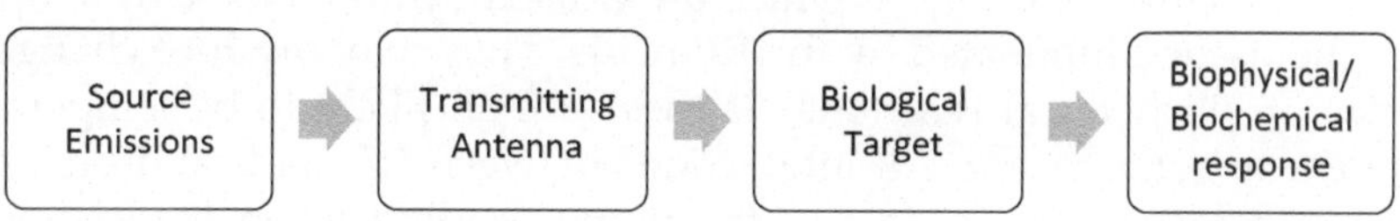

The mechanism(s) by which this proceeds is not fully understood, though the physical laws of EM field theory can be applied to investigate and explain the observed phenomena. This is true in general for the non-ionizing part of the EM radiation, with which we are presently concerned (RF and microwaves).

Since biological tissues consist 75–80% of water and hence once the microwaves fall upon these objects, the dielectric behavior of water becomes important to know the amount of power deposited. Water is a broadband attenuator of microwaves and its absorption behavior is frequency dependent, so that $\epsilon_{static} = 80$ and then decreases with the increasing frequency, signifying change in the mode of EMF biointeraction and thereby making the issue complex.

The ICNIRP (International council on Non-ionizing Radiation Protection) guidelines for the head or trunk for frequencies between 100 KHz and 10GHz require the average specific absorption rate (SAR) in any contiguous 10 g region to be less than 10 W/kg (occupational) or 2 W/kg (public). However, to discuss mechanisms, it is usually more convenient to translate these SARs into rms RF electric fields E_{inside}, say, the tissue of the head that gives rise to these values. For tissue of density 1×10^3 kg/m^3 and resistivity 1Ω.m, a SAR of 10 W/kg corresponds to E = 100 V/m and the magnetic field B accompanying such an E field would be around 0.3μT. This assumes the relation between E and B that applies in the far field and may be incorrect by a small factor in the near field of a mobile phone.

2.2 Physical Aspects of RF Reflection and Absorption in Tissue

When EM fields propagate from one medium to another, they can be reflected, refracted, transmitted, or absorbed, depending on the complex conductivity of the exposed body and the frequency of the source. Absorbed EM energy can be converted to other forms of energy and cause interference with the functioning of the living system. Most of this energy is converted into heat: absorption. However, not all EM field effects can be explained by this mode of energy transfer. At frequencies well below 100 kHz, it has been shown that induced electric fields can stimulate nervous tissue. At the microscopic level, other types of interaction have also been observed.

Interaction can take place either by thermal or non-thermal mechanisms. Thermal mechanisms are those which are caused by an increase in temperature of the tissue illuminated by the RF fields. They may produce changes in the rates of biochemical reactions, as these are all likely to be temperature dependent to some extent. All interactions between RF fields and biological tissue result in energy transfer to the tissue, leading to an increase in its temperature. On the other hand, non-thermal mechanisms are those that are not directly associated with the rise in temperature. These may be due to the changes caused in the tissue by the RF electric or magnetic field. The electromagnetic radiations as it penetrates the biological body cause the change in the pattern of internal field distribution. This is dependent upon a variety of external environmental parameters. This then establishes the cause and the observed biological effects. The established biophysical mechanisms, underlying the interaction of RF radiation with cells, tissue, and entire bodies, include induced charge and dipole relaxation, enhanced attraction between cell for pearl chain formation and other RF-induced force effects, microwave auditory phenomenon, and may be some more.

Polar molecules such as water and other cellular components of biological materials can undergo translational and rotational motion in response to an applied sinusoidal electric field. The motion is impeded by inertia and by viscous forces. Since reorientation of polar molecules does not occur instantaneously, this gives rise to a time-dependent behavior known as the relaxation process in biological tissues. Under the influence of RF electric fields at frequencies up to 100 MHz, molecules and cells would rearrange and form chains along the direction of the field. Threshold electric field strength between 2 and 10 kVm^{-1} is needed to produce the non-thermal effects which depend on frequency, cell or particle size, and pulsing wave parameters of the applied field. Both pulsed and CW fields are known to cause alignment of cells and larger molecules. However, the reversible and irreversible changes in membranes require much stronger fields.

Exposure due to low-frequency electric and magnetic fields results in negligible energy absorption and consequently causes no measurable temperature rise in the body. On the other hand, exposure due to electromagnetic fields at frequencies above about 100 kHz can lead to significant absorption of energy and a consequent temperature rise. In general, exposure to a uniform (plane-wave) electromagnetic field results in a highly non-uniform deposition and distribution of energy within the body, which must be assessed by dosimetric measurement and calculation.

Another mode of energy dissipation in biological tissues is through the eddy currents generated by microwave absorption by magnetite particles (Fe_3O_4) present in biological tissues. These particles are also present in brain tissue causing absorption in the frequency range of 500 MHz–10 GHz (Kirschvink 1996).It is speculated that exposure of such particles to mobile phone frequencies may cause cell death. However, a small amount of particles are present in the tissue, though these are unlikely to generate SAR high enough to affect guidelines for safe exposure.

The attenuation of EM wave in a homogenous tissue is given as

$$E = E_0 \exp(-\mu d) \qquad (2.1)$$

Where E is the electric field at a distance d and μ is the attenuation coefficient. It is predicted that for a 12 cm (2.5 GHz) wavelength, the depth of penetration is 1 cm. This wavelength is presently used in microwave diathermy. For a wavelength of 3 cm (10 GHz), the penetration is 0.1 cm.

As regards absorption of energy by the human body, range of electromagnetic fields can be divided into four parts (Johnson & Guy 1972; Durney et al. 1986), depending upon the mode and the quantum of absorption (Figure 2.1):

1. For frequencies between 10 kHz and 20 MHz, the absorption in the trunk portion rapidly increases with the increasing frequency. Because of their curvature, significant amount of microwave absorption occurs in the neck and legs.

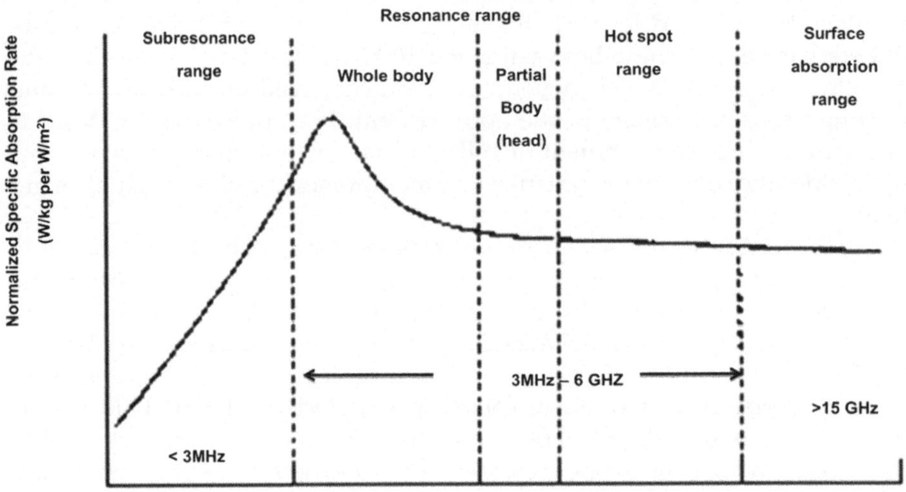

FIGURE 2.1
Absorbed power in W/kg variation of SAR with frequency.

Notes: RF-MW standards are frequency specific and based on resonances

- Subresonant (<3 MHz)—Body and parts are not antennas. As is characterstic of low frequencies, current flow considerations follow.
- Resonant (3 MHz–6 GHz)—Body becomes good antenna which maximizes energy absorption.Current flow and SAR are both important considerations. Absorption falls of in proportion to square of frequency (3–30 MHz).Because of resonance absorption, the criteria for safe exposure are most stringent in the range of 30–300 MHz(human resonant frequency).In the subsequent range (300 MHz–3 GHz), absorption drops off linearly as frequency increases.
- Superesonant (6 GHz–300 GHz)—Body again ceases to be a good antenna, absorption declines (~1/10 peak absorption). Most of the energy is absorbed in the skin (penetration is <1 cm). Skin absorption is dominant (>15 GHz).

2. For frequencies in the range from about 20 MHz to 300 MHz, the resonance for whole body and partial body exposure exists, at which relatively high absorption can occur in the whole body and to even higher values if partial body (e.g., head) resonances are considered.
3. For frequencies in the range from about 300 MHz to several GHz, significant local, non-uniform absorption occurs; and for frequencies above about 10 GHz, where the penetration depth is low, energy absorption is mainly confined to the surface of the body.

In tissue, SAR is proportional to the square of the internal electric field strength (Equation 3.4), and consequently values of SAR depend on the following parameters:

(i) The incident field parameters, i.e., the frequency, intensity, polarization, and source configuration (near or farfield);
(ii) The characteristics of the exposed body (i.e., its size and internal and external geometry) and the dielectric properties of its various components; and
(iii) Ground effects and reflector effects of other objects in the field near the exposed body.

When the long axis of the human body is parallel to the electric field vector, and under plane wave exposure conditions (i.e., far-field exposure), whole-body SAR reaches maximal values. For taller individuals, the resonant absorption frequency is somewhat lower. For shorter adults, children, babies, and seated individuals, it may even be greater than 100 MHz. The values of electric field reference levels are based on the frequency dependence of human absorption; in grounded individuals, resonant frequencies are lower by a factor of 2 (WHO 1993).

2.3 Mechanism of Energy Transfer

Non-thermal

(i) While considering non-thermal biointeraction, an important consideration is the magnitude of the energy of RF photons. The energy of a photon of an electromagnetic wave is hν, where h is Planck's constant and ν is the frequency of the electromagnetic field. Non-thermal effects are usually explained as: the energy quanta of radiation at 0.9 and 1.8 GHz equal 4 and 8 μeV, respectively. Both these values are extremely small and possible changes can arise occur only if the effect of the electric field within the biological system exposed to RF fields is not masked by thermal noise (i.e., the Brownian motion). These values are much smaller than 1eV, which is required to ionize a typical molecule (by a factor of approximately 2×10^5). So if exposure to RF fields were to damage DNA, it cannot be caused due to ionization or excitation due to the absorption of a single photon. So if the phenomenon like DNA strand break is to occur, it would have to be through some other non-thermal phenomenon, which at present is not fully understood.

(ii) Another mechanism involving cells concerns the attraction between them in the presence of an electric field (Adair 1994). The electric field polarizes the cell, that is to say charges in the cell move so that one side of it becomes positive with respect to the other. The cell is then an electric dipole and attracts similarly polarized cells. For typical cells and frequencies below 100 MHz, the energies involved are calculated to become comparable to thermal noise in electric fields of E = 300 V/m. Other possible biological effects are associated with cell membranes and the movement of currents through the membrane in either direction. When a voltage is applied across the membrane, the current that flows is not always proportional to the voltage (non-linearity). This may, partly, be due to the effect of the electric field on the proteins either in the membrane or localized nearby, which results in the flow of the currents through the membrane, which can also act as a rectifier (non-linearity) (Montaigne & Pickard 1984).

(iii) The phenomenon which is also non-thermal (not related with rise in temperature) is the pearl chain formation. Molecules and cells under the influence of RF electric fields at frequencies up to 100 MHz would rearrange and form chains along the direction of the electric field (Schwan 1957, 1982; Takashima & Schwan 1985). This is due to the forces acting on particles causing cordless pearl chain effects. This occurs when suspended particles are placed in a continuous RF field (1–100 MHz), which occurs when electrical charges tend to accumulate on opposite cell surfaces to form induced dipoles, whose orientation tends to change with oscillations of the field. A dipole-dipole attraction occurs in the process. The attractive forces between the dipoles are enhanced when the cells are in close proximity to each other. The particles cause chain formation parallel to the electric lines of force. The chain formation occurs due to the attraction between particles in which dipole charges are induced by RF fields. Pearl chains are formed with biological materials (with cells or molecules, such as erythrocytes or bacterial suspensions). The chain could be single stranded or multi-stranded as well. At low frequency, the threshold is proportional to the square root of the frequency, but above 1 MHz, it is nearly independent of frequency. The effect can be produced both by pulsed and by continuous fields, with a time proportional to the square of the electric field (E^2). A minimum amount of energy—proportional to τE^2 (τ and E is the minimum pulse width and threshold field strength, respectively)—is required to overcome the Brownian motion caused by the random thermal motion. Since this is the same for pulsed and continuous fields, it is suggested that both are equally effective in inducing this effect.

(iv) In addition to the alignment of the cells and larger molecules, other RF field-induced effects such as shape changes and permeabilization of cells have also been reported (Weaver 1993; Gehl 2003).

(v) Another non-thermal effect is the dielectric saturation occurring in solutions of proteins and other biological macromolecules due to intense microwave fields. It is suggested (Schwan 1958) that such field can cause polarized side change of the macromolecule to line with the direction of the electric field (polarization).

The microwave auditory phenomenon is another example of non-thermal effect. The minuscule but rapid rise in temperature as a result of the absorption of pulsed microwave energy launches an acoustic wave of pressure that travels to the cochlea by the hair cells and relayed to the central 7kHz and 15 kHz, which falls within the audible range of humans and has been verified experimentally (Lin 1978). Peak amplitude of thermo-elastic pressure waves have been computed for spherical head models approximating that size of rats, cats, infants, and adult humans exposed to 10 μs plane wave pulses at 1 $kW.kg^{-1}$. The corresponding incident peak power density is about pressure varying from approximately 350 to 1,000 mPa. (The threshold pressure is 20 mPa for perception of sound at the cochlea by humans.) Besides this, the effect of amplitude modulated (16 Hz) RF field on bone causes fracture healing and bony reunion, suggesting possibilities of high-frequency (≥14MHz) bone responses and ultrasonic transaction phenomena at such frequencies (Ray & Behari 1987a; Behari 2009a). As of now, the biological effects of low-level RF/microwave frequencies are well documented (Polk & Postow 1986; Behari 2009b; Bioinitiative 2012).

For a single pulse or brief application of RF energy, the exposure duration may not be long enough for significant conductive or convective heat transfer to biological tissues. For longer exposure durations, RF energy-induced temperature rise depends on the tissue target (in vivo/vitro) and their thermal regulatory behavior and active compensation process. For local or partial body exposures, if the amount of RF energy absorbed is excessive, there could be a rise in local tissue temperature. Under moderate conditions, a temperature rise on the order of 1°C in humans and laboratory animals can result from an SAR input of 4 W/kg. However, this temperature rise is within the normal range of human thermoregulatory capacity, and correspondingly the SAR is also within the limits of safe exposure and any biological damage seems unlikely.

Low-level radiofrequency (RF) waves interact with biological tissue through varied mechanisms, even at fields below the accepted guidelines for safe exposure, indicating certain bioparameters pointing to definite adverse health effects. Adair (2003) noted that the interactions were all weak compared with the endogenous interactions and concluded that it is most unlikely that RF fields of intensity less than 100 W/m^2 incident on humans could affect its physiology to any significant extent. However, it is now reported that the bioeffects indeed exist (Behari 2009) and it is explored if there could be health effects caused due to such exposure from RF fields below guidelines (e.g., AGNIR 2001, 2003).

Thermal

Biological tissue heating due to microwave exposure is more widely acceptable. These are mainly associated with the absorption of the RF energy resulting from the electrical conductivity (σE^2) of biological tissue. The RF electric field generates an oscillating current and the rapid transfer of the energy of this current into the molecular motion is responsible for most of the heat capacity resulting in an increase in the local temperature. The electrical conductivity is in fact only partly contributes to the translational motion of charged particles (ions). The other main contribution arises from the hindered rotation of molecules (mostly water). The water molecule has a large permanent dipole moment, which is randomly oriented because of thermal energy. With the application of an applied electric field E, dipole moments are partially oriented along the direction of the field. Because of the viscosity of the water, the field has to do work to rotate the dipoles resulting in energy transfer into the system. This dissipation mechanism is most effective over a fairly broad range of frequencies, ν, close to those given by $\omega\tau = 1$ (resonance condition), where $\omega = 2\pi\nu$ and τ is the average time the dipoles take to re-orient. Since $\tau = 4 \times 10^{-11}$ s for water, $\omega\tau \sim 0.25$ at 1 GHz, so this mechanism is very effective at the frequencies of mobile phones. The power dissipated is proportional to E^2 in both cases and defined as σE^2 per unit volume (Joules Law).

It may be stated that the thermal energy of microwave heating is the sum of a molecule's dielectric loss, magnetic loss heating, and conduction loss heating (De la Hoz & Loupy 2013). Compared to the conventional heating, microwave heating is much rapid. Bohr and Bohr (2000a, 2000b) have performed a series of experiments on globular proteins. They applied RF in a microwave oven (2.45 GHz, 800 W) for a period of

5 s (~0.3°C temperature increase) in the protein solution. Using optical rotational dispersion, the authors showed that exposure accelerated conformational changes of the protein and further an enhancement of folding and denaturation of the protein. The results were interpreted as evidence of coherent RF excitation of vibrational or torsional modes leading to altered conformation of protein molecules. De Polimeri et al. (2003) considered the exposure of solutions of bovine serum albumin at 1 GHz (15 mW/kg), exposure lasting for 3–48 hours and temperature from 25 to 45°C, enhanced the aggregation of the protein at a time and in a temperature-dependent manner. Copty et al. (2006) reported some specific effects on a solution of green fluorescent protein exposed to 8.5 GHz. At maximum RF power, the calculated SAR was 4 W/kg and increase in temperature was ~3°C. These authors reported that heating produced a decrease in the protein fluorescence intensity. It was noted that as compared to resistive heating, the alteration in fluorescence is larger in RF heating (for the same rise in temperature). In the latter case, it was interpreted as indicative of non-thermal effect due to RF heating. However, in either case the spectrum is red-shifted.

Limitations to the Effects of RF Radiation Imposed by Thermal Energies (k_BT)

The components of living systems are constantly subjected to the fluctuations of electric and magnetic fields (incident field) that are associated with the random motion of charges at the body temperature (Brownian motion (thermal noise). These random fields impose a limit on the sensitivity of the system to respond to applied RF fields. Hence, the search is for the requirement allowing us to predict magnitude and type of the applied field required to produce a given biological effect. Obviously this need to be greater than the one required to overcome the internal random field. The thermal energy of each mode of a component has an average value of around k_BT, so at body temperature, the thermal energy is around 26 μeV per mode. The oscillatory motion of an ion or other charged component in an RF field could possibly lead to biological effects. The average energy of a singly charged object of mass m and mobility μ in an rms electric field E oscillating at frequency ν is $m\ \mu^2E^2/2$. For a chloride ion, this is around 10^{-17}eV (for E = 100 V/m). This is much smaller than the thermal energy of 26 μeV.

In the light of the above it is suggested that the oscillatory motion of ions in fields below guidelines cannot possibly cause biological effects. However, since the oscillatory energy is proportional to the mass of the charged component, energies comparable to the thermal energy might be acquired by the oscillations of a large charged cell of diameter 50 μm containing 10^{15} atoms or more. The condition is valid to all systems that are well coupled thermally with respect to their surroundings.

2.4 Microwave Interaction with Biological Structure

Resonance Absorption in Head and Human Body

The human body has been variously examined as an antenna model, exhibiting whole and partial body resonances, with energy absorption based on physical dimensions and orientation of its parts with respect to planes of polarization of incident RF fields. In the upright position, the grounded body has a longitudinal resonance around 35 MHz (Gandhi 1975). However, without being grounded, this resonance gets doubled, i.e., around 70 MHz. In the transverse and anteroposterior axis, maximum absorption occurs at higher frequencies (from 135 to 163 MHz) (Gandhi et al. 1994, 1996). Although these configurations may be realized in far-field exposures, by contrast, near-field patterns of energy absorption, as in the user of cellular phone near the head, will be dominated by regional peaks determined by proximity of the transmitting antenna to specific body parts. For the head, the resonant frequency is a function of head size, varying from about 700 MHz in the infant to 400 MHz in adults (Gandhi & Hagmann 1977). The human head resonates between 400 and 500 MHz.

Whole-body rates of energy absorption for models of human and for animals subjected to incident fields of 10mW/cm^2 show that rates of energy deposition at resonant frequencies in the presence of a ground plane or a reflector are very different (Dimbylow & Mann 1994). With grounding and reflection combined, they are very high. Energy deposition rates for models of humans subjected to fields at a power density of 10mW/cm^2 predict SAR values as high as 35–70 times the basal metabolic rate for adults at resonant frequencies. The time-to-time convulsion of 100-g rats exposed to power densities of 3–20 mW/cm^2 confirms some of these predictions of enhanced absorption in the presence of reflecting surfaces. Early studies using thermalizing far-field exposure levels described "hot spots" of increased energy absorption within the head. These hot spots occur inside lossy spheres that model brain tissue with radii 8 cm<r>0.1 cm for frequencies between 300 MHz and 12 GHz (Kritikos & Schwan 1975). However, at lower frequencies (where the wavelength is much larger than that size of the object) and at much higher frequencies, heating occurs primarily at the surface of the sphere facing the source. Heat conduction and convection from a central brain hot spot have also been modeled, with inclusion of a factor for blood flow (Kritikos & Schwan 1979). For a spherical head 10 cm in diameter, exposed to a 1.0 GHz, 10 mW/cm^2 field with a central hot spot 2 cm in diameter, the expected temperature rise would be 0.5°C with normal blood flow and heat conduction being the means of heat removal.

For a given incident field flux, the heating potential in the hot spot decreases rapidly with increasing head radius (Kritikos & Schwan 1972,

1975, 1976). Also, there are strong differentials in convective capacities between cerebral gray and white matter, attributable to substantially higher densities of blood vessel capillary beds in cerebral cortical gray matter (Ranck 1964).

The wave length of a 3,000-MHz signal is 10 cm and is closely related to the length of mice or rats (~8 cm), making "hot spots" at some point along the body. A hot spot for a mouse or rat may occur near the tip of the tail and may be along the neck. For the human head, simulated as a sphere 15 cm in diameter with three layers representing brain, fat, and skin, a 2,450-MHz microwave beam is rapidly absorbed at the surface of the head. There is a maximum SAR for energy of 2.0 W/kg in the outer1.0 cm of the phantom for an incident power density of 1.0 mW/cm^2, although the average heating for the whole head is only 0.121 W/kg. In a small zone in the center of the head, curvature and a high tissue refractive index produce an SAR of 0.2 W/kg for the monkey head. This picture for humans is sharply changed at a lower frequency of 918 MHz, where energy absorption at the center of the head for an incident field of 1.0 mW/cm^2 is 0.45w/kg, which is significantly higher than that calculated at the surface.

Intracranial Fields Induced by Mobile Phones

For some devices that operate at frequencies above 10 MHz (e.g., dielectric heaters, mobile phones), human exposure occur under near-field conditions. The frequency dependence of energy absorption under these conditions is very different from that described for far-field conditions.

There have been numerous experimental assessments and numerical simulations of intracranial fields induced by mobile phones held against the head. Initial studies were based on FM transmitters (Cleveland & Athey 1989). The energy absorption mechanisms for lossy bodies in close proximity to antennas have been well described by Kuster & Balzano 1992; Gandhi et al. (1994), although levels of energy deposition reported in these simulations differ significantly. However, this is a near-field situation, where energy deposition is largely induced by the magnetic field component, i.e., generation of eddy currents.

Presently, the most important parameter determining the amount of energy absorbed in the tissues of the head is the distance separating the antenna or radiating structure. Absorption decreases approximately as the inverse square of increasing distance between the antennas or radiating structure and tissues. Depth of penetration is basically determined by carrier frequency, with more rapid attenuation as the frequency increase. At frequencies of 10–20 GHz, typical attenuations are in the range of 20 dB/mm from the skin surface.

These near-field conditions differ sharply from far-field exposures, defined as occurring 20–30 wavelengths from a radiating source, where the far-field scenario exists. In conformity with near-field models having strong magnetic coupling to tissues immediately adjacent to the transmitting antenna, there is a consensus that maximum field levels occur in skin, subcutaneous tissues, bone, and immediately subjacent brain tissue (interfaces where dielectric discontinuously occurs) (Bach Andersen et al. 1995).

The usefulness of numerical modeling calculations, as well as measurements of induced body current and tissue field strength, for assessment of near-field exposures has been demonstrated for mobile phones, walkie-talkies, broadcast towers, shipboard communication sources, and dielectric heaters (Kuster & Balzano 1992; Dimbylow & Mann 1994; Gandhi 1995; Jokela et al. 2004). The importance of these studies lies in their having shown that near-field exposure can result in high local SAR (e.g., in the head, wrists, ankles) and that whole-body and local SAR are strongly dependent on the separation distance between the high-frequency source and the body. Finally, SAR data obtained by measurement are consistent with data obtained from numerical modeling calculations. Whole-body average SAR and local SAR are convenient quantities for comparing effects observed under various exposure conditions (World Health Organization 1993).

2.5 Layering Resonances near the Body Surface

Mammalian body has layering of skin, fat, muscle, and bone and absorbed energy has a spatial distribution over it. The energy deposited in different body layers would be different owing to its differencing dielectric properties. Layering resonances in the vicinity of the body surface emphasize the need for caution in the use of SAR in terms of averaged values. The layering is associated with a resonance for three-dimensional bodies that is quite distinct from the geometrical resonance. Calculations for a multilayered prolate spheroidal model of man predicted a whole-body layering resonance at 1.8 GHz with an SAR 34% greater than predicted by a homogeneous model (Barber et al. 1979). However, for a specific skin-fat-muscle cylindrical model of man predicted a layering resonance frequency of 1.2GHz, with an "averaged" SAR double that calculated for the corresponding homogeneous model. The layering resonance frequency was the same for incident waves polarized parallel or perpendicular to the cylinder axis. The energy deposited in different body layers would be different.

2.6 Relaxation Phenomena

Relaxation refers to that part of polarization that is due to the ordering of permanent dipoles. The polarization caused by this mechanism is called electronic polarization or optical polarization.

Three relaxation processes are mainly responsible for the dielectric properties of tissues: dipolar orientation, interfacial polarization, and ionic diffusion. The theories summarized below apply to linear responses to weak fields. As the field intensity is increased, above a certain level, the response ceases to be linear. The threshold, at which non-linearity occurs, depends on the system and the investigated dielectric effect.

The interaction of molecules and fields is described by quantum mechanics (Stratton 1941). Individual molecules have discrete energy states and they absorb energy from an alternating field of frequency f, so that

$$\Delta W = hf \tag{2.2}$$

where ΔW is the energy difference between two quantum levels and h is Planck's constant. The molecule can take up or radiate energy only at the frequencies and in the quantum of the amount given by Equation (2.2). Each molecule have thus characterized by a spectrum with a number of discrete frequencies, corresponding to various excited states (in multiples of hf). The energy differences (in the multiple of hf) are extremely small and the smallness of ΔW may be understood when it is compared with kT. For f = 10 GHz, ΔW is only $(6 \times 10^{-3})\ kT$ at room temperature while the energy per degree of freedom is ½ kT in equilibrium condition.

2.7 Macromolecular Resonance

When collisional perturbations are very brief in comparison with the field period, every collision is quite effective in interrupting the molecule's radiation absorption-emission process. In a fluid with a large rate of collision, a collisional broadened relaxation type spectrum results. On the other hand, for collisions of long duration compared to the EMF period, the spectrum becomes resonant, even for a high rate of collisions, because each collision causes, statistically, little disruption. The collision time in a macromolecular fluid is a fixed function of temperature, and therefore the EMF frequency determines the kind of spectrum (rotational or resonant). Attenuation of MW fields is dominated by the presence of water, which also shields other possible bimolecular absorption processes.

The RF exposure effects structure and function of biological macromolecules such as proteins and DNA. The hypothesis being investigated is that absorption of RF energy by these molecules could modify their structure and also their behavior (Frohlich 1968). Experiments suggest resonant absorption in growing cells at 41 GHz fields and in DNA at 11 GHz (Azanza et al. 2002).

2.8 Radiation Effects

When the wavelength is on the order of the size system, energy can be efficiently beamed through the air, as well as transmitted through coaxial cables and waveguides. A typical system for transmitting EM signals through the air consists of a source, such as a radio transmitter or microwave generator, a transmission line or waveguide, and an antenna. The source produces EM fields that propagate along the transmission line or waveguide to the antenna, which launches the propagating wave into space, where it propagates similar to as free wave propagation. Such antennas are called transmitting antennas. EM radiation is propagated along a transmission line to a receiver. An antenna can usually be used as either a transmitting antenna or a receiving antenna.

Radiation patterns can be either field patterns or power patterns. Field patterns show either the E field or the H field as a function of position, and power patterns show the power as a function of position. The distance (R) from the center of the antenna to where the far fields begin is given by the Equation (1.9), i.e.,

$$R = 2D^2/\lambda \tag{2.3}$$

which gives the far-field pattern for a thin half-wavelength dipole. The plot is called a polar plot. In a polar plot, each point in the plane is located by two coordinates, the distance out from the origin (center) and the angle from a vertical line. In the radiation pattern, the angle of each point on the curve is the angle at which the magnitude of the E field is calculated, and the distance out from the origin represents the relative magnitude of the E field at that given angle. The magnitudes of the E field are all calculated at a given far distance from the antenna. In the far fields, the angular dependence of E does not depend on the distance away from the antenna.

Indirect Coupling Mechanisms

There are two indirect coupling mechanisms:

(i) Currents that result when the human body comes into contact with an object at a different electric potential; and
(ii) Coupling of EMF to medical devices implanted in humans.

When an individual and a conducting object is exposed to a strong field come into close proximity, transient discharges (sparks) can occur (Tenforde & Kaune 1987; World Health Organization 1993). The magnitude and spatial distribution of such currents depend on frequency, the size of the object, and the size of the person, and the area of contact.

2.9 Interaction of Radiofrequency Fields with Tissues

Quantification of internal fields induced inside the biological bodies is required for the purpose of dosimetric studies. The biological effects of microwaves depend both on the external power density and consequently on the field inside the tissue or the body. Hence, the knowledge of internal field is important. A biological body is assumed to be an inhomogeneous and lossy dielectric. Both the inhomogeneity of the dielectric properties and the complexity of the shape make the understanding difficult. Experimental approaches are also subject to enormous difficulties. The intensity of the internal fields depends on a number of parameters of the external field, e.g. frequency, intensity, and polarization of the external field; size, shape and dielectric properties of the body; spatial configuration between the exposure source and the exposed body; and the presence of other objects in its proximity. With a complex dependence on so many parameters, it is apparent that the internal fields in a mouse and a man exposed to the same external field can be dramatically different and hence their biological response. Conversely, it is apparent that different exposure conditions, pertaining to different frequencies, may induce similar fields inside such diverse shape as a mouse and a man. This offers challenges in the procedure of determination of criteria for the safe exposure.

The electric and magnetic fields produced in the body by a nearby electromagnetic source may cause both thermal and non-thermal biological effects. Thermal effects caused by the rise in temperature produced by the energy absorbed from oscillating electric fields. The force produced by an electric field on charged objects, such as the mobile ions present in the body, causes them to move, resulting in electric currents and the electrical resistance of the material in which the currents follow the heating effects. This heat input causes the temperature to rise and it continues to do so until the heat input is balanced by the rate at which it is removed, mostly by blood flowing to and from other parts of the body. It has not yet been made possible to measure these small changes in temperature directly, except those at the outer skin (Adair et al. 2003). Despite the fact that a number of sophisticated probes have been designed for its measurements, yet the challenges remain.

For dosimetric purposes, theoretical studies target the computation of one parameter, the specific absorption rate/ratio (SAR). The relationship between the SAR and the resulting temperature rise is a complex issue and is significantly dependent on the energy received by the biological body, which in turn is dependent upon antenna configuration, location, and frequency. Another possible mechanism is the effect of the electric field on the proteins either in the membrane or localized nearby, which assist in the flow of the product currents through the membrane, which can also act as a rectifier.

Microscopic Phenomena in Biological Matter

The overall interaction mechanism of electric field interaction at the microwave frequencies with biological matter is dependent upon the dielectric behavior of its constituents, which is dominated by water and the suspensions therein. In this context the discussion on electric properties of tissue and cells becomes relevant. Suppose a step function potential is applied to a sample of matter. The corresponding behavior in the frequency domain is given by Debye equation:

$$\epsilon^* = \varepsilon'((\epsilon_0 - \epsilon_\infty)/1 + jw\tau) + \epsilon_\infty \tag{2.4}$$

(where ε^* is the complex permittivity of the medium and is $=\varepsilon'$ -ε'',ε' and ε'' being its real and imaginary part) with the time constant τ that characterizes the exponential behavior in the time domain. $w = 2\pi f$ is the angular frequency of the applied field, while the subscription 0 and ∞ refers to the dielectric constant at low and high frequencies. The phenomenon of dielectric dispersion is established by practically all tissues following the relaxation equations of the type:

$$c' - \epsilon_\infty = (\epsilon_0 - \epsilon_\infty)/(1 + f//f_c)^2 \tag{2.5}$$

$$\sigma - \sigma_0 = (\sigma_\infty - \sigma_0)(f/fc)^2/(1 + f/fc)^2 \tag{2.6}$$

The cell membranes, with a capacity of approximately $1\mu F/cm^2$, act as insulating layers at low frequencies. The charging time constant is small to completely charge and discharge the membrane during single cycle, resulting in high tissue capacitance and hence a high dielectric constant. When frequency is increased, the capacitive reactance of the cell decreases. This causes an increase in currents in the intracellular medium with a resulting increase in total conductivity of the tissue (Figure 2.2 a, b, c). At high frequencies (≥100 MHz), the cell membrane capacitive reactance becomes sufficiently low so that the cell can be assumed to be short-circuited. This increase in frequency will subsequently prevent the cell from becoming totally charged during a complete cycle, resulting in a decrease in ϵ_H at such frequencies and above. In the frequency range of 100 MHz–1GHz, the ion constant of the electrolyte medium has no effect on the dispersion of the dielectric constant, thereby indicating that the values of ϵ_H and σ_H are independent of frequency. It is seen that the amount of the current passing through the cell is variable. The final decline of ϵ_H or corresponding increase in σ_H at frequency above 1 GHz can be attributed to the polar properties of water molecules, which have a relaxation frequency around 22 GHz (Daniel 1967, Figure 2.3). This also shows that an increase in conductivity with frequency is associated with a decrease in permittivity.

In the RF range, the tissues can be considered to be electrically equivalent to suspensions of non-conductive protein (and other solids) in electrolyte.

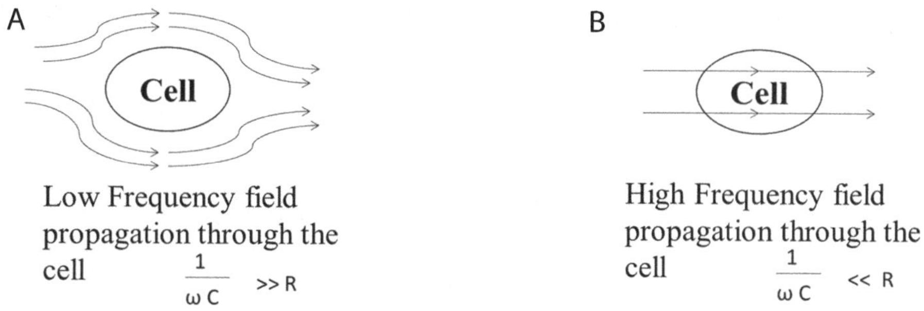

FIGURE 2.2a, b
Change in cellular behavior in transit from low-frequency to high-frequency electromagnetic field.
An electric current passing through the cell divides it into two parts. One part of it will bypass the cell by means of the surrounding fluid (Figure 2.2a). This is characterized by R_0 (extracellular resistance) and C_0 (cell membrane capacitance). For the current passing through the cell interior, (Figure 2.2b) R_I is the intracellular resistance and M is the capacitance (Figure 2.2c). Since the ratio of the two current changes with frequency, the dielectric constant is the function of frequency.

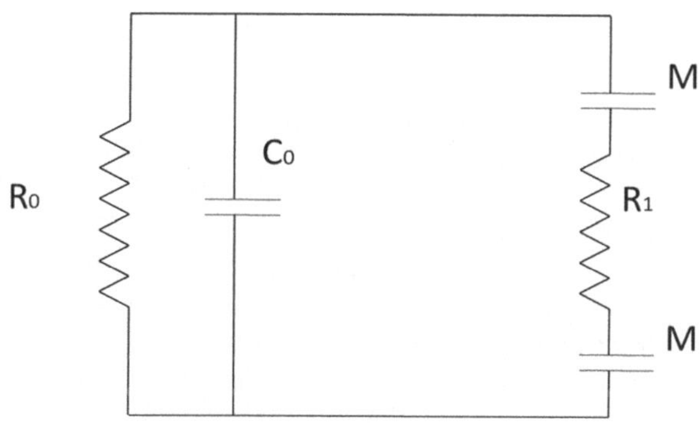

FIGURE 2.2c
Equivalent of a cell.

The conductivity of most tissues approaches a plateau between 10 and 100 MHz. Considering this, it may be mentioned that dielectric dispersion (variation of the dielectric constant with frequency) is a major issue in understanding the mechanism of EMF biointeraction.

Dielectric properties of biological tissues are frequency dependent (dispersive). A significant variation in dielectric properties over a given frequency range is called as dielectric dispersion. Permittivity values can exceed 10^5–10^6 at sub audio frequencies and can be expected to reach limiting values of 4–5 at frequencies approaching 100 GHz. At microwave frequencies, the

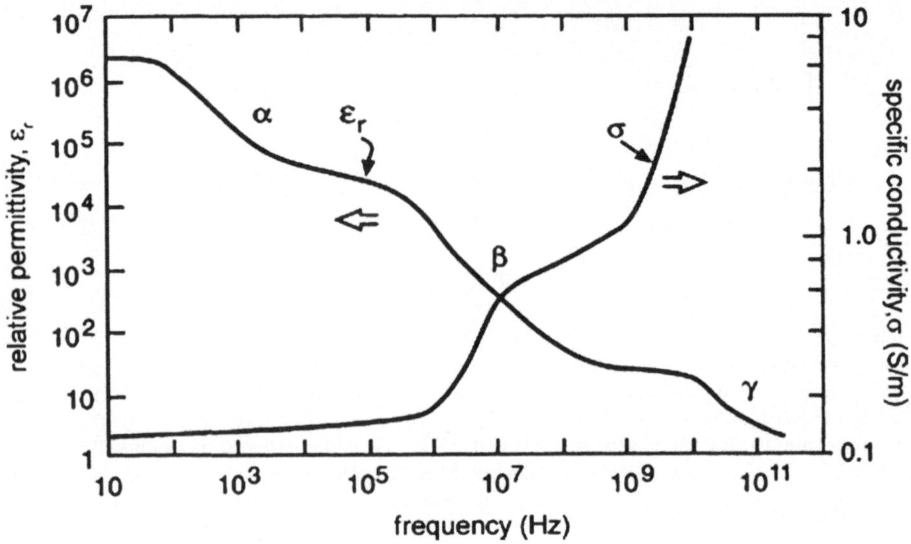

FIGURE 2.3
Variation of dielectric permittivity and conductivity follows an inverse relationship. While permittivity follows a sharp decline by many orders of magnitude (behavior changes in various frequency ranges), that of conductivity is much less.

dielectric dispersion can be attributed to arise from the dipolar relaxation of the bulk tissue water. Dipolar relaxation of water is a dominant effect in tissues at microwave frequencies. Some authors have called delta (δ) dispersion a small dispersion occurring in tissues and other biological materials between 0.1 and 3 GHz. The lack of a single dominant mechanism makes the interpretation of the dispersion region difficult.

Three major dispersion regions can be identified, which would correspond to separate relaxation processes. Schwan and Foster (1977) introduced three dispersions regions to characterize the anomalous electric properties of biomaterials. The three frequency ranges in which the dielectric characteristics can be divided are as follows:

(i) **α′ Dispersion:** Alpha dispersion is found in the low frequency (Hertz) range and it lasts till about a few kHz. Heterogeneous structure and composition and ionic activities inside the tissue dominate the low-frequency dielectric behavior of the tissue. In this region, large permittivity values are produced by ionic diffusion processes in micron- and large-sized objects. According to Foster and Schwan (1986), the alpha dispersion is due to surface admittance (lateral to the membrane surface). This is due to a frequency-dependent impedance of the folded inner membrane system of the cell or tubular system (Falk & Fatt 1964). At low frequencies, the current penetrates deeply into the sarcotubular system, leading to an increase in the total capacitance between the sarcoplasm and the extra cellular medium. Consequently, the relaxation time constant is determined by a combination of the sarcotubular capacitance and resistance of the fluid with these tubules. The dispersion resulting from the charging of the sarcotubular system would be associated with an increase in the bulk permittivity of the tissue, corresponding to the increase in apparent membrane capacitance from that of the outer cell membrane plus sarcotubular system. The total capacitance of the sarcotubular system can exceed that of the outer cell membrane by an order of magnitude or more. This access is ionic and hence its temperature coefficient is equal to that of the conductivity of the electrolyte, i.e., about 2%/°C.

At very low frequencies, the permittivity value is very large (10^6, Haines 1992), largely due to counterion diffusion. The alpha dispersion also results from other contributions active membrane conductance phenomena, charging of intracellular membrane bound organelles that connect with the outer cell membrane, and frequency dependence in the membrane impedance itself (Bardy & Sawyer 1990). Although alpha dispersion is dominantly visible in the permittivity, it is not so visible in the conductivity. Assuming a dielectric constant (10^6) and a relaxation frequency of 100 Hz, the Kramer and Kronig relation yields an increase in conductivity of about 200 times larger. These values of dielectric constant and frequency yield a total increase in conductivity of about $70Sm^{-1}$ (Walinsky et al. 1987). At RFs, the conductivity of tissue is essentially that of intracellular and extracellular fluids. This data further suggests that at low frequencies, tissues are resistive despite their high permittivity values.

This discussion refers to dielectrics with a single relaxation time, a phenomenon that is not common in biological tissues. Single relaxation time phenomena are found in certain dilute solutions of large polar molecules in non-polar solvents. For some materials (e.g., water) permittivity is close fit by a first-order Debye equation. For biological media, which involves multiple relaxation times, higher order terms are also necessary (Dubois et al. 1966, Schwan & Foster 1980).

(ii) **β Dispersion:** This region signifies where membrane filters low-frequency currents and permits high-frequency currents to pass through and exists in the frequency range from tens of kHz to tens of MHz. This arises from interfacial polarization (Maxwell-Wegner effect) of biological membrane systems. The βdispersion occurs at RFs mainly due to the capacitive charging of cellular membranes in tissue. Some minor contributions are also expected from dipolar relaxation of proteins in the tissue. This dispersion range is caused by Maxwell-Wagner polarization effects in which the cellular membranes are charged through the electrolytes. For tissues, total change in permittivity through the βdispersion approaches 10^4 relative to free space value, while the relaxation frequency value is about 500 kHz.

For fibers, orientation parallel to the field, β dispersion will be produced by the charging of the outer cell membrane, although it will occur at sub audio frequencies. At audio frequencies, the conductivity of the tissues in the parallel orientation should be close to that of the cytoplasm. In the perpendicular orientation, the outer cell membranes are charged with much smaller time constants. Hence, the membrane charging time constant varies inversely with the conductivity of the electrolyte, i.e., 2%/°C.

A small contribution might also come from dipolar orientation of tissue proteins at high RFs. As an example, blood exhibits a total dielectric increment of 2,000 and a β relaxation frequency of 3 MHz (Walinsky et al. 1987). The associated increase in ion conductivity is about 0.4 Sm^{-1}. For tissues, the static permittivity and relaxation times of this dispersion are typically larger than in blood.

Collins and Leadbeater (2007) hypothesized that MW-effects on enzymatic digestion could be due to the increasing dipole moments of the α-helices of proteins. They speculated that the interaction between the dipole moment of α-helix and the three-dimensional structure of protein. They further hypothesized that if the microwave energy interacts with the dipole of α-helix, the perturbation of the protein structure could facilitate the previously enclosed areas of the protein.

There is a smaller, though not well-defined δ dispersion in the range of 0.1–3 GHz, for which no single, dominate relaxation process has been identified. In tissues, the total observed changes in relative permittivity between 0.1 and 1 GHz are associated with it. It was examined for hemoglobin (Pennock & Schwan 1969), albumin (Grant et al. 1968), and bone (Behari 2009a, p. 140). In case of bone, the role of bound water is important emphasized. This dispersion (δ) is suggestive of a broad spectrum of characteristic frequencies extending from some hundred to some thousand MHz. Its magnitude is considerably smaller than that of the other two dispersions, and it is thought to be caused by a corresponding dispersion of the protein bound water and/or partial rotation of polar subgroups.

(iii) **γ Dispersion:** The gamma (γ) dispersion occurs in the microwave frequency range with a center frequency near 25 GHz at body temperature, due to dipolar relaxation of the water, which accounts for 80% of the volumes of most soft tissues, yielding a total dielectric constant of 50. γ dispersion arises from mobile counterions associated with fixed charges on cell membranes. This follows from the theory proposed by Schwarz (1972), suggesting that the characteristic frequency is proportional to the mobility of these counter ions and hence giving temperature coefficients similar to that of the conductivity of electrolytes. Here the relaxation frequency is close if not identical to that of free water and, hence, its temperature dependence is equal to that of water, i.e. close to 2%/°C. The contribution of the tissue water to the permittivity at microwave frequencies can be estimated by fitting the complex permittivity data about 5 GHz to the Debye equations and assuming a relaxation frequency identical to pure liquid water ($\varepsilon_\infty = 4$). In order to understand the dielectric behavior of the biological tissues, it is necessary to know the relaxation frequency (fs, corresponding to the relaxation wavelength λs), the dielectric constant at the low frequency end of the dispersion (Ɛs), the dielectric constant at the high frequency (ε_∞), and α the measure of spread of relaxation time. Following the Cole-Cole distribution formula, this can be written in the form (Grant 1979):

$$\frac{\lambda\varepsilon''}{\varepsilon' - \varepsilon\alpha} = \lambda\left(\frac{\lambda g}{\lambda}\right)^{1-\alpha}\left[1 - \left(\frac{\lambda s}{\lambda}\right)^{1-\alpha} \cdot \frac{\alpha\pi}{2}\right], \tag{2.7}$$

where λ_s and λg and are the free space and guide wavelength, respectively. In this way, the dielectric dispersion can be interpreted by Cole-Cole function with spread in relaxation time.

Assuming tissue to be a suspension of low permittivity, non-conducting sphere in water, the volume fraction solid (P) can be estimated from Maxwell's relation:

$$\frac{\varepsilon \text{ mixture}}{\varepsilon \text{ water}} = \frac{1 - P}{1 + \frac{P}{2}} \tag{2.8}$$

Using dielectric value at 1.2 GHz (>> the relaxation frequency), one can undertake estimation of the protein content of the tissue.

While dispersion due to charging cell membrane clearly exhibited in tissues as well as in cell suspensions, tissues exhibit a much broader range of relaxation time constants that is evident in suspension of individual cells. In the microwave frequency range, the following parameters contribute to the dispersion:

(1) Presence of bound water,
(2) Protein suspended in electrolyte exhibit Maxwell dispersion, and
(3) The suspended protein may also exhibit relaxation.

Following the Rayleigh formulation, connecting the dielectric constant of the solid tissue (Ɛα) with that of protein (ƐP) and the suspending fluid (Ɛw) is related through:

$$\varepsilon s = \varepsilon w \frac{\varepsilon P\,(1 + \phi) + \varepsilon w\,(1 - \phi)}{\varepsilon w\,(1 + \phi) + \varepsilon P\,(1 - \phi)} \tag{2.9}$$

where ϵ_∞ refers to the dielectric constant much above the relaxation frequency and ϕ is the volume fraction of the protein in the solution, which can be determined from the value of the solid content of the tissue.

Lin (1976) has considered a homogenous tissue with dielectric properties appropriate for brain tissue or some concentric sphere representing skull, brain, etc. With this concept, cerebrum and cerebellum are identified as to portion possessing differing dielectric properties. It is computed from the data of Ray and Behari (1987) that a value of 317±16 MHz for cerebrum and a different value for that of cerebellum 264±10 MHz. Shape factor is almost the same in the two cases. Further ε_s, ε_∞ turns out to be (35.0, 33.0, cerebrum) and (50.0, 40.0, cerebellum) respectively.

In the above discussions, possible changes in membrane impedances have not been considered. This is justified because of small change in the membrane capacitance with temperature (0.3%/°C) for erythrocytes (Schwan 1948). For each of the three dispersions, the dielectric constant exhibits a small negative temperature coefficient at low and high frequencies and a positive coefficient in-between which results from the strongly shifting dispersion. Prediction of temperature coefficient is difficult if there is a spread of relaxation time, but it may be possible by assuming only one time constant. Hence, near the characteristic frequency, it may take the following form:

$$d\epsilon/\epsilon = d\sigma/\sigma[(\epsilon_0 - \epsilon_\infty)/(\epsilon_0 + \epsilon_\infty)] \tag{2.10}$$

where $d\epsilon/\epsilon$ is the relative change in dielectric constant due to relative change in conductivity = $d\sigma/\sigma$. Here ϵ_0 and ϵ_∞ are nearly independent of temperature, with ϵ_0 much larger than ϵ_∞. It may be concluded that the temperature coefficient varies with increasing frequency, with the dispersion ranging from about –0.3 through a maximum of +2 and back to –0.3%/°C.

Similar considerations apply for the conductivity, however, with some difference. For one relaxation process, the expression for conductivity is as given by Equation (2.7), and the corresponding infinite frequency (>> f_c) value is:

$$\sigma_\infty = \sigma_0 + (\epsilon_0 - \epsilon_\infty)/f_c \,.\, 18 \times 10^{11} \text{ mohs/cm} \tag{2.11}$$

Since $\sigma_\infty >> \sigma_0$, σ_∞ is proportional to f_c which has a temperature coefficient of about 2 percentage/°C. If f is close to f_c, the numerator of the ratio $\{(f/f_c)^2/[1+(f/f_c)^2]\}$ decreases with increasing temperature twice as quickly as the denominator, so that the ratio itself changes with a temperature coefficient of about –1%/°C. Thus conductivity temperature coefficients of about 2%/°C at frequencies well above and below f_c change by only 1%/°C in the dispersion range (Schwan & Foster 1980). These three are the three major relaxation phenomena in biological tissues.

Relaxation in Dielectrics

The relaxation frequency (characteristics frequency $f_c = (2\tau\pi)^{-1}$) is the frequency at which the permittivity is halfway between its low- and high-frequency values. All living matter contains electrical charges (ions, electrically polarized polarized molecules such as water, etc.) and insulating materials such as lipids. It is therefore a weakly conducting medium (called a dielectric). The dielectric properties of tissues determine the net electromagnetic energy absorbed (SAR), which ultimately results in increased translational and rotational kinetic energy, thus converting into heat. A better knowledge of the dielectric properties of biological tissues enables a more accurate derivation of the dosimetric relationship between exposure, SAR, and the rise of tissue temperature.

In the first approximation, the Debye equation is the best possible description of a relaxation process. The relaxation process consists in the approach to equilibrium of a system which is initially not in thermodynamic equilibrium. Such a process is irreversible and not covered by equilibrium thermodynamics. Most relaxation processes fulfill the conditions for which irreversible thermodynamic is applicable. Relaxation occurs when the free energy stored in the system is degraded into heat, i.e., if entropy is created irreversibly. The irreversibility is related to the fact that the free energy of the field is used to increase the total amount of heat stored in the dielectric plus the heat reservoir surrounding it.

Conductivity

Above 100 MHz, conductivity resulting from dielectric loss becomes increasingly significant.

In the Equation (2.6) $\sigma = \omega\varepsilon''$ and σ_0 is low-frequency conductivity.

The dispersion magnitude $\varepsilon_0 - \varepsilon_\infty$ and $\sigma_\infty - \sigma_0$ are related by

$$\sigma_\infty - \sigma_0 = (C0 - \varepsilon_\infty)\, \varepsilon_r \bullet 2\pi f_c \tag{2.12}$$

One may also say that they relate the conductivity of materials, including to their permittivity. It may be concluded that for the imaginary part to exist, the permittivity has to vary as a function of frequency. On the other hand, when a material has a non-zero imaginary part of the permittivity, it exhibits losses and is said to be dissipative (or lossy). This property is called dissipation and it induces dispersion.

Another common definition is that of effective conductivity is:

$$\sigma''_{\text{eff}} = (\sigma + \omega\varepsilon_0\, \varepsilon'') \tag{2.13}$$

where σ''_{eff} has the unit of (siemens/meter, S/m).

The action of electromagnetic fields on tissues produces two types of effects that control the dielectric behavior. One is the oscillation of the free charges or ions and the other the rotation of dipole molecules at the frequency of the applied electromagnetic energy. The first gives rise to conduction currents with an associated energy loss due to electrical resistance of the medium, and other effects the displacement current through the medium with an associated dielectric loss due to viscosity. These effects control the behavior of the complex dielectric constant, given as

$$\varepsilon * /\varepsilon_0 = (\varepsilon' - \varepsilon''), \tag{2.14}$$

where

ε_0 = permittivity of free space,

ε' = real part of the complex dielectric constant,

ε'' = loss factor of the medium.

The effective conductivity σ (caused due to conduction current and dielectric losses) of the medium is related to

$\varepsilon'' = \sigma/\omega\varepsilon_0$ and the loss tangent is given by

$\tan\delta = \varepsilon''/\varepsilon = \sigma/\omega\varepsilon'\varepsilon_0$.

The quantity ε^* will be dispersive due to the various relaxation processes associated with polarization phenomena.

The decrease in dielectric constant ε_H and a corresponding increase in conductivity σ_H for tissues having high water content with increasing frequency (Table 2.1) are due to interfacial polarization across the cellular membrane.

The values of dielectric constant determine the amount of total power a given biological specimen will absorb when placed in an electromagnetic field.

At microwaves, above 100 MHz, three effects (free charges of ions, rotation of dipole molecules, interfacial polarization) add significantly to the conductivity.

It also introduces some dispersion at several hundred MHz because of the difference in the electrical properties of tissue protein and electrolyte. Maxwell-Wagner effects typically are dominant at RFs (Foster & Schwan 1986).

> The time constant for dipolar relaxation of globular proteins varies as the cube of the protein radius (Walinsky et al. 1987). Thus, small molecules relax at higher frequencies than larger ones. Since the maximum conductivity increase is proportional to the mean relaxation frequency, a small component with a high relaxation frequency may contribute noticeably to the total conductivity at these high frequencies.

TABLE 2.1

Frequency (MHz)	Wavelength in Air (cm)	Dielectric/ Constant ϵ_L/ϵ_H	Conductivity σL (mmho/m)	Wavelength λL (cm)	Depth of Penetration (cm)
915	32.8	5.6/51	55.6–147/1.60	13.7/4.46	17.7/3.04
1,500	20	5.6/49	70.8–171/1.77	8.41/2.81	13.9/2.42
2,450	12.2	5.5/47	96.4–213/2.21	5.21/1.76	11.2/1.70
3,000	10	5.5/46	110–234/2.26	4.25/1.45	9.74/1.61
5,000	6	5.5/44	162–309/3.92	2.63/0.89	6.67/0.79
5,900	5.17	5.05/43.3	186–338/4.73	2.29/0.775	5.24/0.72
8,000	3.75	4.7/40	255–431/7.65	1.73/0.528	4.61/0.41
10,000	3	4.5/39.9	324–549/10.3	1.41/0.464	3.39/0.34

(Partially obtained from Johnson & Guy 1972)
$\epsilon L/\epsilon_H$ = Low water/high water dielectric constant.
$\sigma_L/\sigma_{L\,H}$ = Low water/high water conductivity.

$$\lambda_{LH} = \lambda_0/\sqrt{\epsilon_{L,H}}.$$

Parameters of low and high water content tissue.

Dielectric Relaxation of Water. Water plays an important role in controlling the bioelectric phenomena in biological tissues. The dielectric properties of pure water have been well established from dc (direct current) up to microwave frequencies, approaching the infrared (Afsar & Hasted 1977). Temperature static and frequency-dependent permittivity values at room temperature are close to 80 and 5, respectively. Hence, the microwave conductivity is close to 0.8 mho/cm above 20 GHz, much larger than typical low-frequency conductivities of biological fluids which are about 0.01 mho/cm.

Three dielectric parameters are characteristic of the electrical and viscous properties of water: a) the static dielectric permittivity ε_0 observed at $f << f_c$ = 20 GHz, b) the relaxation frequency f_c, and c) the conductance of ions in water. A detailed study of the internal conductivity of erythrocytes revealed the intracellular ionic mobility to be identical with that of ions in dilute electrolyte solutions if appropriate allowance is made for internal friction with suspended macromolecules (Pauly & Schwan 1966). Tissue conductivities near 100 or 200 MHz, sufficiently high that cell membranes do not affect tissue electrical properties, are comparable to the conductivity of blood and to somewhat similar protein suspensions in electrolytes of physiological strength. Hence, it appears that the mobility of ions in the tissue fluids is also not noticeably different from their mobility in water.

Characteristic frequencies may be found from dielectric permittivity data or even from conductivity data. There is no difference between the relaxation frequency of tissue water and that of the pure liquid (Schwan & Foster 1977). The static dielectric permittivity of electrolytes of usual physiological strength (0.15 N) is about two units lower than that of pure water (Hasted 1973), a negligible change.

1. Dipolar relaxation of water is a dominant effect in tissues at microwave frequencies. Pure water undergoes nearly single time constant relaxation centered at 20 GHz (at room temperature, 25GHz at 37°C). Water associated with protein surfaces has a lower relaxation frequency than that of the bulk liquid, and this water fraction is responsible for the dielectric dispersion at frequencies near 1 GHz. For typical high-water-content tissues, the conductivity at 3–5 GHz is due in roughly equal proportions to ionic conductivity and to dipolar loss of water. It can be estimated that its conductivity will rise nearly quadratically with frequencies below about 10 GHz.
2. Theory predicts a dielectric increment of the order of 10^6 (Haines 1992).

The alpha dispersion also results from other contributions: active membrane conductance phenomena, charging of intracellular membrane bound organelles that connect with the outer cell membrane, and perhaps frequency dependence in the membrane impedance itself (Bardy & Sawyer 1990). Although alpha dispersion is very striking in the permittivity, it does not appear in the conductivity. Assuming a dielectric increment of 10^6 and a relaxation frequency of 100 Hz, the Kramer and Kronig relations yield an increase in conductivity, about 200 times larger. Thus, at low frequencies, tissues are essentially resistive despite their tremendous permittivity values.

These values of dielectric increment and frequency yield a total increase in conductivity of about 70 Sm^{-1} (Walinsky et al. 1987). At RFs, the conductivity of tissue is essentially that of its intracellular and extracellular fluids. The above description refers to the dielectrics with a single relaxation time, which is not common in biological media. In fact, three classes of dielectrics can be identified:

(i) Dielectrics with Single Relaxation Time. These are rare and are found in certain dilute solutions of large polar molecules in nonpolar solvents. For some materials, such as water, permittivity is closely fit by a first-order Debye equation, while for others, such as biological media, where several relaxation times are involved, higher order terms are also necessary (Dubois et al. 1966, Schwan & Foster 1980).

(ii) Dielectrics with Approximate Debye Behavior. The peaks of ε″ are wider and have a somewhat different shape. This is a large class which contains many simple compounds and solutions of dipolar compounds in non-polar solvents.

(iii) There are dielectrics for which Debye peaks cannot be recognized.

Protein Solutions

Water is the major constituent in most tissues, and because of its origin, this is also called biological water. Dielectric relaxation, conductivity, and diffusion have been further investigated for seeking a comparison. For instance, Cole-Cole representations show a relaxation time of the water in muscle tissue 1.5 times longer than that of pure liquid water, which is not much of a difference (Walinsky et al. 1987). The question of relaxation time of tissue water is, more precise, than that of the distribution of relaxation time. At microwave frequencies, the dielectric properties of tissues are dominated by their water content, the relaxation centered near 20 GHz. The magnitude of this water dispersion in tissues is typically diminished by some 20 dielectric units due to the proteins which displace a corresponding volume of water.

The dielectric properties of proteins and nucleic acids have been reviewed by several workers (Takashima 1969; Takashima & Minikata 1975). Protein solutions exhibit three major dispersion ranges. One occurs at RFs and is believed to have been arisen from molecular rotation in the applied electric field. Typical characteristic frequencies range from about 1 to 10 MHz, depending on the protein size. Dipole moments are of the order of 200–500 Debyes and low-frequency increments of dielectric permittivity vary between 1 and 10 units/g protein/100 ml of solution. The high-frequency dielectric permittivity of this dispersion is lower than that of water because of the low dielectric permittivity of the protein leading to a high-frequency decrement of the order of 1 unit/g protein/100 ml. This RF dispersion is quite noticeable in pure protein solutions. However, in tissues and cell suspensions, it only contributes slightly to the large β dispersion found in these materials.

Dielectric saturation for proteins can be predicted from the Langevin equation and occurs in the range of 10–100kv/cm. Indeed, onset of saturation has been experimentally observed in PBLG[1] at 50kV/cm, which agrees with the results obtained from Langevin formulation. Any irreversible changes in protein structure that accompany its rotational responses to an electrical field are unlikely to occur at field levels smaller than required for complete orientation, i.e., dielectric saturation. The thermal energy kT (where k is the Boltzmann constant and T is the absolute temperature) is in this case greater than the product μE (where μ is the dipole moment and E is the field strength), representing the change in potential energy that occurs with rotation. Thus changes in protein structure caused by non-saturating electric fields would probably occur spontaneously in the absence of any exciting field at normal temperatures.

Illinger (1977) has discussed the possibilities of vibrational and torsional substructural effects at microwave or millimeter wave frequencies. A calculation of internal vibrations in an alanine dipeptide in water, using a molecular dynamics approach, has been previously discussed (Rossky et al. 1979). In this model, the lowest frequency internal oscillations which occur (dihedral angle torsions at 1,500 GHz) are strongly damped. Conceivably, large proteins might exhibit lower frequency internal vibrations. But one would expect that any macromolecular vibration which displaces the surrounding water will be over damped by the water medium, which is quite lossy at frequencies below 100 GHz. Langevin equation predicts that saturation for smaller polar units requires higher field and strength values (Frohlich 1949). Thus we would expect that biologically critical field strengths are, for the various modes, probably well above the levels required by the Langevin equation for the complete rotational orientation of the total molecule.

Schwarz (1972) has discussed additional relaxation mechanisms which might be anticipated from the polarization of the biopolymer's counter ion cloud and from chemical relaxation processes including proton transfer and zwitterions. Counterion redistribution caused by the applied field is difficult to experimentally distinguish from thc rotational response and could contribute significantly to the biopolymer's dielectric properties. Evidence for dielectric relaxation due to fast conformational changes has also been discussed by (Schwarz & Seelig 1963). These considerations largely pertain to low field levels where the dielectric permittivity is independent of field strength. The field strengths at which non-linearity becomes significant are not well known, but field induced conformational changes are indicated at a level of 30 kV/cm near the temperature at which a conformational transition spontaneously occurs.

Cells and Membranes: Mechanism of Signal Amplification

Amplification process at the membrane site is by far the least understood issue in relation to non-ionizing radiation with biological systems. Amplification of extremely weak electric field can be provided by highly cooperative non-equilibrium biomolecular processes at the membrane level, viz. cell membrane behaves as extremely efficient energy amplifier under weak stimuli (Figure 2.4). In the process, the trigger or input signal to the system is amplified—by many orders of magnitude. In this regard, many processes can be considered in organized biomolecular systems.

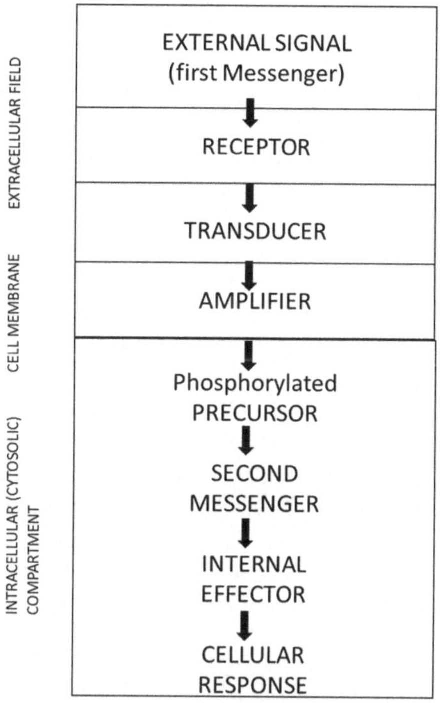

FIGURE 2.4
Diagrammatic representation of signal transduction pathway by membrane receptors.

While considering non-thermal effects, the use of weak EM fields to study the sequence and energetics of events that couple humoral stimuli from surface receptor sites to the cell interior has identified cell membranes as a primary site of interaction with low-frequency fields in the pericellular fluid. Circumscribing ELF-EMF or ELF-modulated high-frequency field interaction will play their role in the process of transmembrane coupling of the signal to the cytoplasm. It is suggested that soliton waves are responsible for such coupling. Such solitary waves involve a high degree of non-linearity in the molecular binding. Field modulation of cell surface chemical events indicates a major amplification of initial weak trigger associated with bindings of hormones, antibodies, and neurotransmitters to their specific binding sites. Calcium ions play a key role in this stimulus amplification, may be through highly cooperative alterations in binding to surface glycoprotein, with spreading waves of altered calcium binding across the membrane surface. Fields millions of times weaker than the membrane potential (gradient of 10^7 Vm^{-1}) modulate cell responses to surface-stimulating molecules. The evidence supports non-linear, non-equilibrium processes at critical steps in transmembrane signal coupling.

Cancer-promoting phorbol esters act at cell membranes to stimulate ornithine decarboxylase (ODC), which is essential for cell growth and DNA synthesis. This response is enhanced by weak microwave fields, also acting at cell membranes. There is strong evidence that cell membranes acts as powerful amplifiers of weak EM fields in their vicinity (Adey 1988). A point to mention is that equilibrium thermodynamics processes do not hold in cooperatively effects to explain the effects of ELF-EM (Frohlich 1968).

Cell Signaling

Signal transduction could be of two types: extracellular or intracellular. The former of the two is an example common to the endocrine, immune, and nervous system of mammals. Cells produce mediators (e.g., ligands and hormones) that can be detected by other cells via specific receptors located at the periphery of the cell on the plasma membrane and which induces responses in these cells. The signal can be transmitted inside the cell via a change in conformation of the receptor. This transformation may initiate various intracellular pathways via secondary messengers. Here either the ligand penetrates into the cell to bind to a cytoplasmic receptor, which will then generally act at the nuclear level as a transcription factor, or it binds to the extracellular part of a transmembrane receptor, thus modifying its conformation including the intracellular part of the receptor will have an increased enzymatic activity or bind to other proteins (e.g., kinases or G proteins). These reactions induce intracellular signaling such as protein phosphorylation cascades, which trigger specific cellular responses of the cell: Signal transduction has three stages: communication, transduction, and signaling. RF exposures affect calcium ion concentrations, intracellular gap junctions, and the clustering of receptors at the cell surface.

Calcium Signaling

This is an important species in intra-and inter-cellular signaling, as it plays a major role as a second messenger. Intracellular calcium is an important intracellular messenger. Calcium ions (Ca^{2+}) relay electrochemical messages to the cell surface and its biochemical mechanisms. Calcium is preferred over other neighboring ions (Mg^{2+}, Na^{+}, K^{+}, Cr^{+}) because this is able to bond without causing deformation to either membrane proteins or solute proteins of cytoplasm or organelles. Calcium is known to regulate processes such as cell division, differentiation, exocytosis, and differential gene transcription. AGNIR (2001, 2003) has reported that very low levels of ELF-amplitude modulated RF exposures (too low to cause heating) increased calcium efflux from isolated brain hemispheres. This efflux was assessed by measuring the movement of radiolabelled calcium ions out of the brain tissue both in vitro (Lin-Liu & Adey 1982; Dutta et al. 1984, 1989) and in vivo (Adey 1981).

It may be mentioned that very complex field distributions can occur, both inside and outside the biological systems exposed to EM fields. Refraction within these systems can focus the transmitted energy, resulting in markedly non-uniform fields and energy causing deposition. Different energy absorption rates can result in thermal gradients causing biological effects that may be generated locally and are difficult to anticipate (World Health Organization 1993). The geometry and electrical properties of biological systems will also be determining factors in the magnitude and distribution of induced currents at frequencies below the microwave range.

Interfacial Relaxation

If a material is electrically heterogeneous, charges do appear at the interfaces within the material because of boundary conditions at the interfaces. Interfacial effects typically dominate the dielectric properties of colloids and emulsions.

The bulk permittivity and conductivity of the composite material can easily be calculated. When the bulk material properties of the constituent phase vary with frequency, the frequency dependence of the heterogeneous material can no longer be characterized by a single relaxation time.

The conductivity of a dilute suspension of spherical particles has been calculated by Maxwell as a function of the volume fraction of the suspended particles. His analysis has been extended by Wagner to the case of alternating currents, which led to a set of dispersion equation in the form of Equation (2.5). These results clearly show that the presence of heterogeneity introduces dispersion in the material. This is often termed the Maxwell-Wagner theory. Asami et al. (1980) extended Fricke's (1924) formulation to the case of prolate or oblate spheroids for which the introduction of shape factor is termed as the Maxwell-Fricke mixture theory. It has also been extended to cover the cases of a spherical particle contained within a larger sphere and of a suspension of spheres surrounded by a thin shell of a material with different dielectric properties. These structures are membrane-covered spheres, such as cell suspended in physiological fluids. It is shown that the dielectric properties of the suspension are rather insensitive to the membrane conductance at RFs. An approximate analysis might not be valid for small cells or concentrated cell suspensions or at high frequencies. A more detailed analysis shows that there is a second dispersion, generally at frequencies in the range of 100–1,000 MHz. This gives rise to a dispersion whose relaxation frequency corresponds to the midpoint of the transition between these two limiting situations and is determined by the time constant for charging the cell membrane capacitance through the extracellular and intracellular fluids. This shows three types of dispersion behavior (α, β, and γ) and in-between β and γ, there is δ dispersion. This time constant is of the form RC, where R is a resistance, inverse to the conductivity, and C is the capacitance of the permittivity. In measurements by Ray and Behari (1987a) in the frequency range of 400–1,300 MHz, a relaxation phenomenon due to bound water attached to protein molecules was observed. This is identified as δ dispersion, which is usually smaller than β dispersion (Schwan & Foster 1977, 1980). The relaxation lies in the range of 800 MHz–1,000 MHz for wet and dry bone (Behari 2009a). The contributions from these two adjacent dispersions (β and δ dispersions) cannot be separately assessed due to the complexity of the system. For pure collagen, relaxation frequency turns out to be 500 MHz.

Ionic Diffusion: Counterion Polarization Effects

Counterion phenomena are due to ionic diffusion in the electrical double layers adjacent to charged surfaces. Counterion polarization effects have been reported in a variety of systems containing charged surfaces: emulsions, suspensions of charged polystyrene spheres, microorganisms, and long-chain macromolecular polyions such as DNA. The time constants for such effects are of the form L^2/D, where L is the length over which diffusion occurs and D is a diffusion coefficient. On the other hand, the time constant for the Maxwell-Wagner effect is of the form of RC or $\varepsilon\varepsilon_0/\sigma$, where R (or $1/\sigma$) is a resistance and C (or $\varepsilon\varepsilon_0$) is a capacitance. Counterion effects contribute to the alpha dispersion that is found in tissues at low frequencies. They are dominant in biological systems at kilohertz frequencies and below. Suspensions of submicrometer-sized polystyrene spheres have permittivity values approaching 10^4 with relaxation frequencies in the kilohertz range (Foster & Schwan 1986).

Grosse (1988) assumes that the counterion layer is very thin and the diameter of the particle is much larger than the Debye screening length of the electrolyte (Grosse & Foster 1987). The model also assumes that the counterion layer contains only ions that are opposite in sign to that of the fixed charges on the particles, and the counterions can exchange freely only with ions of the same sign in the bulk electrolyte. When an electric field is applied, the ions redistribute under the influence of both the field and diffusion. A set of coupled differential equations are obtained for the ion concentration and current densities, which yields a broad, asymmetrical, low-frequency dispersion in the permittivity of the particle. The dispersion is broad and can be fitted to a Cole-Cole relaxation function with $\alpha = 0.4$ [Equation (2.7)].

The physical interpretation of counterion polarization is rather simple (Polk & Postow 1986). The motion of an ion in the bulk electrolyte near the particle depends greatly on whether its sign is the same or opposite than of the ions in the counterion layer. Ions of the same sign can enter the counterion layer and their charge is quickly conducted to the opposite side of the particle: The particle acts as a good conductor. Those of opposite sign are excluded from the layer and must travel around the particle in the bulk electrolyte surrounding the particle: The particle acts as an insulator. As a result, charges accumulate in the electrolyte near the particle, giving rise to an induced dipole moment of the system and hence a large permittivity of the suspension.

Another problem comes arises from the uncertainty about the underlying mechanism, which makes a judgment about endpoints used in human studies, whether or not they can be considered as adverse effects, difficult. Consider for example the studies on effects of pulsed high-frequency EMFs on human sleep (Mann & Rösch-ke 1996; Wagner et al. 1998; Borbely et al. 1999): The occurrence of several other effects could be attributed to an interaction of the field with basic functions of the central nervous system and therefore viewed as an indication of a possible hazard, because this interaction will not be confined to structures guiding the architecture of sleep. Hence, the interpretation with regard to health will depend on the details of the unknown mechanism and not on the observed endpoint.

2.10 Free Radical Mechanisms in Biological Thresholds

It has been generally believed that non-thermal effects are unsustainable because observed sensitivities relate to field that lack sufficient energy to break chemical bonds. This perception that bond rupture represents a benchmark as an essential first step in biological transduction of electromagnetic fields is countered by growing theoretical and experimental evidence pointing to free radical mechanisms as one possible substrate. This model processes that magnetic fields may interact with free radicals produced in on-going chemical reactions, rather than inducing their formation (Adey 1993). It is generally accepted that OH^- ions are more severe than the others.

Grissom (1995) has set perspective on his studies of the much enzymatic sensitivity to static magnetic fields in the milli tesla range. But in the context of mobile phone users, interest centers on possible effects of much weaker fields oscillating at GHz frequencies. But even at these frequencies, interactions of tissue free radicals with cell phone fields during their typically brief nanosecond lifetimes may resemble those occurring in static fields. McLauchlan and Steiner (1991) attribute the highest level of free radical sensitivity to hyperfine-dependent singlet-triplet state mixing in radical pairs with a small number of hyperfine states (i.e., a small number of nuclear spins) or with a high degree of nuclear spin degeneracy, "with the implication that even very low fields may have significant effects on radical reactions".

Communication between brain cells is mediated by a spectrum of chemical substances that excite and inhibit transaction and transmission of information between them. These substance acts by binding to their specific receptors on cell surfaces. This process is also sensitive to modulated microwave fields. Kolomytkin et al. (1994) studied specific receptor binding to rat brain synaptosomes of three neurotransmitters: gamma-aminobutyric acid (GABA), an inhibitory transmitter; and acetyl choline and glutamate, both excitatory. Microwave exposures used 880 MHz or 915 MHz fields at power densities from 10 to 1,500 µW/cm^2. It was found that with incident field densities of 1.5 mW/cm^2, binding were observed at 3, 5, 5 or 30 Hz. Conversely, with 16 pulse per second (pps) modulation induced a significant increase in glutamate receptor binding. For acetyl choline receptors, binding decreased by 25% at 16 Hz, with similar trends at higher and lower frequencies; that is, as a function of field intensity as low as 50 µW/cm^2 at 16 Hz with 915 MHz fields.

Microwave exposure under athermal conditions occurs when no temperature rise can be measured by conventional thermometry. The existence of biological effects arising from the athermal exposure is still controversial, partly because of a lack of the linear dose-response relation. A model has proposed in which pulsed microwave radiation causes a triggering of the heat shock or stress response by altering the conformation of proteins through a transient heating of the protein and its close environment. This is supported by using the model of heat diffusion equation and shows that pulsed exposure even when a thermal can lead to transient temperature excursions outside the normal range. It is proposed that the power window phenomenon in which biological effects are observed at low power levels may be caused by an incomplete triggering of the heat shock response.

References

Adair ER (1994) Effects of weak high-frequency electromagnetic fields on biological systéme. In: *Radiofrequency Radiation Standards* (Klauenberg BJ, Grandolfo M & Erwin DN eds.). New York: Plenum Press, p. 207.

Adair RK (2003) Biophysical limits on athermal effects of RF & microwave radiation. *Bioelectromagnetics*, 24: 39.

Adey WR (1981) Tissue interactions with nonionizing electromagnetic fields. *Physiol. Rev.*, 61: 435.

Adey WR (1988) Cell membrane: the electromagnetic environment & cancer promotion. *Neurochem. Res.*, 13(7): 671.

Adey WR (1993) Electromagnetics in biology & medicine. In: *Modern Radio Science* (Matsumoto Hed.). Oxford: Oxford University Press, p. 231.

Afsar MN & Hasted JB (1977) Measurements of the optical constants of liquid H_2o & D0 between 6 & 450 cm^{-1}. *J Opt. Soc. Am.*, 67: 902.

AGNIR (2001) Possible health effects from terrestrial truncked radio (TETRA) Report of an Independent Advisory Group on Non-ionizing Radiation. *Docs NRPB*, 12(2), 86. China (National Radiological Protection Board) NRPB.

AGNIR (2003) Health effects from radiofrequency electromagnetic fields. Report of an Independent advisory group on non-ionising radiation. *Doc NRPB (National Radiological Protection Board)*, 14(2): 1.

Asami K, Hanai T & Koizumi N (1980) Dielectric approach to suspensions of ellipsoidal particles covered with a shell in particular reference to biological cells. *Japanese J. Appl. Phys.*, 19(2): 359.

Azanza MJ, Perez BRN, Lederer D, Calvo AC, Vander Vorst A & Del Moral MA (2002) Reversability of effects induced on the spontaneous bioelectric activity of neurons under exposure to 8.3 & 217 Hz low intensity magnetic. *2nd Int Workshop: Biol. Effects of EMFs*, Rhodes, p. 651.

Bach Andersen J, Johansen C, Pedersen GF et al. (1995) *On the Possible Health Effects Related to GSM & DECT Transmissions. A Tutorial Study*. Copenhagen, Denmark: Center for Personkommunikation, Institute of Electronic Systems, Aalborg University, p. 60.

Barber PW, Gandhi OP, Hagmann MJ et al. (1979) Electromagnetic absorption in a multilayer model of man. *IEEE Trans. Biomed. Eng.*, 26: 400.

Bardy GH & Sawyer PL (1990) Biophysical & anatomical considerations for safe & efficacious catheter ablation for arrhythmias. *Clin. Cardiol.*, 13: 425.

Behari J (2009a) *Biophysical Bone Behavior: Principles & Applications*. Singapore: John Wiley & Sons Asia Pvt. Ltd., p.140, 173.

Behari J (2009b) Biological correlates of electromagnetic field exposure. In: *General & Applied Toxicology* (Ballantyne B, Marrs TC & Syver T eds., 3rd Edition), Chapter 106, p. 1.

Bioinitiative (2012) *A Rationale for Biologically-Based Exposure Standards for Low-Intensity Electromagnetic Radiation*. Bioinitiative Working Group 2012.

Bohr H & Bohr J (2000a) Microwave enhanced kinetics observed in optical rotational dispersion of a protein. *Bioelectromagn.*, 21: 68.

Bohr H & Bohr J (2000b) Microwave enhanced folding & denaturation of globular proteins. *Phys Rev.*, E61: 4310.

Borbely AA, Huber R, Graf T, Fuchs B, Gallmann E & Achermann P (1999) Pulsed high frequency electromagnetic field affects human sleep & sleep electroencephalogram. *Neurosci Lett.*, 275: 207.

Cleveland RF & Athey TW (1989) Specific absorption rate (SAR) in models of the human head exposed to handheld portable radios. *Bioelectromag.*, 10: 173.

Collins JM & Leadbeater NE (2007) Microwave energy: a versatile tool for the biosciences. *Org. Biomol. Chem.*, 5(8): 1141.

Copty AB, Neve-Oz Y, Barak I, Golosovsky M & Davidov D (2006) Evidence for a specific microwave radiation effect on the green flouresence protein. *Biophys. J*, 91: 1413.

Daniel VV (1967) *Dielectric Relaxation*. New York: Academic Press.

De la Hoz A & Loupy A (eds.) (2013) *Microwaves in Organic Synthesis*, Vol 1 & 2. Wein heim: Wiley-VCH.

De Polimeri DI, Smith B, Dawe A, North A, Smith T, Archer DB, Duce IR, Jones D & Candido EP (2003) Microwave radiation can alter protein confirmation without bulk heating. *FEBS Lett.*, 543(1–3): 93.

Dimbylow PJ & Mann SM (1994) SAR calculations in an anatomically realistic model of the head for the mobile communication transreceivers at 900 MHz & 1.8 GHz. *Phys. Med. Biol.*, 39: 1537.

Dubois L, Sozanski JP, Tessier V, Camart JC, Fabre JJ, Pribetich J & Chive M (1966) Temperature control & thermal dosimetry by microwave radiometry in hyperthermia (In: Rosen A, & Vander Vorst A (Eds.) Special Issue on Medical

Applications & biological effects of RF/Microwaves). *IEEE Trans. Microwave Theory Tech.*, 44(10): 1755.

Durney CH, Massoudi H & Iskander MF (1986) *Radiofrequency Radiation Dosimetry Handbook*, 4th Edition, Report USAFSAM-TR-85-73. TX: USAF School of Aerospace Medicine, Aerospace Medical Division (AFSC), Brooks Airforce Base, 78235-5301.

Dutta SK, Ghosh B & Blackman CF (1989) Radiofrequency radiation induced calcium efflux enhancement from human & other neuroblastoma cells in culture. *Bioelectromagnetics*, 10(2): 197.

Dutta SK, Subramoniam A, Ghosh B & Parshad R (1984) Radiofrequency radiation induced ion efflux from human neuroblastoma cells in culture. *Bioelectromag*, 5: 71.

Falk C & Fatt P (1964) Linear electrical properties of striated muscle fibers observed with intracellular electrodes. *Proc. Roy. Soc. Lond. B.*, 160: 69.

Foster KR & Schwan HP (1986) Dielectric properties of tissues. In: *Handbook of Biogical Effects of Electromagnetic Fields* (Polk C & Postow E eds.). BocaRaton, FL: CRC Press, p. 27.

Fricke H (1924) A mathematical treatment of the electrical conductivity and capacity of disperse system. *J. Physical Review*, 24: 575.

Frohlich H (1949) *Theory of Dielectrics*. Oxford: Oxford University Press.

Frohlich H (1968) Long range coherence & energy storage in biological systems. *Int. J Quant Chem.*, 2: 641.

Gandhi OP (1975) Strong dependence of whole animal absorption on polarization & frequency of radio frequency energy. *Ann. N Y Acad. Sci.*, 247: 532.

Gandhi OP (1995) Some numerical methods for dosimetry: extremely low frequencies to microwave frequencies. *Radio Sci.*, 30: 161.

Gandhi OP, Chen Y & Wu D (1994) Electromagnetic absorption in the human head for cellular telephones. *Bioelectromagnetics Society, 16th Annual Meeting, Proceedings*, p. 64.

Gandhi OP & Hagmann MJ (1977) Some recent results on deposition of electromagnetic energy in animals & models of man. In: *The Physical Basis of Electromagnetic Interactions with Biological Systems* (Taylor LS & Cheung AY eds.). College Park: University of Maryland, p. 243.

Gandhi OP, Lazzi G & Furse CM (1996) Electromagnetic absorption in the human head & neck for mobile telephones at 850 & 1900 MHz. *IEEE Trans. Microwave Theory Tech.*, 44: 1884.

Gehl J (2003) Electroporation: theory & methods, perspectives for drug delivery, gene therapy & research. *Acta Physiol. Scand.*, 177: 437.

Grant EH (1979) Determination of bound water in biological materials. *Proc. Workshop: Physical Bases of Electromagnetic Interactions with Biological Systems*, University of Maryland, p. 113.

Grant EH, Keefe SE & Takashima S (1968) The dielectric behavior of aqueous solutions of bovine serum albumin from radio wave to microwave frequencies. *J. Phys. Chem*, 72: 437.

Grissom CB (1995) Magnetic field effects in biology: a survey of possible mechanisms with emphasis on radical-pair recombination. *Chem. Rev.*, 95: 3.

Grosse G (1988) Permittivity of a suspension of charged spherical particles in electrolyte solution II: influence of the surface conductivity & asymmetry of the electrolyte on the low & high frequency relaxations. *J. Phys. Chem.*, 92: 1905.

Grosse G & Foster KR (1987) Permittivity of a suspension of charged spherical particles in electrolyte solution. *J. Phys. Chem.*, 91: 3073.

Haines DE (1992) Current & future modalities of catheter ablation for the treatment of cardiac arrhythmias. *J. Invas. Cardiol.*, 4: 291.

Hasted JB (1973) *Aqueous Dielectrics*. London: Chapman & Hall.

Illinger KH (1977) Millimeter wave & far infra red absorption in biological systems. In: *The Physical Basis of Electromagnetic Interactions with Biological Systems, Proc. Workshop* (Taylor LS & Cheung AY eds.). University of Maryland, p. 43.

Johnson CC & Guy AW (1972) Nonionizing electromagnetic wave effects in biological materials and systems. *Proc. IEEE*, 60: 692.

Jokela K, Puramen I & Shivonen AP (2004) Assessment of the magnetic field exposure due to the battery current of digital mobile phones. *Health Phys.*, 86: 56.

Kirschvink JL (1996) Microwave absorption by magnetite: a possible mechanism. *Bioelectromagnetics*, 17: 187.

Kolomytkin O, Yurinska M, Zharikov S et al. (1994) Response of brain receptor systems to microwave energy exposure. In: *On the Nature of Electromagnetic Field Interactions with Biological Systems* (Frey AH & Landes RG eds.). Austin, TX, p. 195.

Kritikos HN & Schwan HP (1972) Hot spots generated in conducting spheres by electromagnetic waves & biological implications. *IEEE Trans. Biomed. Eng.*, 19: 53.

Kritikos HN & Schwan HP (1975) The distribution of heating potential inside lossy spheres. *IEEE Trans. Biomed. Eng.*, 22: 457.

Kritikos HN & Schwan HP (1976) Formation of hot spots in multilayered spheres. *IEEE Trans. Biomed. Eng.*, 23: 168.

Kritikos HN & Schwan HP (1979) Potential temperature rise induced by electromagnetic field in brain tissue. *IEEE Trans. Biomed. Eng.*, 26: 123.

Kuster N & Balzano Q (1992) Energy deposition mechanism bybiological bodies in the near field of a dipole antenna above 300MHz. *IEE Trans. Vehicular Tech.*, 41(1): 17.

Lin JC (1976) Eletromagnetic pulse interaction with mammalian cranial structures. *IEEE Trans. Biomed. Engg.*, 23: 61.

Lin JC (1978) *Microwave Auditory Effects & Applications*. Springfield, IL: Charles C Thomas.

Lin-Liu S & Adey WR (1982) Low frequency amplitude modulated fields change change efflux rates from synaptosomes. *Bioelectromagnetics*, 3: 309.

Mann K & Rösch-ke J (1996) Effects of pulsed high-frequency electromagnetic fields on human sleep. *Neuropsychobiology*, 33: 41.

McLauchlan K & Steiner UE (1991) The spin-correlated radical pair as a reaction intermediate. *Molec. Phys.*, 73: 241.

Montaigne K & Pickard WF (1984) Offset of the vacuolar potential of characean cells in response to electromagnetic radiation over the range 250 Hz – 250 kHz. *Bioelectromagnetics*, 5: 31.

Pauly H & Schwan HP (1966) Dielectric properties & ion mobility in erthrocytes. *Biophysical J.*, 6: 621.

Pennock BE & Schwan HP (1969) Further observations on the electrical properties of hemoglobin-bound water. *J. Phys. Chem.*, 73: 2600.

Polk C & Postow E (1986) *Handbook of Biological Effects of Electromagnetic Fields*. Boca Raton, FL: CRC Press.

Ranck JB (1964) Specific impedance of cerebral cortex during spreading depression & an analysis of neuronal, neuroglial & interstitial contributions. *Exp. Neurol.*, 9: 1.

Ray S & Behari J (1987) Dielectric dispersion in brain tissue. Proceedings of first Asia-Pacific microwave conference. In: *MicrowaveTechnology & Applications* (Srivastava GP & Sharma MK eds.), p. 496.

Ray S & Behari J (1987a) Electrical conductivity in bone in frequency range 0.4–1.3 GHz. *Biomat. Med. Dev. Art. Org.*, 14(3 & 4): 153.

Rossky PJ, Karplus M & Solvation A (1979) Molecular dynamics study of a di peptide in water. *J. Am. Chem. Soc.*, 101: 1913.

Schwan HP (1948) Temperature dependence of the dielectric constant of blood at low frequencies. *Z. Naturforsch*, 38: 361.

Schwan HP (1957) Electrical properties of tissue & cell suspensions. In: *Advances in Biological & Medical Physics* (Lawrence JH & Tobias CA eds.). Academic Press, Vol. 4, p. 147.

Schwan HP (1958) Molecular response characteristics to ultrahigh frequency fields. In: *Proceeding 2nd Tri serv. Conf. on Biol. Effects of Microwave Energy*, Rome, NY, p. 33.

Schwan HP (1982) Nonthermal cellular effects of electromagnetic fields AC-field induced ponderomotoric forces. *Br. J. Cancer*, 5(S): 220.

Schwan HP & Foster KR (1977) Microwave dielectric properties of tissues: some comments on the rotational mobility of tissue water. *Biophys. J.*, 17: 193.

Schwan HP & Foster KR (1980) RF-field interaction with biological systems: electrical properties & biophysical mechanisms. *Proc. IEEE*, 68(1): 104.

Schwarz G (1972) Dielectric relaxation of biopolymers in solution. *Advan. Mol. Relaxation Processes*, 3: 281.

Schwarz G & Seelig J (1963) Kinetic properties & the electric field effect of the helix-coil transition of poly(r-benz1 L-glutamate) determined from dielectric relaxation measurements. *Biopolymers*, 6: 1263.

Stratton JA (1941) *Electromagnetic Theory*. New York: McGraw-Hill.

Takashima S (1969) Dielectric properties of proteins. I. Dielectric relaxation. In: *Physical Principles & Techniques of Protein Chemistry* (Leach JS ed.). New York: Academic, p. 291.

Takashima S & Minikata A (1975) Dielectric behavior of biological macromolecules. *Dig. Diel. Lit.*, (Nat. Res. Council, Washington, DC), 37: 602.

Takashima S & Schwan HP (1985) Alignment of microscopic particles in electric fields & its biological implications. *Biophys. J.*, 47: 513.

Tenforde TS & Kaune WT (1987) Interaction of extremely low frequency electric & magnetic fields with humans. *Health Phys.*, 53: 585.

Wagner P, Röschke J, Mann K, Hiller W & Frank C (1998) Human sleep under the influence of pulsed radiofrequency electromagnetic fields: a polysommnographic study using standardized conditions. *Bioelectromagn.*, 19: 199.

Walinsky P, Rosen A & Greenspon AJ (1987) Methods & apparatus for high frequency catheter ablation. U.S. Patent 4,641.

Weaver JC (1993) Electroporation:ageneral phenomenon for manipulating cells & tissues. *J. Cell Biochem.*, 51(4): 426.

World Health Organization (1993) *Electromagnetic Fields (300 Hz to 300 GHz)*. Geneva: WHO.

3

Dosimetry

3.1 Introduction

A biological body is an inhomogeneous, lossy dielectric, whose macroscopic electrical properties are described by the complex permittivity. Following this, the fields inside biological bodies exposed to known external electromagnetic (EM) fields have been computed by solving Maxwell's equations subjected to a set of boundary conditions. The inhomogeneity of the dielectric properties and the complexity of the shape make a solution difficult, or sometimes even a full formulation of the problem is a formidable task. Only much simplified models can be analyzed. The other approach appears to be an experimental one, which is also constrained with considerable limitations.

The characteristics of the internal fields depend on the parameters of the external fields, (frequency, intensity, polarization, size, shape, dielectric properties of the exposed body, spatial configuration between the exposure source and the exposed body, and the presence of other objects in the vicinity). With a complex dependence on so many parameters, it is apparent that the internal fields in a mouse and a man exposed to the same external field can be dramatically different, and so will be their biological response. On the other hand, different exposure conditions, for example, different frequencies, may induce similar fields inside such diverse shapes as a mouse and a man. These are the major cause of uncertainty in deciding the criteria for safe exposure in various biologic species (Stuchly 1978).

Dosimetry (dose–effect relationship) plays an important role in risk evaluation of human exposure to radio-frequency (RF) fields, for example, induced fields and evaluation of specific absorption ratio (SAR), and current density. This also defines the criteria for safe exposure on living systems. It is important to carefully select appropriate methods of dosimetry in each case. It is also highly recommended to validate the dosimetry by comparing with the results obtained with other methods. In addition to the experimental techniques (with whatever limitations), it is customary to revert to mathematical methods to arrive at an estimation of dosimetric parameters along with possible experimental data on phantoms.

3.2 Fundamentals

In an attempt to collect basic information and their interpretation, one falls back on laboratory investigations. Reliability of these studies, while reporting biological effects of RF/MW exposures on animal experiments depends, though not limited to the following parameters:

1. Selection of an animal model with consideration of its physiologic responses
2. Methods applied for investigation of biological processes
3. Extrapolation of data from animals to man

It is apparent that SAR variability is thus implied and so its uncertainties.

We now consider the following parameters and the mechanisms involving dosimetry:

Energy Absorption

Electromagnetic field interactions with biological system and subsequent energy transfer in the process are a matter of prime concern. While falling on biological objects, the energy absorbed by an object exposed to incident EM fields, the E-field can transfer energy to electric charges through the forces it exerts on them, but the B-field does not transmit energy. The forces that B exerts on the charges can merely change their directions, but not their energy. This follows from the fact that B-field exerts forces in a direction perpendicular to the velocities of the charges. The B-field can, however, transfer energy through forces on permanent magnetic dipoles, but biological tissue is mostly nonmagnetic (contains very few permanent magnetic diploes). Hence, this effect is not prominent in EM biological interactions.

The absorption is dependent on the size and geometry of the biological body relative to the wavelength. This wavelength-to-body size relationship (λ/L, where L is one-half the longest axis dimension of the body) is a critical factor in the relative absorption cross section, besides the ratio of the absorbed energy per second to the power incident on the geometrical cross-sectional area of the animal (Anne et al. 1962). At longer wavelengths, the orientations of the animal with respect to the **E** and **H** vectors also affect the relative absorption cross section (Gandhi 1975).

Specific Absorption Ratio

A dosimetric measure that has widely adopted nonionizing biointeractions is the SAR defined as "the time derivative of the incremental energy (dW) absorbed by, or dissipated in an incremental mass (dm) contained in a volume element (d*V*) of a given density (ρ)." The average SAR is expressed in watts per kilogram (W/kg). The average SAR is defined as a ratio of the total power absorbed in the exposed body to its mass. The local refers to the value within a defined unit volume or unit mass, which can be arbitrarily small. Hence, SAR is written as:

$$\text{SAR} = \mathrm{d}/\mathrm{dt}(\mathrm{d}W/\mathrm{d}m) = \mathrm{d}/\mathrm{dt}[\mathrm{d}W/\rho(\mathrm{d}V)] \tag{3.1}$$

It is understood that in low level exposure, induced fields primarily cause the biological effect of RF exposure, though its mechanism remains to be fully understood. Thus, to achieve a quantitative understanding of biological response in a quantitative manner, knowledge of induced electric field (SAR) and current density is of importance. This is interpreted in relation with the observed phenomenon. In addition, it may be understood that the field induced in a biological body due to the radio-frequency exposure is usually specified in terms of such physical characteristics as modulation (continuous wave (CW) or pulsed), and also duration of exposure, besides several other factors. Further, the coupling of RF energy into biological systems may be quantified by the induced electric and magnetic fields, power deposition, and the distribution and penetration into biological tissues. These quantities are in turn all functions of its relationship to the physical configuration and dimension of the biological body.

The internal fields can be quantified in various ways. The magnetic permeability of most tissues is practically equal to that of free space, and all known and anticipated interactions at higher RFs occur mainly through the E-field (including the currents induced by the H-field). Therefore, the E-field vector, or its distribution throughout the exposed body, fully describes the exposure field–tissue interaction. Neglecting the possible thermal losses, the absolute electric power can be expressed as the power generated by internal electric current within the organ.

For the special case of sinusoidal steady-state EM fields, the time rate of energy transferred to charges in an infinitesimal volume element ΔV of a material is given by

$$P = (\sigma + \omega\varepsilon_0\varepsilon'')E^2_{\text{rms}}\Delta V(\text{W}) \tag{3.2}$$

where ω is the radian frequency in radians/second (r/s) and E_{rms} is the root-mean-square (rms) value of the magnitude of E at that point. Thus, Equation (3.1) is a point relation because it applies only at the given point where E has the given value. Since ΔV (volume) has units of m^3, the quantity $(\sigma + \omega\varepsilon_0\varepsilon'')$ E^2_{rms} has units of W/m^3, which is the density of absorbed power.

$$\text{SAR} = (\sigma + \omega\varepsilon_0\varepsilon'')E^2{}_{\text{rms}}/\rho(\text{W/kg}) \tag{3.3}$$

The term within the bracket is defined as effective conductivity, by which the expression for SAR is defined below:

$$\text{SAR} = \sigma_{\text{eff}}E^2{}_{\text{rms}}/\rho(\text{W/kg}) \tag{3.4}$$

σ_{eff} is often referred to as just "conductivity."

$$\sigma_{\text{eff}} = (\sigma + \omega\varepsilon_0\varepsilon'')$$

where ρ is the mass density in kg/m^3. The quantity σ in Equation (3.3) shows a spatial relationship, so the computed SAR has a local significance. The space average SAR for a body can be obtained by calculating the local SAR at each point in the body and then can be averaged over the whole body. In nonionizing biointeraction, complicating factor is that exposure of the whole body to a given field strength could have outcomes far different for partial body or whole body exposure at the same strength. The spatially averaged field strength, depending on the region of space over which the fields are averaged, may vary widely for a given body. SAR values are tissue-type dependent (different tissue conductivities), and require a region of specific tissue mass for averaging. This then defines correlation with corresponding biological response. It is obvious that smaller the average region size, the greater is the precision. The sensitivity and resolution of present-day computational algorithms and the computer time available and precision of experimental measurement devices can provide dosimetric values accurate with a spatial resolution on the order of 1mm in dimension or sometimes even better.

Losses are associated with power absorption σ (ε''), hence the greater the values of σ or the ε'', the greater the loss in the material; that is, the more power is absorbed for a given E. This is then suggestive that tissue with higher water content, such as muscle, is more lossy than tissue with lower water content, for example, bone and fat. Equation (3.4) expresses the rate at which the electromagnetic energy is converted into heat through well-established interaction mechanisms. This then provides a quantitative measure of all the interaction mechanisms that are dependent on the intensity of the internal E-field (Guy 1979; Durney & Christensen 2000). However, should the direction of the internal E-field with respect to the biological structures be of importance for a given interaction mechanism, the SAR would not provide full quantitative information. This is because SAR provides only average information. SAR so obtained enables comparison of experimentally observed biological effects for various species under various exposure conditions. This also provides the means of extrapolating the animal data into potential hazards to humans exposed to RF radiation.

Equation (3.4) has severe limitations. From this equation for the computation of SAR, it is obvious that the quantities j (generated current density), E (generated internal electric field), ρ (tissue density), and σ (tissue conductivity) are assumed to be constant within an organ (e.g., eye) or a group of organs (e.g., head) of a living body. This is an oversimplification of the true scenario, since every organ or group of organs consists of many different types of biological tissue and all these quantities vary significantly between different biological tissues and even within a single type of tissue and within a single cell. This is obvious because conductivity shows not only spatial dependence but also is frequency dependent. For example, at a frequency of 1 GHz, conductivity in different tissues of the human body can vary from about 0.04 S/m (bone marrow) to about 2.45 (cerebrospinal fluid). Moreover, the conductivity of a given tissue type increases considerably and nonlinearly with frequency (up to a hundred times for a frequency range between 10^5 and 10^{10} Hz) (Gabriel et al. 1996). Even within a single cell, conductivity can have large variations from 10^{-7} S/m (cell membrane) to 0.5–1 S/m (cytoplasm, extracellular aqueous solution) (Foster & Schwan 1989).

However, experimental data on energy dependency of biological effects by EMF have shown that the present SAR formulation, very often, neither adequately explains the real value of (a) the nonlinear character of EMF-induced bio effects due to the existence of amplitude, frequency, and "exposure time windows." A plausible explanation put forward for the reported increased bioactivity of the ELF components of a microwave field is given by the "ion-force doscillation theory" (Panagopoulos et al. 2000, 2002). According to this, the bioactivity of oscillating EMFs is inversely proportional to the frequency of the field and directly proportional to the amplitude of the force doscillation induced on free ions in the vicinity of cell membrane electro sensitive channels within the exposed biological tissue. Moreover, according to the same theory, pulsed fields are twice as much bioactive than the corresponding CW fields with other identical parameters and this explains the results of several studies (Franzellitti et al. 2010). Also the (b) EMF-induced bio effects significantly depend on physical and chemical composition of the surrounding medium.

Dielectrics are materials having negligibly small conductivity (σ). The properties of dielectrics are described in terms of the loss tangent (dissipation factor), which is defined as

$$\tan \delta = \varepsilon'' / \varepsilon' \tag{3.5}$$

Data of dielectric properties are often presented in terms of ε' and $\tan \delta$ (Table 2.1).

However, the measurements of the internal fields are beset with difficulties, because biological materials (e.g., phantom materials) are having high impedances. This demands specially designed high input impedance probes for measurements of induced fields. This needs special instruments and techniques. For instance, since some effects of radio waves modulated in amplitude at extremely low frequencies (ELF) are dependent on the E-field intensity (Adey 1981). However, should the direction of the internal E-field with respect to the biological structures be of importance for a given interaction mechanism, the SAR would not provide full quantitative information. Similarly, for the interactions directly through the H-field.

Precise measurements of the external fields and the evaluation of the exposure conditions are a part of experimental dosimetry (IEC 2005; IEEE 2003). Therefore, to prevent potentially hazardous exposure to man, the knowledge of external fields is necessary and hence their measurements. Data on the intensities of external fields that potentially constitute a hazards to man are obtained through experimental evaluation of the intensities of the internal fields (SARs) that cause damage to animals. It is estimated that this may produce similar internal fields (SARs) in man.

Variation of SAR

Frequency Scaling

It is customary to perform exposure experiments on animals and extrapolating the results to humans. For this the conditions of EM similitude can be applied (Stratton 1941; Vander Vorst 1994). These conditions are often used in a reduced form termed frequency scaling. They enable us to use results obtained with a given object and adapt them to predict the results to be obtained with another object, similar in form to the first but differing only by a scale factor.

It is often said that the conditions of EM similitude are satisfied when a smaller size model is submitted to a correspondingly smaller wavelength, that is, a correspondingly higher frequency. From this, it is often understood that two times smaller model will yield the same results as the original one if the frequency is doubled. The reason lies in the Maxwell's equations: In the presence of losses, there is one more term to take into account. This modifies the factors that have to remain constant when shifting from one model to another to keep the equations dimensionless. However, keeping the ratio size to wavelength a constant is not a sufficient condition anymore. There are circumstances where frequency scaling is very inaccurate (and inadequate), may indeed be in biological systems, because these are lossy dielectrics.

From Equation (4.3), it is apparent that internal SAR distribution in the rat-sized spheroid at 600 MHz would be similar to the internal SAR distribution in the man-sized spheroid at 80 MHz, since the wavelength-to-object size ratio is about the same in both cases. To get similar internal SAR distributions in two objects of different size sizes, each object should be irradiated at a frequency for which the ratio of object size to wavelength is approximately the same.

Thermal Methods to Quantify SAR

Thermal effects have been a subject of investigation for a long time. SAR as defined before actually refers to thermal effects. However, the vast number of recorded biological effects from man-made nonionizing environmental radiation is accounted for by nonthermal phenomena. Even if SAR could be accurately estimated for a whole tissue, organ, or body, the biological/health effect is determined by tiny amounts of energy/power absorbed by specific biomolecules, which cannot be easily calculated or even be estimated. Moreover, it depends upon field parameters not taken into account in SAR calculation.

Thermal measurements are important, in particular on human beings. A comprehensive database is available, mainly concerning animal studies and in vitro studies. Methods of biological effect determination based on thermal measurements can be divided as follows:

1. Calorimetric methods particularly suited for in vitro measurements, in which heating and cooling data can be analyzed to estimate the energy absorbed by an exposed sample.
2. Thermometric methods, used to measure the temperature due to microwaves with particular types of nonperturbing thermometers (fiber optic probe).
3. Thermographic techniques, used to measure temperature with thermographic cameras.

Technique (3) is essentially noninvasive and, as a consequence, especially attractive for thermal measurements on human beings.

If Pm is the metabolic heating rate and Pc and Pb are the rate of heat lost per unit volume due to thermal conduction and blood flow, respectively, the rate of temperature change in the subcutaneous tissue in vitro exposed to RF or microwave energy is related to the SAR as follows (Stuchly & Stuchly 1986):

$$\Delta T/\Delta t = (\mathrm{SAR} + P_\mathrm{m} - P_\mathrm{c} - P_\mathrm{b})/C \tag{3.6}$$

where ΔT is the temperature increase, Δt the exposure duration, and C is the specific heat.

If before the exposure a steady-state condition exists such as

$$Pm = P_c + P_b \tag{3.7}$$

then during the initial period of exposure one has

$$\Delta T/\Delta t = \mathrm{SAR}/C \tag{3.8}$$

and the SAR can be determined from measurements of an increase in the tissue temperature over a short period of time following the exposure. For tissue phantoms and tissues in vitro, Equation (3.6) may be used as long as the thermal conductivity can be neglected, that is, for short durations of exposure. Several methods of SAR determination are developed to make thermal measurements.

Frequency Dependence of SAR

The E and B-fields are approximately uncoupled at low frequencies, that is, at frequencies low enough that the wavelength is large compared with size that of the object. In this frequency range, dosimetry consists of determining the internal fields due to the incident E and B-field acting alone alternately.

The general characteristics of the average whole-body SAR as a function of frequency for a model of an average man irradiated by an incident plane wave with a power density of 1 mW/cm^2 are shown in Figure 3.1 (adopted from Durney et al. 1986). The calculated results shown in this figure are the results of work using a combination of simple models (prolate spheroid, cylinder, capped cylinder), empirical techniques, and for part of the graph, interpolated estimations. Several methods of calculation were used over various parts of the frequency range. At low frequencies, a long-wavelength approximation was made. The extended boundary condition method (EBCM) was used up to approximately the resonant frequency. Above that, the iterative EBCM (IEBCM) method was used.

Calculation in models with more realistic shapes show additional bumps on the average whole-body SAR graph that are caused by local resonance effects of the head, arms, and legs. The overall shape of the SAR graph is similar to that obtained for simpler models. Inhomogeneous models have also been used to simulate the presence of organs and other details of the body. From Equation (3.4), it is apparent that the spatial variation of the conductivity (σ) of the various tissues of the body can cause the SAR to vary over the body. This local variation is strongly frequency dependent. Even in homogenous models, the SAR can vary significantly over the body. In some cases, areas of intense local SARs can occur. These are often called "hotspot" or a site for preferential absorption of thermal energy.

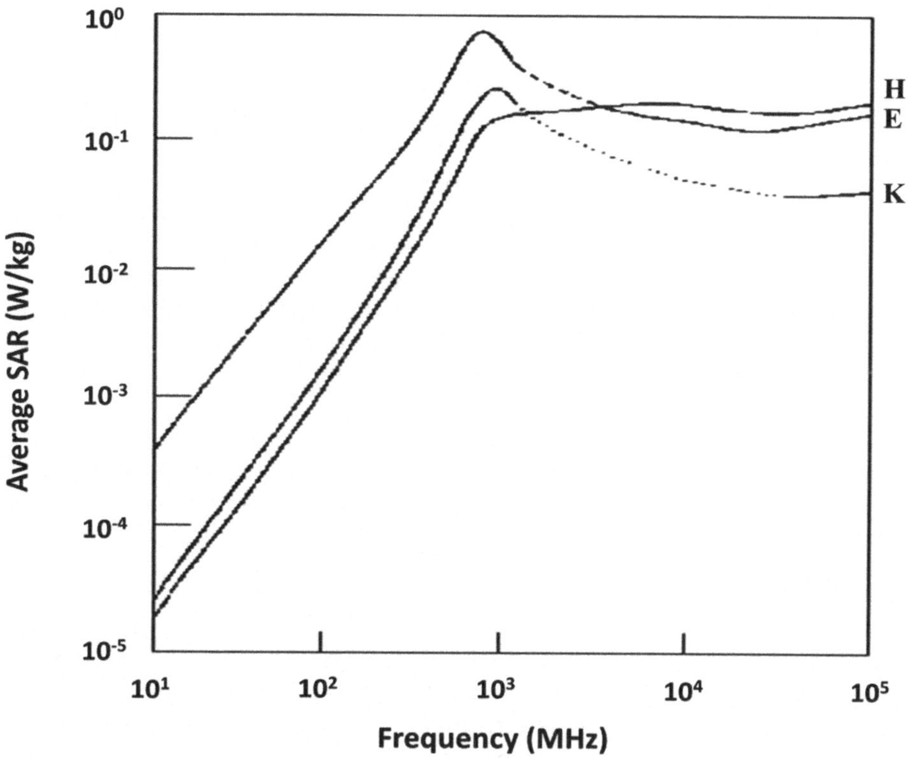

FIGURE 3.1
SAR values at a given frequency are polarization dependent. (Adopted from Durney et al. 1986).

Whole-body SAR is maximal when the long axis of a body is parallel to the E-fields vector and is four-tenths the wavelength of the incident field. At 2.45 GHz (λ = 12.5 cm), for example, standard man (long axis L = 175 cm) will absorb about half of the incident energy. If the human whole-body SAR is divided by the basal metabolic rate (BMR) for man, a ratio is obtained that provides a measure of the thermal load incurred due to a known incident power density (Stuchly 1978). In the region of human whole-body resonance (60 to 80 MHz), this ratio reaches a maximum value (about 0.16 for an incident far-field power density of $10 W/m^2$). The ratio drops off rapidly on either side of this peak, and at 0.01 GHz and below, the ratio would be less than 0.001 (Johnson et al. 1976).

At frequencies that result in maximal absorption (defining whole-body resonance), the electrical cross section of an exposed body increases. This increase occurs at a frequency near 70 MHz for standard man and results in an approximately eightfold increase in absorption relative to that in a

2.45 GHz field. At frequencies above resonance, the SAR varies approximately as the inverse of the frequency. On the other hand (Figure 3.1), at frequencies below resonance, the SAR for E-polarization is highest, for H-polarization it is lowest, and for K-polarization it is in between the other two. This suggests the variation of the induced field with frequency.

Models with realistic shapes are often used in both experimental measurements and in computations. For experimental measurements, phantom materials are used, while for calculations, some block models are used. These block models consist of cubical mathematical cells arranged to approximate the shape and volume of human and other animal bodies. Because of the complexity of the realistic biological structures, analytical solutions cannot be obtained for these models. In the absence of this, instead, numerical methods are used to calculate the internal fields. These numerical methods essentially consist of solving Maxwell's equations using some computer technique that gives the E and H-fields in each defined cell.

Polarization and L/λ Ratio

Polarization of the incident field has a strong influence on both coupling and homogeneity and hence the induced field (SAR). There are three types of polarizations possible, E, H, or K. This relates to the orientation of the electric field, magnetic field, or direction of propagation with respect to the long dimension of the exposed object.

Another is the SAR frequency dependence ($1/\lambda$) on the object size (L). For a model of human being irradiated by a microwave beam of intensity 1 mW/cm^2, average whole-body average SAR for free space for three polarizations (E,H, and K) (Figure 3.1) along with Figure 3.2 shows the difference in SAR values (13 W/kg for rat and 0.4 W/kg for human, frequency 2 GHz) (Guy 1979). This shows the difference in SAR values average whole-body SAR for a model of a medium-sized rat. The resonant frequency for E-polarization in this case is about 600 MHz, considerably higher than for the average man. This is because the rat is much shorter than the man. For the rat, the SAR also varies approximately as the frequency squared below resonance and above it as the inverse of the frequency.

f (MHz)	H (A/m)	σE^2_{tr} (W/kg)	σE^2_{tm} (W/kg)
2000	0.5	12	0.4

We see that for E-polarization, $\mathbf{E}_{inc}$ is mostly parallel to the body, and the cross-sectional area intercepted by $\mathbf{H}_{inc}$ is large compared with that of

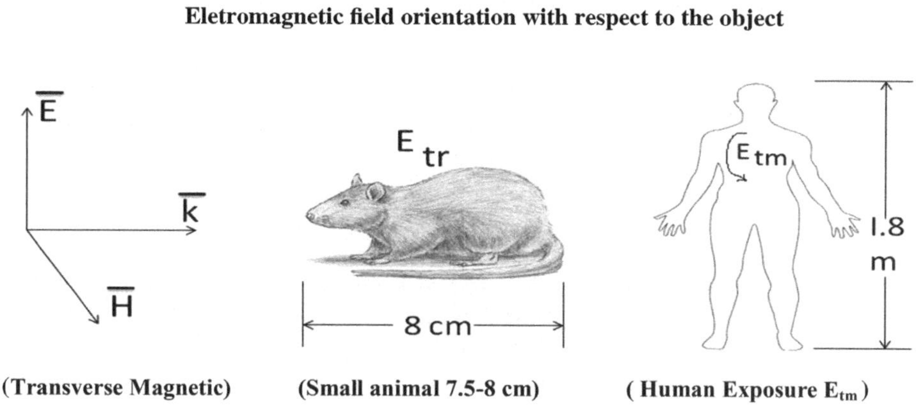

FIGURE 3.2
Field induced in biological objects of different sizes.

the other polarizations. Thus for E-polarization, both $\mathbf{E}_{Eint}$ and $\mathbf{E}_{Hint}$ are relatively strong. For H-polarization, on the other hand, $\mathbf{E}_{inc}$ is normal to the body, and the cross-sectional area intercepted by $\mathbf{H}_{inc}$ is smaller than that for E-polarization. Therefore, both $\mathbf{E}_{Eint}$ and $\mathbf{E}_{Hint}$ are relatively weaker than for E-polarization. The SAR for E-polarization is thus greater than that for H-polarization. For K-polarization, $\mathbf{E}_{inc}$ is mostly normal to the body, but the cross-sectional area intercepted by $\mathbf{H}_{inc}$ is large. $\mathbf{E}_{Eint}$ is therefore weak, but $\mathbf{E}_{Hint}$ is strong. This explains the trend in SAR variation (Figure 3.1, Table 3.1).

Effects of Object Size on SAR

Even for objects of the same basic shape but of different size size, the internal SAR distribution can be quite different, depending on the frequency. For example, consider two prolate spheroids, one man-sized. At 80 MHz, the internal SAR inside the man-sized spheroid would vary significantly over the volume of the spheroid. On the other hand, at 80 MHz, since the

TABLE 3.1
Effect of incident field direction with respect to the body on SAR

Type of the Incident Field	Polarization	SAR
E	Parallel to the incident field ($E_{induced\ maximum}$)	Maximum
H	Perpendicular to E ($E_{minimum}$)	Minimum
K	Perpendicular(to E H) (field induced between the above two)	Between E&H

wavelength is much larger than the object size (rat), SAR inside the rat spheroid would be relatively constant, depending upon the ratio of the object size compared with the wavelength. It is also dependent upon the size of the object (Morgan et al. 2014).

The SAR in an object can also be affected by the presence of other objects and the resonant frequency is dependent on a number of parameters. For example, when an object is placed on a perfectly conducting plane, the resonant frequency is approximately reduced to half as compared to that of the object in free space. Thus, for a man standing on a perfectly conducting plane in good contact, the resonant frequency would be about 40 MHz. This effect occurs because the conducting plane has the effect of mirroring or imaging, making the man appear to be twice as tall. For a man standing on the ground, which is not perfectly conducting, the resonant frequency would be lower than for free space, but not half, as it would be for a perfectly conducting plane. Also, a person standing on an insulating plane would insulate it from the ground, thus again affecting the resonant frequency.

3.3 SAR Measurements

It is clear from discussions before that SAR is the key parameter for dosimetric purposes. Experimental dosimetry includes the following areas: measurements of the total SAR and its distribution in live or in cadavers and measurements in models of animals and humans. Design and development of exposure systems for animals and in vitro preparations with quantification of the exposure conditions and internal fields can be controlled.

As is obvious from Equations (3.3) and (3.8) that SAR can be measured in two different ways:

a. Measurements of induced fields (Figure 3.3a) and
b. Measurements of temperature increase due to microwave exposure (Figure 3.3b,c).

It is suggestive from above that the two equivalent definitions emerge: one from definition of induced field inside the biological body and other from the increase in temperature of the exposed tissue material. However, the two do not arrive at the same result and the former yields data smaller than the latter.

In an attempt to obtain a realistic estimate of SAR values in a simulated medium, an automated measurement system was developed that uses mobile phone as source and can be used for compliance testing at 1718.5 MHz. The system is capable of angular movement in the range 0°–90° using a computer-controlled stepper motor. This is fitted with a miniature tip monopole probe,

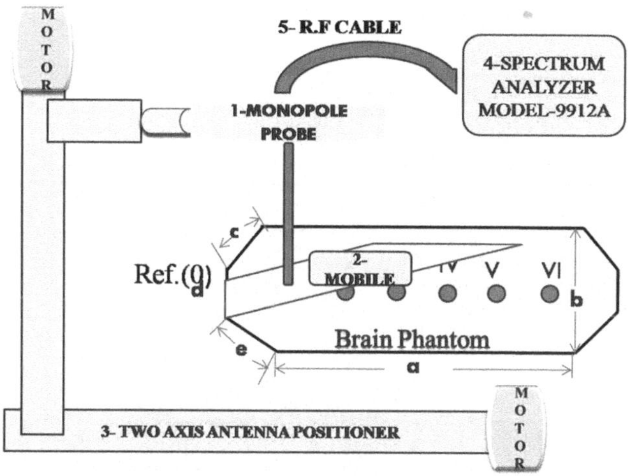

1- Monopole Probe 1718 MHz
2- Mobile Phone (Nokia 2730 Classic)
3- Two axis antenna positioner
4- Spectrum Analyzer Agilent N9912A
5- R.F Cable (Low loss)
6- Perspex Box
a = 120 mm
b= 45 mm
c= 25 mm
d= 20 mm
e= 25 mm
f= 50 mm

0→ Reference point
0→I = 25mm
0→II = 50 mm
0→III = 75 mm
0→IV = 100 mm
0→V = 125 mm
0→VI = 150 mm

FIGURE 3.3a
A schematic presentation of a two-axis antenna positioner, to measure induced field in a brain phantom.

used to measure induced field, which in turn is used to compute angular SAR variations.

Induced Fields

Knowledge of the E-field, or its distribution throughout the exposed body, fully describes the exposure field–tissue interaction and suggests that internal field measurements are vital. Some additional parameters may be needed for full quantification, for example, frequency characteristics of the exposure field, modulation characteristics, and modulation frequency.

Phantoms have usually been employed for experimental dosimetry of human exposure; correspondingly, animal cadavers have been used for dosimetry in laboratory studies. Measurements carried out with an electric field probe are standardized for compliance tests of cellular phones to satisfy the RF safety guidelines requiring high reproducibility.

Experimental Setup

A phantom, a surrogate of a human body (total or part of it), is placed in a Perspex box and exposed to RF fields. The phantom has equivalent electrical properties of those of the human body. Various materials have

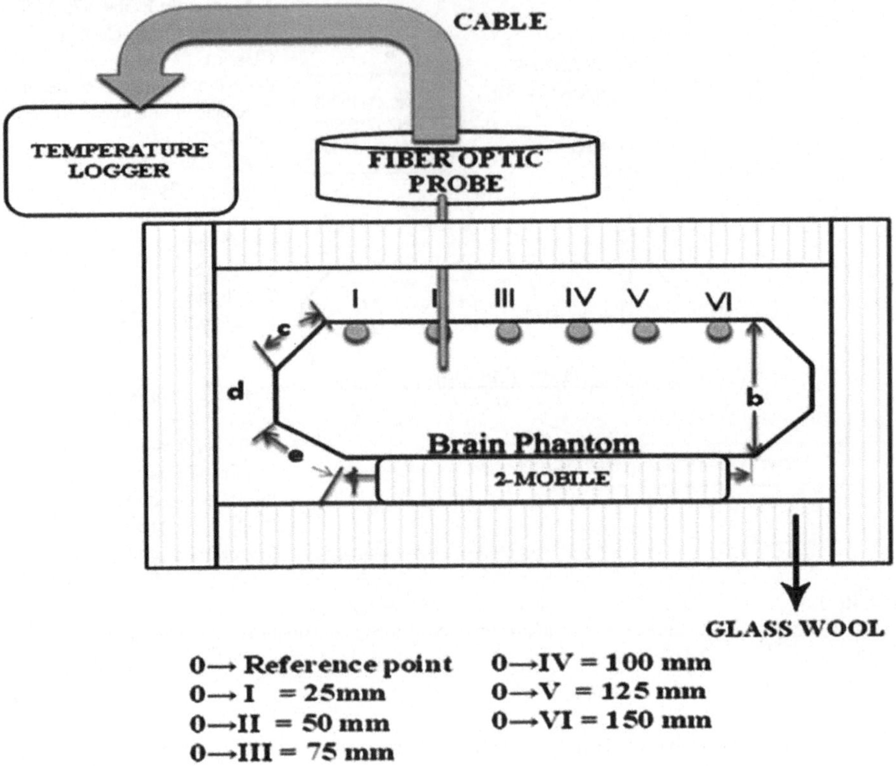

FIGURE 3.3b
A fiber optic probe to measure the temperature increase in a brain phantom exposed to mobile phone frequency.

been attempted (e.g., Okano et al. 2000) to simulate the electrical properties (Tables 3.2 and 3.3). Procedures for SAR measurements have been mentioned previously (IEC.IEC 62209-1-2005 2005).

The schematic diagram of the experimental setup for measuring the induced electric field in the simulated biological bodies is shown in Figure 3.4 (Guru 1976). For simulated biological bodies, a number of experimental models are constructed with plexiglass and filled with saline solutions of various concentrations. These models were placed inside the anechoic chamber and illuminated by electromagnetic wave with frequencies ranging from 1.0 to 3.0 GHz (with 1 kHz modulation). A horn antenna is used as a radiating source. The anechoic chamber is first probed in the y-and z-directions to find a region where there is no variation in SWR (SWR being inversely proportional to the electric field intensity) under free space conditions. These regions are 4 cm from the center in y-direction and greater than 17 cm away from the

TABLE 3.2

Approximate composition of brain-equivalent phantom. These values are adjusted to reproduce electrical data

Material	Amount (% by volume)
Deionized water	84
Agar	2.6
Sodium chloride	0.54
Sodium azide	0.05
TX-151	1.43
Polyethylene	11.4

TABLE 3.3

Composition of skull-equivalent phantom

Material	Amount (%) By volume
Silicone emulsion	50
Glycerol	40
TX-151	2.4
Agar	4.0
Polyethylene powder	3.6

central location along z-direction. The central location used as reference here is approximately 3 feet away from the horn antenna. The induced electric field inside the saline solution is measured by small dipole type probe loaded with microwave detector. The output of the detector loaded probe is connected to SWR meter. A vertical dipole probe was used to detect the vertical component of the induced electric field, E_x, and a horizontal probe was used to measure the horizontal components E_y and E_z.

In an attempt to see the variation of SAR in a stimulated scenario, a system was developed (Behari & Nirala 2013). In this setup, a Perspex box (wall thickness 2 mm) equal to the volume (150 × 50 × 50 mm) of a small Wistar rat (200–250 g) was chosen for measuring field distribution due to mobile phone exposure. Measurements were carried out in brain phantom, while restricting the mobile phone movement within the range (0°–20°), simulating the normal usage in humans. The phantom characteristics are used to simulate the impedance characteristics in human tissues

(Okano et al. 2000). As a test case, measurements were confined to inclination values at 10° and 20° only. A similar set of measurements were performed by measuring increase in temperature due to mobile phone exposure and data compared (Behari & Nirala 2012, 2013).

Induced field measurements: Plexiglass material is used in fabricating box used for containing brain phantom, irradiated by mobile phone (Figure 3.3a). Platform supporting mobile phone is tied by a thread and is carried over a pulley, whose movement was controlled by a computer-controlled stepper motor programmed to a predetermined rate of angular movement variation (2°/min) limited to 10° and 20°. A monopole probe was positioned to measure induced fields at various locations in the phantom material. Induced field measurements were carried out in two configurations. In the first instance, the mobile phone antenna was positioned parallel to the phantom.

An automated measurement system was developed that uses mobile phone as source and can be used for compliance testing at 1718.5 MHz. The system is capable of its angular movement in the range (0°–90°) using a computer-controlled stepper motor. This is fitted with a miniature tip monopole probe used to measure induced field, which in turn is used to compute angular SAR variations.

The probe was moved parallel to the plane of mobile phone, beginning at location I (25 mm) pierced into phantom material to a depth of 37 mm. The probe was horizontally moved from location I to VI (25–150 mm). Induced field in each location was measured and SAR value computed. In the second scenario (configuration in Figure 3.3a), the mobile phone was placed by the side of the box and the probe was vertically positioned at various depths (2, 10, 15, 25, 37, and 46 mm, from the top) in the phantom material, controlled by the two-axis antenna positioner. Field induced was computed by the same monopole probe connected to a spectrum analyzer. The plane of the mobile phone was moved to 10° and 20° with respect to the horizontal plane and stationed, respectively, to each position to measure values of the induced fields. Values of the induced fields so obtained were used to compute SAR values at two positions (10° and 20°).

Total depth of the box was 45 mm, where the probe was lowered up to a depth of 35 mm. The data at each position were averaged by repeating each measurement thrice, whereby the variation is found to be less than 5%. The mobile phone antenna radiates maximum power in the direction of the phantom contained within the box. The measurements were performed at the mobile phone frequency of 1718.5 MHz in all the three locations (10° and 20° and one parallel to the phantom surface (for maximum exposure)), and the data compared. It is apparent that the SAR is maximum when the mobile phone is placed parallel to the wall and decreases subsequently (Figure 3.3c).

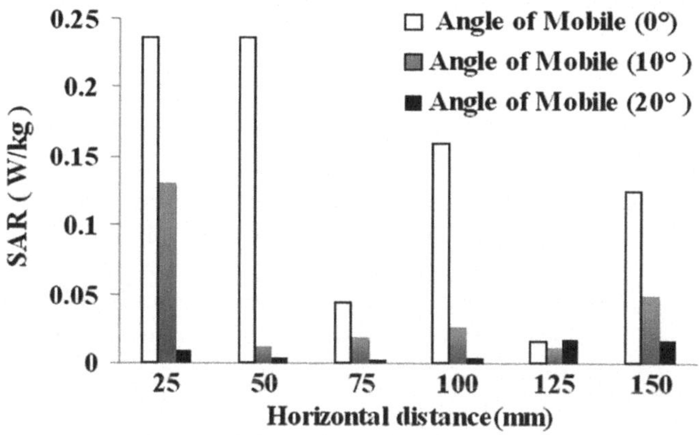

FIGURE 3.3c
Temperature variation (SAR) in various mobile locations with respect to the illuminated phantom. The power deposited is maximum when the mobile is placed (in contact) parallel to the box containing brain phantom (0°).

Thermal Methods to Measure SAR

Detailed SAR distribution in a human head exposed to the near-field of a cellular phone has been derived from finite-difference time domain (FDTD) calculations. It is found that the antenna current distribution is one of the important factors to determine the SAR distribution and the position of the maximum local SAR. From Equations (3.4) and (3.8), two equivalent definitions emerge: one from definition of induced field inside the biological body and other from the increase in temperature of the exposed tissue material.

It is observed that:

$$\mathrm{SAR} = \sigma_{\mathrm{eff}} E^2{}_{\mathrm{rms}}/\rho \mathrm{W/kg} \neq C(\Delta T/\Delta t) \tag{3.11}$$

Temperature Measurement (ΔT/Δt)

From Equation (3.8), it is apparent that the rate of change of temperature with time is the unknown that needs to be determined. Several optical temperature sensors take advantage of the fact that optical fibers, being low loss dielectrics, are neither directly heated by an electromagnetic field nor do they perturb it. In the liquid crystal, optical fiber probe with a strong temperature dependence of the reflectance of red light by the liquid crystal is used. The liquid crystal medium is sealed between a glass lance and a fiber optic catheter. Light (670 nm) emitted by the sensor is carried to a photo detector, which in turn converts light into electrical signal (voltage). An increase in the temperature of the sensor results in an increased reflectance from the crystal and subsequently an increase in the detected voltage. The shape and position of the liquid meniscus vary with temperature. The light beam is carried by optical fibers.

Properties of rare earth phosphor and fiber optics are utilized in another temperature monitoring system. The principle of operation is based on emissions by the phosphorus of well-defined fluorescent lines, whose rations of intensities depend on the temperature of the phosphor only. The ratios of intensities depend on the temperature of phosphor only.

In order to measure the temperature rise due to mobile phone exposure, a thermally insulated chamber was designed. This consists of a rectangular chamber made up of plexiglass sheet and inner lining covered with glass wool. Outer dimension of the chamber is 600 × 300 × 300 mm (length × width × height) and the plexiglass thickness of the wall is 10 mm. Inside walls were covered with glass wool to a uniform thickness all along, leaving a free space of 300 × 100 × 100 mm (Figure 3.3b).

Top of the box was covered with a sliding plate. This tightly fits in with the box. At the top of this box cover, a 2 mm diameter hole was made for introducing a sensor of fiber optic probe inside the chamber containing the phantom material. For making measurements, a Perspex box (wall thickness 2 mm) equal to the volume (150 × 50 × 50 mm) of a small Wistar rat (200–250 g) was chosen for measuring temperature distribution due to the mobile phone exposure, up to a period of 30 min. This box had a material thickness of 1 mm, filled with phantom material. The same mobile phone as used before (Nokia 2730 classic) was lowered inside the chamber and placed in a vertical position touching the wall of the box containing the brain phantom. The system was then used for tracking the temperature data over 30 min, whereby the difference in temperature between inside and outside of the box was measured and the maximum temperature difference recorded was 0.1 °C (sham exposed, passive mode). The temperature rise due to mobile phone exposure in the "receiving mode" (active mode) was estimated by subtracting the data when the mobile phone was in active mode from the one when it was in passive mode.

In a parallel experiment, a rectangular Perspex box (22.5 × 22.5 × 22.5 mm) of wall thickness 2 mm containing phantom material was chosen because SAR values in such amount of tissues are recommended for setting standards for safe exposure. The mobile phone touching the box was kept in a passive mode (not excited) for 30 min and the change in temperature measured after every 2 min. The mobile phone was then activated in "receive" mode and the temperature rise recorded after every 2 min interval over 30 min period. The measurements were carried out in two configurations (induced field measurement and temperature rise) as mentioned before and were chosen to confirm the temperature variations in different volumes and studying the corresponding SAR variations.

Local Parameters Causing SAR Variation

Temperature elevation has been evaluated as a factor in inducing adverse health effects due to exposure to RF fields. Numerical simulation techniques using voxel human models have been developed to include complex thermal properties of a human body. Time constants of temperature elevation at locally exposed region depend on the blood-flow convection and heat conduction while the time constant of body-core temperature due to the whole-body exposure is also affected by thermoregulatory response which results in longer time constants compared with those of partial-body exposure.

Temperature elevation of tissues associated with the localized exposure of the human head to near-field of a cellular phone has been a matter of concern. For this reason, it has been extensively studied. The eye has been investigated using various models for the temperature simulation. It has been found that tissue thermal properties influence temperature elevation inside the eye leading to adverse effects (Stang et al. 2001). Temperature elevation in other organs of the head is an issue of equal importance. Indeed, there exists good correlation between peak spatial-average SAR and maximum temperature elevation in the head (Gandhi et al. 1996). It is likely that metal objects implanted in a human body can cause enhancement of local SAR around the objects although RF exposure guidelines often do not incorporate such complicated situations as well as malfunction of medical implanted devices. However, numerical dosimetry has revealed that the enhancement of the SAR due to the metal objects is limited to a very small area around the tip or corner of the metal objects.

The age dependence related aspect is also of relevance for dosimetry and risk assessment. It is found that the permittivity and conductivity of tissues are higher for young rats than for adult ones. Studies using realistic whole-body voxel models of children suggest that the whole-body averaged SAR (WBSAR) can be higher for children than for adults. However, significant differences in SAR average over 10 g due to a cellular phone have not been found between child and adult head models in a multi laboratory collaboration study, although some research suggest the possibility of significant increase of the child head SAR (De Salles et al. 2006). It remains possible that the distribution of absorption within the child and adult head may be different. Pregnant female voxel models have also been developed (Togashi et al. 2008; Murbach et al. 2016). Although most of the calculated SAR of the fetus or embryo models is similar or lower than that of the mother, temperature simulation is required for a more comprehensive risk assessment of RF exposure of fetuses and embryos.

Above 10 GHz, a direct relationship exists between the temperature elevation and the incident power density. The power absorption is localized within the skin and some thresholds of thermal sensation have been estimated based on present data. However, more detailed dosimetry is needed in this region which offers many challenges.

Microdosimetry is the quantitative study of the spatial and temporal distributions of electromagnetic fields imparted in cellular and subcellular biological structures and their relationship to biological effects (Markov 2017). Although marked field discontinuities exist at microscopic level of cell membrane, micro thermal heating due to RF exposure is negligible. Methodologies for micro dosimetry have been developed for microscopic dielectric theory and biochemical process, as well as the interaction of fields with biological materials, for example, electric field manipulation of cells and electroporation (Waker & Lindborg 2017).

An evaluation of uncertainty in RF dosimetry is necessary for appropriate risk assessment. While international standards exist for the evaluation of uncertainty in the maximum local SAR values for compliance tests of cellular phones, procedures to evaluate the uncertainty of the numerical dosimetry have not been established. The representativeness of the human anatomic voxel models in use is also a limitation for risk assessment. Accurate and repeatable dosimetry is essential in developing laboratory exposure systems.

3.4 Exposure Systems for Laboratory Studies

The main purpose of exposure systems is to provide a highly defined electromagnetic exposure to the study subject. These include all exposure parameters and their variation over time and space. In addition, exposure systems for laboratory studies need to fulfil certain criteria in order to prevent any non-EMF exposure related interference of the system itself with the subject. One such parameter is that exposure systems must be controlled for temperature variations, they have to provide a live-friendly environment (food, air, etc.), and they should not expose the study subject to other physical or chemical agents. In addition, there are biological factors, which influence the design and the performance of an exposure system that needs to be known and considered (Guy et al. 1999; Kuster & Schönborn 2000; Paulraj & Behari 2004).

In Vitro Exposure Systems

An important factor for the design of exposure systems for in vitro studies is the coupling between the incident electromagnetic field and the medium and the controlling parameters (Guy et al. 1999; Schönborn et al. 2001; Schuderer & Kuster 2003; Zhao 2005; Zhao & Wei 2005). One major cause of an SAR uncertainty is the field scattering due to various containers. A large number of containers cause the variation in field pattern in a complex manner.

E-polarization provides the weakest coupling. It has been calculated that for a 60 mm Petri dish the coupling factor increases by approximately one order of magnitude between 1 and 2.5 GHz. It also increases by approximately one order of magnitude when medium height increases from 2 to 5 mm. Depending on the height of the medium, coupling efficiency for an E-polarized standing wave can be up to a factor of four higher than for a plane wave. SAR is highest at the bottom of the dish. Homogeneity of the spatial SAR distribution with respect to a cell monolayer at the bottom of the dish or flask is very good. For a 60 mm Petri dish, a standard deviation of approximately 20% was calculated with only little variation with medium height or frequency. For cell suspensions, however, homogeneity is poor. H-polarization or K-polarization provides a much higher coupling efficiency, but homogeneity of SAR distribution is very weak.

In addition, the meniscus, which forms at the walls of dishes or flasks at the air–liquid boundary, can significantly influence the SAR distribution in the medium (Guy et al. 1999; Schuderer & Kuster 2003). For a cell monolayer at the bottom of the dish, SAR values are underestimated if the meniscus is not taken into account. The magnitude of this effect depends on medium height in the dish and on frequency. In a 35 mm Petri dish with a medium height of 2 mm, the error of ignoring the meniscus at 1800 MHz can be approximately 60%. At much higher frequencies this error is reduced (Zhao & Wei 2005). If cells do not settle from the meniscus in cell suspensions, very high inhomogeneity in the SAR distribution of higher magnitude may result.

In another design for a large-scale in vitro study (Lyama et al. 2004), 49 Petri dishes were exposed employing a horn antenna, a dielectric lens, and a culture case in an anechoic chamber. The average SAR was 0.175 W kg^{-1} per W antenna input power with a standard deviation of 59%. There are methods to reduce the inhomogeneity of this design, for example, by surrounding the flask with a matching box filled with liquid to the same level as the medium in the flasks.

One parameter of concern is the temperature control. For plastic flasks surrounded mainly by air, the thermal coupling between the medium and the temperature-controlled environment is poor, and even SAR values much below 2 W kg^{-1} may result in an unacceptable temperature rise (Pickard et al. 2000; Schönborn et al. 2000).

Animal Exposure System

Bioelectromagnetics research invariably involves exposing animals (mostly small animals, e.g., mice). This needs a chamber which can be used for quantification for dosimetric purposes at various frequencies and power levels. The exposure system uses antennas of two kinds. In some, a directional antenna is used to expose one animal (Figure 3.4). In other applications, antennas with less directionality are used to expose many animals. A basic understanding of the characteristics of antennas is important in designing and interpreting experiments in which antennas are used to expose biological

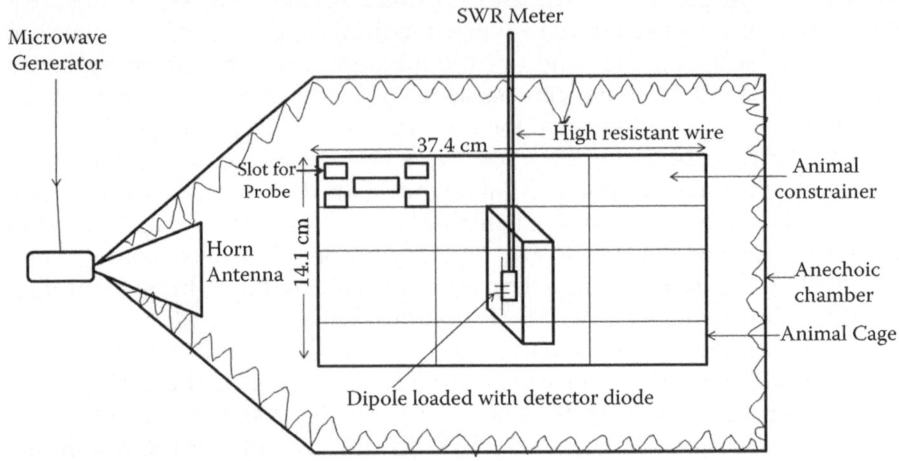

FIGURE 3.4
The schematic diagram of the experimental setup for the measurement of field distribution in the animal cage and the total body exposure.

specimens, thereby computing fields falling on the body and the induced fields and making dosimetry more quantitative.

Transverse Electromagnetic Cell

When the frequency is high enough that the wavelength is comparable to that size of the object, voltage can be defined only in very special cases. One of those special cases is transverse electromagnetic (TEM) modes. TEM cells are now widely used to simulate conditions pertaining to a free-space scenario. The cell comprises a hollow metallic housing having an enlarged center with opposite open ends, and tapering to a distal end of reduced cross-sectional area. A connector is also present at the distal end of each end section, and a stepped septum is mounted within the housing and insulated therein. The cell consists of a section rectangular coaxial connectors. The wave travelling through the cell has essentially a free-space impedance (377 Ω), thus providing a close approximation to a far-field plane propagating in free space. GHz TEM (GTEM) cell forms an enclosed TEM stripline, which acts as either receiving/emissions or transmitting emissions antenna. When measuring radiated emissions, one end of the stripline is connected to a spectrum analyzer, while the other end is terminated with an RF load (e.g., 50Ω).

TEM cell (Figure 3.5a,b) generates modes in transmission systems consisting of two conductors. In each case, a source, such as a voltage source or current source, produces a voltage difference between the two conductors and cause current to flow in the conductors. Other modes can also

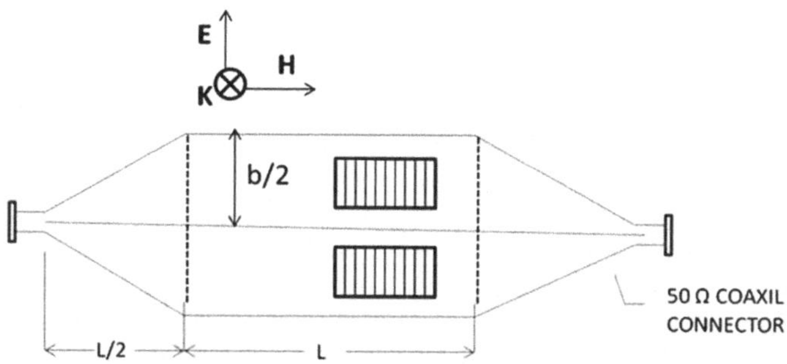

FIGURE 3.5a
Top view of a TEM chamber. The electric field **E**, the magnetic field **H**, and the wave vector **K** are indicated. The two rectangles represent the plastic box in which the rodent can be placed for field exposure.

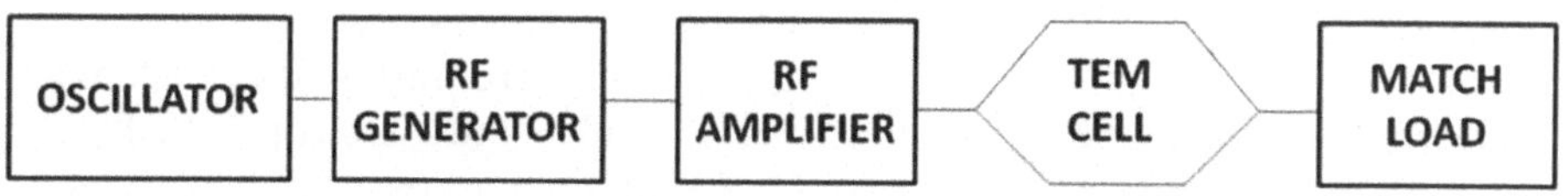

FIGURE 3.5b
Schematic diagram of exposure system.

exist on these transmission systems, but when these systems are used, they are usually designed so that the TEM mode dominates and the other modes are negligible.

A unique potential difference exists between the two conductors because the same amount of work is required to move a charge from one conductor to the other along any path between the two. The same is true for all TEM systems. Since a unique potential difference can be defined for TEM transmission systems, transmission along them is usually described in terms of voltage $V(z)$ between the conductors and current $I(z)$ in the conductors, each described as a propagating wave. These propagating voltage and current waves on all TEM systems are described by the same set of equations, which are called the transmission-line equations. Thus, the characteristic behaviors that result from the solution of these transmission-line equations apply to all TEM systems.

A typical transmission-line configuration is a source applied at the left end of the transmission line, which causes voltage and current waves to propagate along the line, usually to carry information of some kind (a signal) or to transmit energy to some device or system (often called the load, which is represented as load impedance Z_L). When the source is a sinusoidal function of time, the phasor transform is usually used to solve for the voltage and currents. The source generates a voltage wave and a current wave that propagate to the right.

The TEM cell is quite frequently used system, since it is small, self-contained, and exposure items can easily be placed. In addition, the incident field is similar to a plane wave with only transversal electric and magnetic components and do not require frequent calibration. If only few dishes are used per cell, the homogeneity is excellent. In an improved design (Nikoloski et al. 2005), a TEM cell is modified to hold four T25 flasks. They achieved an overall average SAR within the medium of 6.0 W kg^{-1} at 1 Winput power with a standard deviation of less than 52%. However, for larger number of dishes the homogeneity decreases drastically, since the E-field amplitude decreases rapidly toward the wall of the cell, besides the possible field scattering that may possibly occur.

In a design for a large-scale in vitro study (Lyama et al. 2004), 49 Petri dishes were exposed employing a horn antenna, a dielectric lens, and a culture case in an anechoic chamber. The average SAR was 0.175 W kg^{-1} per W antenna input power with a standard deviation of 59%. There are methods to reduce the inhomogeneity of this design, for example, by surrounding the flask with a matching box filled with liquid to the same level as the medium in the flasks.

It is therefore suggestive to use TEM cell in studies with a very low number of dishes. When using TEM cells for ultra wide band exposure, it should be considered that the flasks containing the cells may disturb the field due to refraction and distortion of the incident wave combined with the excitation of resonant modes within the flasks (Ji et al. 2006). The electric field strength (V/m) of the plane wave propagating inside the cell is evaluated by the following relationship:

$$E = \frac{\sqrt{P_i \times Z_0}}{b/2} \tag{3.12}$$

where E is the electric field strength, P_i(W) is the power entering the cell (can be measured by the RF power meter at the input end), Z_0 is the characteristic impedance (50 Ω), and $b/2$ is the distance between the inner and one of the outer plates of the TEM cell. The power density (I, W/m^2) is evaluated using the following equation:

$$I = E^2/Z_0$$

where Z_0 is the characteristic impedance of the medium where the wave propagates (in air: Z_0 = 377 Ω).

Waveguide System

Waveguide systems have also been widely used by several workers (Czerska et al. 1992; Joyner & Bangay 1986; Kumar et al. 2011). The flasks can be oriented in E, H, or K-polarization. If E-polarization is employed to achieve low inhomogeneity for plated cells at the bottom of the flasks, it may be necessary to overcome the poor efficiency due to the weak coupling. One possibility that increases the efficiency by a factor of almost four is to terminate one end of the waveguide with a short-circuiting plate (Schönborn et al. 2000).

Depending on the type of cell culture, the frequency used, and other factors, up to ten 35 mm Petri dishes are located inside a standard L-band waveguide (selected for the frequency used). The efficiency in a nonresonant waveguide setting at 1.62 GHz was 1.6W kg^{-1}W input power and an inhomogeneity of approximately ±30%. In a resonant design, an efficiency of 50 W kg^{-1} per W input power could be achieved with an inhomogeneity of again ±30%. In general, the efficiency of a tuned resonant system is higher than a nonresonant one.

As discussed before, for in vitro exposure systems, different technical solutions include wave guides, TEM cells, RF chambers, or wire patch cells. The characteristics of these exposure systems are dependent on the requirement of the sample type and the corresponding exposure system (Schönborn et al. 2001). A waveguide system (2–10 GHz Figure 3.5c,d) has

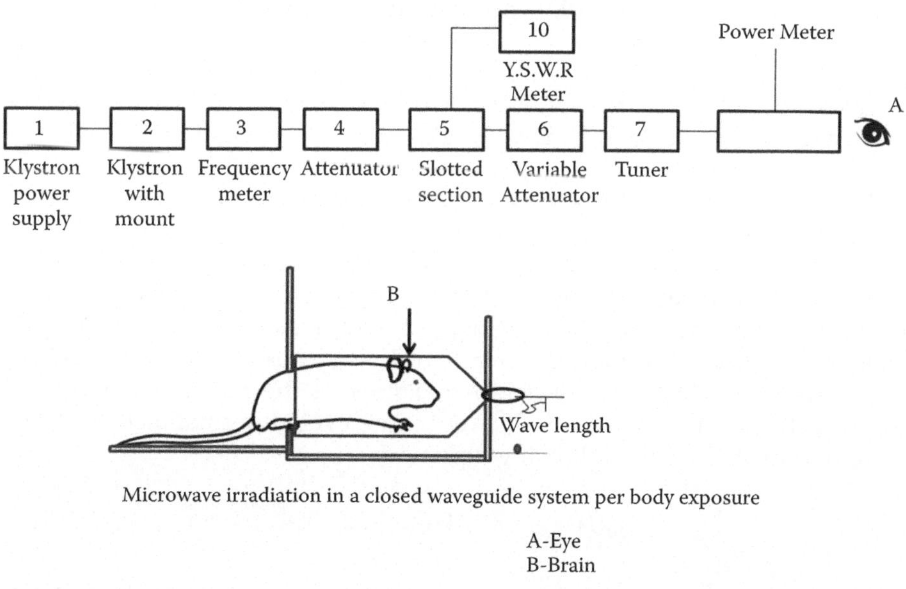

FIGURE 3.5c
Part body/whole body exposure of small animal and insect (Drosophilla).

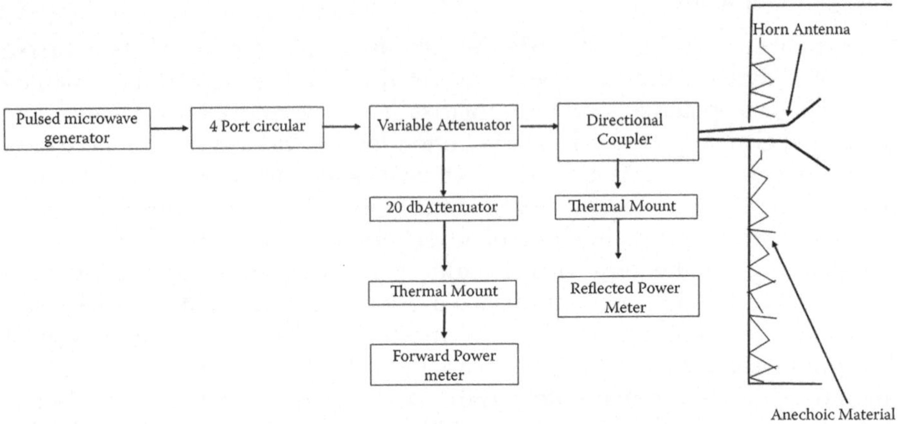

FIGURE 3.5d
A laboratory setup for far-field exposure system and power measurements.

also been used to expose animals (part body or whole body) or may be for insects.

RF Anechoic Chamber

An anechoic chamber meaning nonreflective, nonechoing room designed to completely absorb reflections of either sound or electromagnetic waves (Figure 3.4).

In a RF chamber, an array of flasks or animals with a dimension of several wavelengths can be simultaneously exposed. K-polarization is normally employed, due to the immense power requirements for E-polarization.

A key item for an anechoic chamber is the RF absorber. The absorber treatment must be such that the reflected energy is small and has negligible effect on the measured data. A typical RF absorber is a lossy material shaped to allow for incoming electromagnetic waves to penetrate with minimal reflections. Once the EM energy travels inside the material, the RF energy transforms into thermal energy and dissipates into the surrounding air (Rodriguez 2009). The electrical thickness of the material determines how much energy is absorbed. The reflection level at normal incidence can be approximated by the following equation:

$$R_0(t) = -13.374\ln(t) - 26.515$$

where $R_0(t)$ is the thickness in wave lengths. The equation is valid for $0.25 \geq t \leq 20$. This approximation can be used to get a conservative reflectivity value of an absorber of a given thickness.

Measurement Probe

For induced field measurements, proper design of a field probe is an essential in ingredient. To be satisfactory for microwave near-field measurements, a probe must have desirable polarization characteristics, must have an aperture small enough to measure the field at a point, and must deliver sufficient signal voltage to permit accurate measurement, and yet not significantly distort the fields, which has to be measured. The design of a probe may be simplified if the fields to be measured are known to be almost linear polarized or only of a traveling wave type. Comparison of measurements made with various probes has led to the development of a small open-ended waveguide probe which is simple to construct and has given excellent results.

Construction of Probe

Basic Concept

When a biological body is illuminated by an electromagnetic field, it is difficult to predict the fields induced inside the body. This is because of inhomogeneity of the EM fields induced inside the body, owing to the body composition. It is therefore desirable to have devise an electromagnetic probe to directly detect and measure these induced fields.

Since there is no surrounding surface in a practical SAR measurement system, to enable to use this probe three conditions are assumed: (1) Electromagnetic waves are only incident through the observation plane, which is located within the phantom. (2) No reflection occurs within the phantom. (3) Electric and magnetic fields on the observation plane are assumed to be secondary sources. By applying these assumptions, the SAR distribution can be quantified by measuring electric fields on a 2D plane.

The SAR measurement procedures using an E-field probe comprising diode-loaded dipole sensors. This type of probe can be used in a wide variety of measurements in bio electromagnetics, for example, on the side of the human head irradiated by mobile phone frequency source.

Design of the Monopole Probe

It is presumptive that the basic requirements for such a probe would include: (1) relatively small size (so that it does not perturb the measuring field), (2) high sensitivity, (3) polarization independence (capable of putting the probe in any field configuration), and finally (4) the minimum interference due to the lead lines. The first two requirements are very common in antenna theory and had been incorporated in the design of any impedance-type probe. However, the last two requirements ((3) and (4)) are unique for the measurements in a biological media, and offers great difficulties in designing the probe. The probe was developed by Guru (1976); Chen and Guru (1977); and Chen (1982). This can be simply assembled in the laboratory and is fairly accurate. Its essential features are described next.

This essentially consists of a dipole-type probe mounted with detectors and lossy lead lines. The construction of each probe includes a microwave detector with its axial wires of 5 mm length on each side forming a dipole. A pair of very thin high resistance wires (nichrome V wire of 2 mm diameter) was glued on to the long but thin stick of plexiglass and was wound and soldered on the axial wires of the microwave detector at one end and connected to the output wires at the other end. The high resistance lead wires are needed to minimize the interference of the lead wires with the incident electromagnetic wave. The probe and part of the lead wires are to be immersed in the finitely conducting saline solution or in phantom material for measurement of the induced electric field. It is therefore necessary to insulate the probe and the lead wires (Figure 3.6a). A commercially available transparent spray is used to provide the needed insulation.

After the construction of the probe, it needs pre calibration. A vertical dipole probe and a horizontal dipole probe can be designed, and then calibrated for the measurements of the vertical and horizontal components of the induced electric field.

A major requirement of the experimental setup is that the system be designed such that it gives absorption peaks in good agreement (within ±1 dB) with the values obtained using models in a simulated setup. Keeping

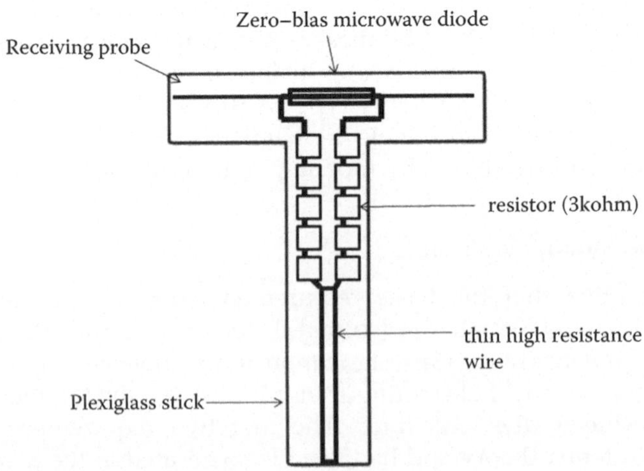

FIGURE 3.6a
Dipole with a detector diode.

this in view, a number of attempts have been made to compute SAR by measuring fields induced in phantom materials by dipole antenna, energized by external sources of varying power (Gandhi 1999). However, these fields are much higher than emitted by cellular devices and they invariably produce heating. Consequently, this may lead to SAR values considerably higher than in a realistic scenario and as such the extrapolation at lower power level is beset with uncertainties. It is possible to generate fields of any frequency or mode of frequencies to make measurements more quantitative, may be in vicinity of mobile phone frequencies sources.

A variant of the above approach is to measure dielectric constants in lossy media (as are the biological systems), using a monopole probe. This has been used for measurements in biological tissues (Ray & Behari 1986, 1987). The principle and the use of this are as follows:

The experimental data available for a monopole antenna fed from a conventional coaxial transmission line (King & South 1981) suggest that a dielectric discontinuity at the plane of the junction will affect the admittance to a degree that is less than the accuracy of most of the measurements. The measured admittance will, however, change with the ratio b/a (ratio of the radii of the inner and outer conductors of the transmission line); the nature of the change will depend on the electrical properties of the media surrounding the antenna. Another way to alter the antenna impedance is, obviously, by changing its length. When the probe length decreases, the configuration approaches that of open-ended coaxial lines. The analysis of an open-ended coaxial line is also approximately applicable to the probe (Figure 3.6b) because the probe lengths are very short (Stuchly & Stuchly 1980; Stuchly & Stuchly 1986). The terminating medium offers some capacitance which actually affects the uncertainty of measurements. Under this condition, following the analysis of an open-ended coaxial line (Stuchly et al. 1974) we can say that in this case also there is an optimum value of capacitance C_0 which assures a minimum uncertainty in determining the permittivity. For a material of certain ε' and ε'' at frequency f, the capacitance C_0 will be approximately $C_0 = [\omega Z_0 (\varepsilon'^2 + \varepsilon''^2)^{1/2}]^{-1}$ (Gajeda et al. 2002). For dielectric measurements of biological tissues, a monopole probe is connected to a spectrum analyzer (Figure 3.6b).

Fiber Optic Probe

Fiber optic temperature sensors are essentially light pipes which are mainly employed for measurement of temperature in a complex environment. They are constructed of thin glass fibers. They make use of the same type of fiber which is used in communication systems. There are basically two approaches by means of which one can easily measure temperature. These are as follows:

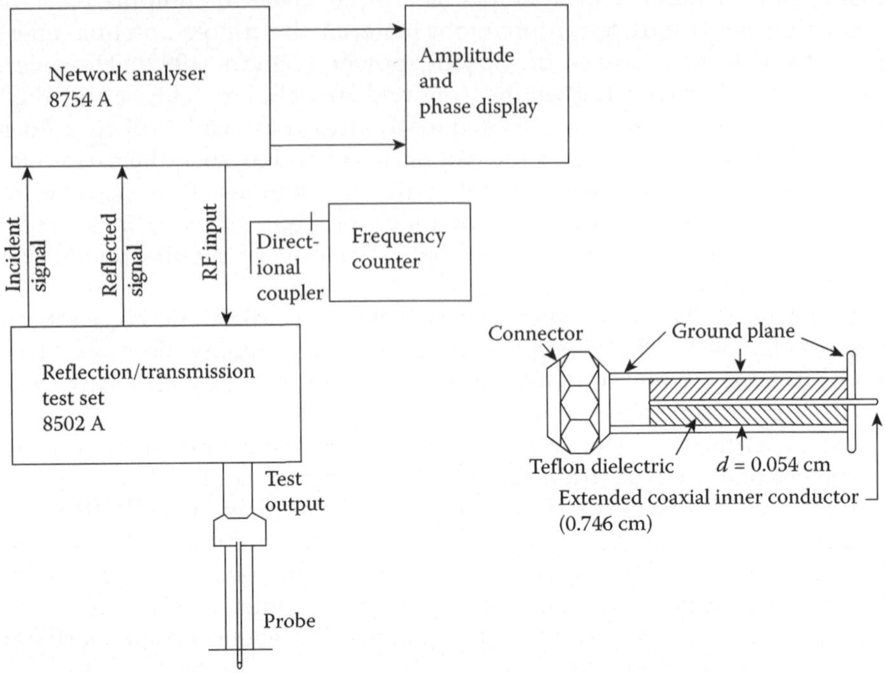

FIGURE 3.6b
Block diagram of the system for measuring dielectric properties, consisting of a probe, a network analyzer, and associated instrumentation. The probe configuration is shown on the right.

Phase Interference: Fiber optic temperature measurement using this technique is shown in Figure 3.7a. In this method, the material used for temperature sensing is applied directly on the cleaved portion of the optical fiber. A transparent temperature-sensitive layer is also present there. Hence, the incoming light will be reflected back in two parts. By measuring the phase difference between two reflected beams of light, one can easily determine temperature.

Fiber Deformation: Another way is to employ a conventional temperature sensing mechanism like bimetallic strip as shown in Figure 3.7b for creating deformation of the optical fiber. This deformation or bending of the fiber must be adequate to produce a considerable difference.

These probes have advantage that these are impervious to electromagnetic interferences caused due to RF signal.

However, compared with monopole probe the cost of fiber optic sensors is much higher.

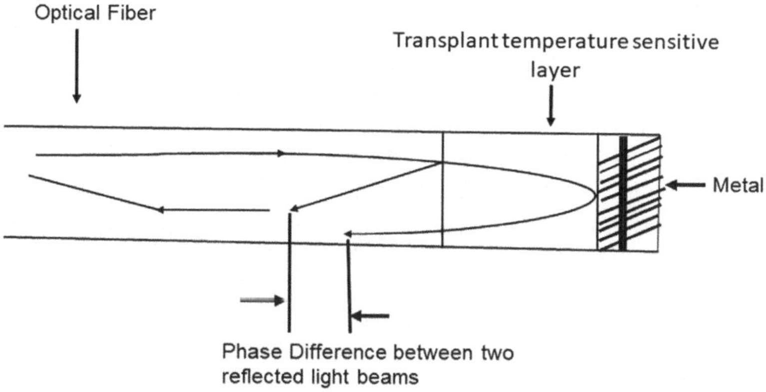

FIGURE 3.7a
Basic concept in fiber optic temperature sensor (Phase interference).

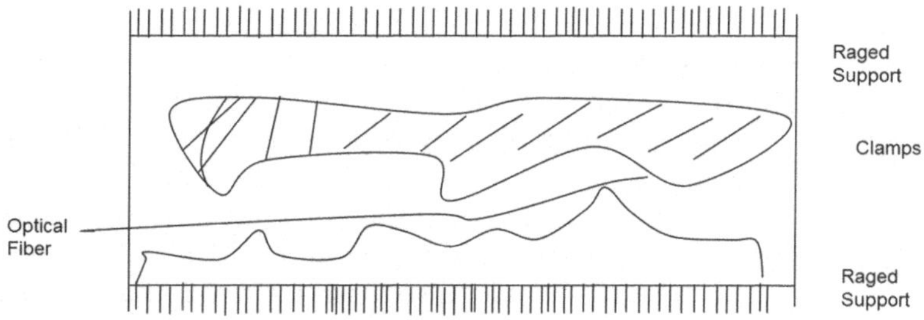

FIGURE 3.7b
Fiberoptic temperature sensor (Fiber deformation).

3.5 Mathematical Formulation: Numerical Methods in SAR Computation

Experimental measurements, which are often beset with experimental uncertainties, have inherent limitations associated with such efforts. It is therefore customary to fall back upon theoretical models. This approach has an advantage for it takes into account the anatomy of physical dimensions of the body. To support/supplement experimental results, computed data are needed. Computational techniques are employed to compute SARs in various biological models, including humans, for a preset field distribution (Durney Carl 1980). This helps to evaluate a wide variety of applicators used to administer microwave hyperthermia for cancer treatment both noninvasively and interstitially. Computational methods can also be used to examine the feasibility of using microwaves in medical diagnosis and imaging. In biomedical applications, both near- and far-field radiations are modeled and incident radiation from single and phased array antennas are used. These techniques were used to calculate electromagnetic SARs in various biological models, including humans, and to evaluate a wide variety of applicators used to administer microwave hyperthermia for cancer treatment both noninvasively and interstitially. Computational methods were also used to examine the feasibility of using microwaves in medical diagnosis and imaging. In these biomedical applications, both near- and far-field radiations were modeled and incident radiation from single and phased array antennas were utilized.

One such theoretical approach to compute fields inside the biological bodies illuminated by microwaves is that of the method of moments (MoM). In this method and several others, the bodies are divided into many tiny blocks and were specified with values of dielectric constants correspondingly (Livesay & Chen 1974; Chen & Guru 1977).

This method is based on solving linear simultaneous equations for unknown electric fields in the blocks so that its computational scale is proportional to the number of blocks squared. Also the block number is inversely proportional to the dimension size of the blocks. This limits its application at frequencies higher than several hundred MHz because smaller size blocks are required for higher frequencies, that is, shorter wave length. Reference levels of incident electric field or power density in various guidelines are derived mainly from the MoM calculations of the whole body average SAR. This was also demonstrated that an incident electric field or power density under the reference levels never yield a whole body average SAR larger than the basic restrictions.

Method of Moments

To develop its mathematical formulation, we consider that when a biological body is interrogated by a beam of electromagnetic radiations, a field is induced inside the body, and also an electromagnetic wave is scattered by the body in the region exterior to the body. Biological body has an irregular shape with permittivity and conductivity, both being frequency dependent, the field induced inside the body and the scattered wave will depend upon the physiological parameters, geometry, frequency, and polarization of the incident electromagnetic field. The field induced inside the biological body is the key parameter to be computed and measured, for it involves the calculation of SAR and the total power deposited inside the biological body. From the Maxwell's equations, both for the incident and the total electromagnetic field, a tensor integral equation is established. This equation provides a link between the three electric and magnetic fields.

$$\mathbf{E}(\mathbf{r}) = \mathbf{E}^{\mathrm{i}}(\mathbf{r}) + \mathbf{E}^{\mathrm{s}}(\mathbf{r}) \tag{3.11}$$

Similarly for total magnetic field **H(r)** can be expressed as follows:

$$\mathbf{H}(\mathbf{r}) = \mathbf{H}^{\mathrm{i}}(\mathbf{r}) + \mathbf{H}^{\mathrm{s}}(\mathbf{r}) \tag{3.12}$$

where $\mathbf{H}^{\mathrm{s}}(\mathbf{r})$ is the scattered magnetic field maintained by the induced current and charge in the biological system. Since $\mathbf{E}^{\mathrm{i}}(\mathbf{r})$ is known, one has to obtain expression for $\mathbf{E}^{\mathrm{s}}(\mathbf{r})$.

Once the expression for the scattered field is obtained, the expression for the total electric field at any point **r** can be obtained. In the method of MoM, the basic equation for the total induced field **E**(**r**) inside the biological body of volume V with conductivity (r), and the expression for the total electric field at any point **r** is written as follows:

$$\left[1 + \frac{\tau(\vec{r})}{3j\omega\varepsilon_o}\right]\vec{E}(\vec{r}) - \text{P.V.}\int_V \tau(\vec{r}')\vec{E}(\vec{r}')\,.\,\overleftrightarrow{G}(\vec{r}\,.\,\vec{r}')\mathrm{d}V' = \vec{E}^{\mathrm{i}}(\vec{r}) \tag{3.13}$$

Here, **E**(**r**) is the incident electric field at any point inside the biological body and is a known quantity. **E**(**r**) is the unknown total electric field at any point inside the body, and ($\mathbf{E}^{\mathrm{s}}$) is the scattered electric field, where P.V. is the principal value of the integral.

In the actual calculation, due to the complex nature of the tensor Green's function **G**(**r**, **r′**), it will be formidable to solve Equation (3.13) without introducing some simplification and approximation. The moment method using the pulse function expansion provides some simplification and approximation in solving this equation numerically. The details of this method are presented by Livesay and Chen (1974).

Following the method of moments, the body is divided into N cubic sub volumes or cells in which the conductivity and the dielectric permittivity are constant. The integral equation is then transformed into a system of $3N$ equations.

Transformation of Integral Equation—Moment Method

The integral involved in evaluating the electric field **E**(**r**) at any point inside the volume V, Equation (3.13), is very difficult to be performed in problems of practical interest. A simple way to obtain approximate solution is to require that the equation be satisfied at certain discrete points in the region of interest. This procedure is called as point matching technique.

In the moment method, the total volume of the biological body is partitioned into N sub volumes or cells. These sub volumes are assumed to be electrically small and in each cell $\mathbf{E}(\mathbf{r})$ and $\boldsymbol{\tau}(\mathbf{r})$ are assumed to be constant. Therefore, the accuracy of this method depends upon the dimensions of the cell. From experience, it is found that any physical dimension of the cell should not be greater than $1/4\lambda_0$, where λ_0 is the free-space wavelength of the incident EM field. On the other hand, due to the limited storage capacity of the modern computers, the number of small sub volumes cannot be increased drastically because in each cell there exists three components (E_x, E_y, and E_z) of the total electric field $\mathbf{E}(\mathbf{r})$. This increases the total number of known quantities to $3N$. These unknowns are to be determined from $3N$ simultaneous equations obtained by transforming Equation (3.13) through the point matching techniques. These simultaneous equations can be grouped into a matrix form symbolically as follows:

$$\begin{bmatrix} [G_{XX}] & [G_{XY}] & [G_{XZ}] \\ [G_{YX}] & [G_{YY}] & [G_{YZ}] \\ [G_{ZX}] & [G_{ZY}] & [G_{ZZ}] \end{bmatrix} \begin{bmatrix} [E_X] \\ [E_Y] \\ [E_Z] \end{bmatrix} = - \begin{bmatrix} [E_X^i] \\ [E_Y^i] \\ [E_Z^i] \end{bmatrix} \tag{3.14}$$

where matrix [G] represents a $3N \times 3N$ matrix and [E] and [E^i] are $3N$ column matrices expressing total electric field and incident electric field at the central locations of N cells.

In condensed form, the same can be written as follows:

$$[G][E] = [-E'] \tag{3.15}$$

The elements of [G] matrix can be numerically evaluated.

From the 1970s, MoM calculations with relatively coarse block human models demonstrated various characteristics of human-body SAR.

Finite-Difference Time Domain Method

Apart from MoM, detailed SAR distribution in a human head exposed to the near-field of a cellular phone has been derived from FDTD calculations (Hagmann et al. 1979; Gandhi 1980; Dimbylow et al. 2008). It is found that the antenna current distribution is one of the important factors to determine the SAR distribution and the position of the maximum local SAR. A significant advance in RF dosimetry is due to the availability of numerical voxel models. Realistic numerical human models are developed with medical diagnostic data, that is, magnetic resonance imaging (MRI), computer tomography (CT), etc. A most favored FDTD calculation using the voxel models provides millimeter-order SAR distribution. It is noted that the detailed SAR distributions derived from the voxel models are generally consistent with the basic SAR characteristics previously obtained with more coarse or simple human models. The FDTD algorithm being simple and efficient is the most versatile numerical method for bio electromagnetic simulations. It is particularly well suited to these applications because it can efficiently model the heterogeneity of the human body with high resolution (often on the order of 1mm), can model anisotropy and frequency-dependent properties as needed, and can easily model a wide variety of sources coupled to the body. It has been used to analyze whole-body or partial-body exposures to spatially uniform (far-field) or nonuniform (near-field) sources. These sources may be sinusoidally varying (CW) or time-varying such as those from an electromagnetic pulse (EMP).

Finite-difference time domain method was proposed by Yee (1966) and is based on direct solution of Maxwell's equations. Therefore, the implication of boundary conditions is the main issue. Theoretical analysis using simple human models, such as a dielectric spheroid, shows general characteristics of SAR inside the human body, including whole-body resonance. Since the 1990s, FDTD calculations with millimeter-resolution block models have contributed toward the development of RF dosimetry. These FDTD calculations show whole-body SAR characteristics similar to those obtained from MoM calculations but with wider variations of spatial averaged local SAR. The differences of the shape and structure of the voxel models and of the procedure of spatial averaging of the local SAR over 1 g or 10 g are important causes of this variation. Also the finite element method is used extensively in commercially available software to resolve sub-millimeter-induced currents, electric and magnetic fields, and SAR at lower frequencies.

The FDTD method has been used extensively over the last several decades for bio electromagnetic dosimetry—numerical assessment of electromagnetic fields coupled to biological bodies (Gandhi et al. 1993; Gandhi 1998; Furse et al. 1994; Jensen & Rahmat-Samii 1995; Young 1995; Gandhi & Furse 1997)or Cole–Cole models (Cole & Cole 1942). Values of interest in these computations include induced current or current density and SAR, which is a measure of absorbed power in the body. The FDTD algorithm is extremely simple and efficient, which has made it one of the most versatile numerical methods for bio electromagnetic simulations. It is particularly well suited to these applications because it can efficiently model the heterogeneity of the human body with high resolution (often on the order of 1 mm), can model anisotropy and frequency-dependent properties as needed, and can easily model a wide variety of sources coupled to the body. It has been used to analyze whole-body or partial-body exposures to spatially uniform (far-field) or nonuniform (near-field) sources. These sources may be sinusoidally varying (CW) or time-varying such as those from an EMP. The FDTD method has been used for applications over an extremely wide range of frequencies, from 60 Hz through 6 GHz, and also for broadband applications.

The FDTD method is a direct solution of the differential form of Faraday's and Ampere's laws.

$$\nabla \times E = -\mu \frac{\partial H}{\partial t} \tag{3.16a}$$

$$\nabla \times H = \sigma E + \varepsilon \frac{\partial E}{\partial t} \tag{3.16b}$$

Assuming that ε and μ are isotropic, frequency-independent, and constant over the region where the equation is being solved, (3.16a) and (3.16b) can be divided into six partial differential equations as follows:

$$\frac{\partial H_x}{\partial t} = \frac{-1}{\mu}\left(\frac{\partial E_z}{\partial y} - \frac{\partial E_y}{\partial z}\right) \tag{3.17a}$$

$$\frac{\partial H_y}{\partial t} = \frac{-1}{\mu}\left(\frac{\partial E_x}{\partial z} - \frac{\partial E_z}{\partial x}\right) \tag{3.17b}$$

$$\frac{\partial H_z}{\partial t} = \frac{-1}{\mu}\left(\frac{\partial E_y}{\partial x} - \frac{\partial E_x}{\partial y}\right) \tag{3.17c}$$

$$\frac{\partial E_x}{\partial t} = \frac{1}{\varepsilon}\left(\frac{\partial H_z}{\partial y} - \frac{\partial H_y}{\partial z} - \sigma E_x\right) \tag{3.18a}$$

$$\frac{\partial E_y}{\partial t} = \frac{1}{\varepsilon}\left(\frac{\partial H_x}{\partial z} - \frac{\partial H_z}{\partial x} - \sigma E_y\right) \tag{3.18b}$$

$$\frac{\partial E_z}{\partial t} = \frac{1}{\varepsilon}\left(\frac{\partial H_y}{\partial x} - \frac{\partial H_x}{\partial y} - \sigma E_z\right) \tag{3.18c}$$

The model space is then divided into a lattice of discrete unit cells, which is shown in Figure 3.8. As customary in the space point in the lattice is defined as $(x,y,z) = (i\Delta x, j\Delta y, k\Delta z)$, and any function of space and time is defined as $F^n(i,j,k) = F(i\Delta x, j\Delta y, k\Delta z, n\Delta t)$ where Δx, Δy, Δz are the lattice space resolutions in the x,y,z coordinate directions, Δt is the time increment, and i,j,k, and n are integers.

The differential equations in (3.17) and (3.18) are then converted into difference equations using the central difference approximations. Time-dependent Maxwell's equations (in partial differential form) are dissected using central-difference approximations to the space and time partial derivatives. The resulting finite-difference equations are solved in either software or hardware in a leapfrog manner: The electric field vector components in a volume of space are solved at a given instant in time;

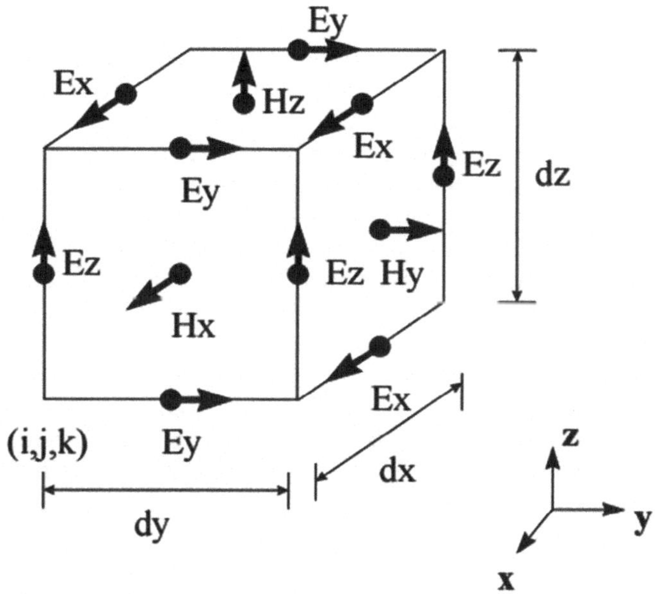

FIGURE 3.8
The "Yee" cell or FDTD lattice showing distribution of the electric and magnetic field components.

then the magnetic field vector components in the same spatial volume are solved at the next instant in time; and the process is repeated over and over again until the desired transient or steady-state electromagnetic field behavior is fully evolved (Figure 3.8).

Following are the steps involved in the solutions using FDTD:

1. Divide the given domain in smallest possible cubicals size (depending upon the body size and the computer memory).
2. Assign values of εr, σ, μr at each central location of the cell, whose location is defined by *i,j,k*.
3. Assume initial conditions (usually that all fields and the source are zero).
4. Specify fields at source.
5. Calculate E^n for all locations.
6. Calculate $H^{n+1/2}$ for all locations.
7. For transient fields, this implies that all of the fields have died away to zero, while for sinusoidal fields, this means that all of the fields have converged to a steady-state sinusoidal value.

There are two constraints controlling what values are defined for the space resolutions, Δx, Δy, Δz, and the time resolution, Δt. The space resolution in bioelectromagnetic simulations is generally controlled by the grid resolution of the human model. Since these models are extremely difficult to create, only some models are available, and while grids can be adjusted somewhat (cells can be combined whereby the resolution is reduced, while correspondingly it can also be subdivided to increase the resolution). It then implies to determine the maximum frequency, at which the available resolution can be accurately used. An underlying assumption is that the largest grid dimension, Δx, for instance, should not be larger than $\lambda/10$, where λ is the smallest wavelength in the model. This limitation comes from the fact that the numerical grid produces a certain amount of artificial (numerical) dispersion which increases with the grid size size and direction of propagation. When the resolution is $\lambda/10$, the numerical dispersion turns out to be approximately 1%. In such cases, demand on antenna type is that it should be highly directional (one large narrow lobe and no side lobes),though this demand is not easy to meet.

Although the FDTD method is suited for bioelectromagnetic simulations, there are some limitations to its use. These include the description of the source (e.g., the mobile telephone) and the fact that the FDTD method demands large amounts of memory and computational power. The size computational space is dependent upon both the physical size dimension of the model and its resolution. Higher frequencies of operation require higher resolutions. Often the telephone has to be represented by a plastic covered metal box, which approximates the shape of the actual device.

The Frequency-Dependent Time Domain Method

For practical bioelectromagnetic applications, such as the interaction of electromagnetic fields with human head and body, accurate simulation of biological tissues is a key factor for reliable results. The characteristics of biological tissues are frequency dependent and thus called dispersive materials. For accurate FDTD simulation of biological tissues, a numerical technique is proposed to derive Debye coefficients from the measured frequency-dependent permittivity of different biological tissues, and then a scattered field FDTD formulation is developed for such dispersive media are characterized characterized by Debye expressions. The proposed scattered field FDTD formulation is valid for three-dimensional analysis of practical EM problems involving combination of dispersive and nondispersive materials (Figure 3.8).

Several methods have been used for the calculation of EM energy absorbed in human tissues. Among the more used different numerical techniques, the FDTD has been used extensively over the last decade for bioelectromanetic dosimetry, that is, the numerical assessment of electromagnetic fields coupled to biological bodies.

With the increase in computing methodology, large and complex problems (as the computation of the SAR induced in a 3D heterogeneous human body) can be easily analyzed. The FDTD method can be very well used, with given tissue properties at a particular frequency, but for broadband simulations this is not sufficient. To circumvent this limitation, the frequency-dependent finite-difference time-domain ($(FD)^2$ TD) method is used. Two general approaches to the $(FD)^2$ TD method have been developed. One approach is to convert the complex permittivity from the frequency domain to the time domain and obtain time-domain electric fields to obtain time-domain fields for dispersive materials.

Based on that, several studies have used 3D human body models to analyze the relationship between the WBSAR induced in a human model and the incident field. Studies have shown that the WBSAR induced by a plane wave with vertical electric field strength set to the reference levels can be nonconservative regarding the BR for some phantoms (Conil et al. 2008). These studies underlines the variability of the WBSAR with frequency due to the variation of the anatomical details.

A high definition, finite-difference time domain (HD-FDTD) method is developed (Zhao et al. 2002) which allows the FDTD method to be efficiently applied over a very large frequency range including low frequencies, which are problematic for conventional FDTD methods. In the method, no alterations to the properties of either the source or the transmission media are required. The method is essentially frequency independent and has been verified against analytical solutions within the frequency range 50 Hz to 1 GHz. As an example of the lower frequency range, the method has been applied to the problem of induced eddy currents in the human body resulting from the pulsed magnetic field gradients of an MRI system. This method only requires approximately 0.3% of the source period to obtain an accurate solution.

Methods of Converting from Time to Frequency Domain

Any signal can completely be described in time or in frequency domain. As both representations are equivalent, it is possible to transform them into each other. This is done by Fourier transformation and the inverse Fourier transformation, respectively.

FDTD and $(FD)^2$TD methods are intrinsically time-domain methods. When frequency-domain information is required, method of conversion is used. Examples of frequency-domain parameters which are calculated are magnitudes of fields (for one or more frequencies), SAR, which is calculated from field magnitudes, currents, or current densities, and integrated properties such as radiation pattern or total power absorbed or reflected. There are several methods which have historically been used to transfer from sampled time domain to frequency domain data for bioelectromagnetic applications.

These are peak detection methods, Fourier transform methods, and a direct calculation method. The goal of all of these methods is to detect the magnitudes and possibly the phases of the time-domain fields.

Uncertainties of RF Dosimetry

The uncertainty of SAR calculations has not been precisely established. One of the important factors to cause uncertainty in FDTD calculation is "staircase modeling" (Holland 1993; Samaras et al. 2006), which means including some portion, while excluding some other, ensuring that the total area remains the same. Boundary conditions that require truncating the region used for FDTD calculations is also a source of uncertainty although reported significance of this effect (PML boundaries) on the whole-body SAR has not been consistent among related studies (Findlay and Dimbylow 2006; Wang et al. 2006; Laakso et al. 2007). A study reported that a standard deviation of 30% was found in 12 separate SAR calculations of heads exposed to the near field of a mobile phone with the same voxel models and exposure conditions (Beard et al. 2006). This may largely be due to uncertainty in the field pattern in the near field due to mobile phone frequency exposure.

For risk assessment, additional uncertainty factors, that is, the generality and/or worst-case situation of human models and exposure conditions should be taken into account. This is especially important when realistic voxel human models are used. Simple models have long been considered as typical worst-case models; some reports of comparison of various realistic voxel models have been published (Kainz et al. 2005). It is however noted that the simple models frequently may provide considerably higher doses (SAR or induced current density) or artificial phenomena such as the appearance of maximum local SAR in the deep region of the model (Lin 2002). It has been reported that the standard deviation of whole-body average SARs from 20 MHz to 2.4 GHz for six adult voxel models can reach up to 40% (Conil et al. 2008).

For in vivo animal studies, there have been several investigations on dosimetric uncertainties (Wang et al. 2004; Kuster et al. 2006; Wang et al. 2006a; Wake et al. 2007). Specifically, estimated uncertainty of SAR was within 15%, that is, 0.6 dB, for a large-scale in vivo study involving 300 rats during the 2-year exposure period. However, in another systematic uncertainty evaluation, the expanded uncertainty was found to be greater than 2 dB (Kuster et al. 2006). Thus, with the expanded uncertainty dosimetry in animal studies is between 1 and 2 dB if the models and exposure conditions are strictly defined although careful consideration of additional uncertainty factors of the models and exposure conditions is necessary for risk assessment.

Experimental dosimetry includes the following areas: measurements of the total SAR and its distribution in live or dead experimental animals, measurements of the average SAR and SAR distribution in models of animals and humans, and development of exposure devices for animals and in vitro preparations in which quantification of the exposure conditions and internal fields is facilitated.

In general, models with more realistic shapes and finer resolution require a larger number of smaller size cells. With a larger number of smaller cells the fields can be calculated with finer resolution, but this also requires more computer memory and computational time. Calculating fields with more resolution is not enough, however. Having huge data files consisting of E and H-fields in each of many mathematical cells does not necessarily provide insight into the characteristic behaviors of these fields. An understanding of this characteristic behavior is important in interpreting and evaluating the interactions of EM fields with biological systems.

References

Adey, WR (1981) Tissue interactions with nonionizing electromagnetic fields. *Physiol. Rev.*, 61: 435.

Anne A, Satio M, Salati OM, &Schwan HP (1962) Relative microwave absorption cross sections of biological significance. In*Proc. 4th Annu. Tri-Service Conf. Biol. Effects of Microwave Radiating Equipment: Biological Effects of Microwave Radiation* (Peyton MF ed.). New York: Plenum Press, p. 153.

Guy AW (1979) Non-ionizing radiation: Dosimetry & interaction, Proc. ACGIH Top. Symp., p. 75.

Beard B, Kainz W, Onishi T, Iyama T, Watanabe S, Fujiwara O, Wang J, Bit-Babik G, Faraone A, Wiart J, Chirst A, Kuster N, Lee A-K, Kroeze H, Siegbahn M, Keshvari J, Abrishamkar H, Simon W, Manteuffel D, & Nikoloski N (2006) Comparisons of computed mobile phone induced SAR in the SAM phantom to that in anatomically correct models of the human head. *IEEE Trans. Electromagn. Comp.*, 48: 397.

Behari J & Nirala JP (2012) SAR measurements due to mobile phone exposure in a simulated biological media. *Electromagn. Biol. Med.*, 31(3): 195.

Behari J & Nirala JP (2013) Specific absorption rate variation in brain phantom due to exposure by a 3G mobile phone: Problemsin dosimetry. *Indian J. Exp. Biol.*, 51: 1079.

Chen KM (1982) Measurement of induced electric field in a phantom model of man. *Radio Sci.*, 17: 5S.

Chen KM & Guru BS (1977) Internal EM field & power density in human torso induced by 1-500 MHz EM waves. *IEEEMTT*, 25: 746.

Cole KS & Cole RH (1942) Dispersion and absorption in dielectrics-II direct current characteristics. *J. Chem. Phys.*, 10(2): 98.

Conil E, Hadjem A, Lacroux F, Wong MF, & Wiart J (2008) Variability analysis of SAR from 20 MHz to 2.4 GHz for different adult & child models using finite-difference time-domain. *Phys. Med. Biol.*, 53: 1511.

Czerska EM, Elson EC, Davis CC, Swicord ML, & Czerski P (1992) Effects of continuous & pulsed 2450-MHz radiation on spontaneous lymphoblastoid transformation of human lymphocytes in vitro. *Bioelectromagnetics*, 13(4): 247.

De Salles AA, Bull G, & Rodriquez CE (2006) Electromagnetic absorption in the head of adults and children due to mobile phone operation. *Electromagn. Biol. Med.*, 25(4): 349.

Dimbylow PJ, Hirata A, & Nagaoka T (2008) Intercomparison of whole-body averaged SAR in European & Japanese voxel phantoms. *Phys. Med. Biol.*, 53: 5883.

Durney Carl H (1980) Electromagnetic dosimetry for models of humans & animals: A review of theoretical & numerical techniques. *Proc. IEEE*, 68(1): 33.

Durney CH & Christensen DA (2000) *Basic Introduction to Bioelectromagnetics*. CRC Press LLC printed in USA, p. 141.

Durney CH, Massoudi H, Massoudi H, & Iskander MF (1986) *Radiofrequency Radiation Dosimetry Handbook*. 4th Edition. Report USAFSAM-TR_85-73. Brooks Air Force Base, TX: USAF School of Aerospace Medicine, Aerospace Medical Division (AFSC).

Findlay RP & Dimbylow PJ (2006) Variations in calculated SAR with distance to the perfectly matched layer boundary for a human voxel model. *Phys. Med. Biol.*, 51: N415.

Foster KR & Schwan HP (1989) Dielectric properties of tissues & biological materials: A critical review. *Crit. Rev. Biomed. Eng.*, 17(1): 25.

Franzellitti S, Valbonesi P, Ciancaglini N, Biondi C, Contin A et al. (2010) Transient DNA damage induced by high-frequency electromagnetic fields (GSM 1.8 GHz) in the human trophoblast HTR-8/SVneo cell line evaluated with the alkaline comet assay. *Mutat. Res.*, 683(1–2): 35.

Furse CM (1997) Application of the finite-difference time-domain method to bioelectromagnetic simulations. *Appl. Comp. Electromagn. Soc. Newsletter*.

Furse CM, Chen JY, & Gandhi OP (1994) A frequency-dependent finite-difference time-domain method for induced current & SAR calculations for a heterogeneous model of the human body. *IEEE Trans. Electromagn. Compat.*, 36: 128.

Gabriel S, Lau RW, & Gabriel C (1996) The dielectric properties of biological tissues: II. Measurements in the frequency range 10 Hz to 20 GHz. *Phys. Med. Biol.*, 41: 2251.

Gajeda GB, McNamee JP, Thansandote A, Boonpanyarak S, Lemay E, & Bellier PV (2002) Cylindrical waveguide applicator for in vitro exposure of cell culture samples to 1.9-GHz radiofrequency fields. *Bioelectromagnetics*, 23: 592.

Gandhi OP (1980) State of knowledge for electromagnetic absorbed dose in man & animals. *Proc. IEEE*, 68: 24.

Gandhi OP, Ben-Qing G, &Jin-Yuan C (1993) A frequency dependent finite-difference time domain formulation for dispersive media. *IEEE Trans. Microwave Theory Tech.*, 41(4): 658.

Gandhi OP & Furse CM (1997) Currents induced in the human body for exposure to ultra wideband electromagnetic pulses. *IEEE Trans. Electromagn. Compat.*, 39(2): 174.

Gandhi OP (1975) Conditions of strongest electromagnetic power deposition in man & animals. *IEEE Trans. Microwave Theory Tech.*, 23: 1021.

Gandhi OP (1998) "Use of FDTD in bioelectromagnetics: Safety assessment &medical applications. In *Advances in Computational Electrodynamics I: The Finite-Difference Time-Domain Method* (Taflove A ed.). Dedham, MA: Artech House, p. 613.

Gandhi OP (1999) An automated SAR measurement system for compliance testing of personal wireless devices. *IEEE Trans. Electromagn. Compat.*, 41: 234.

Gandhi OP, Lazzi G, & Furse CM (1996) Electromagnetic absorption in the human head and neck for mobile telephones at 835 and 1900 MHz. *IEEE Trans.*, 44(10): 1884.

Guru BS (1976). An experimental & theoretical study on the interaction of electromagnetic fields with arbitrarily shaped biological bodies. Ph.D. Thesis submitted to Michigan State University, USA.

Guy AW, Chou CK, & McDuga II JA (1999) A quarter century of in vitro research: A new look at exposure methods. *Bioelectromagnetics*, 20: 21.

Hagmann MJ, Gandhi OP, & Durney CH (1979) Numerical calculation of electromagnetic energy deposition for a realistic model of man. *IEEE MTT*, 27: 804.

Holland R (1993) Pitfalls of staircase meshing. *IEEE Trans. Electromagn. Compat.*, 35: 434.

IEC. IEC 62209-1-2005 (2005) Human exposure to radio frequency fields from hand-held & body-mounted wireless communication devices – Human models, instrumentation, & procedures – Part 1: Procedure to determine the specific absorption rate (SAR) for hand-held devices used in close proximity to the ear (frequency range 300 MHz to 3 GHz).

IEEE. Standard 1528-2003 (2003) IEEE recommended practice for determining the peak spatial-average specific absorption rate (SAR) in the human head from wireless communications devices: Measurement techniques.

Jensen MA & Rahmat-Samii Y (1995) EM interaction of handset antennas & a human head in personal communications. *Proc. IEEE*, 83: 7.

Ji Z, Hagness SC, Bookse JH, Mathur S, & Meltz ML (2006) FDTD analysis of a gigahertz TEM cell for ultrawideband pulse exposure studies of biological specimens. *IEEE Trans. Biomed. Eng.*, 53(5): 780.

Johnson CC, Durney CH, Barber PW, Massoudi H, Allen SJ, & Mitchell JC (1976) *Radiofrequency Radiation Dosimetry Handbook*. SAM-TR-76-35. Brooks Air Force Base, Texas: AFSC, AMD, SAM.

Joyner KJ & Bangay MJ (1986) Exposure survey of operators of radiofrequency dielectric heaters in Australia. *Health Phys.*, 50: 333.

Kainz W, Christ A, Kellom T, Seidman S, Nikoloski N, Beard B, & Kuster N (2005) Dosimetric comparison of the specific anthropomorphic mannequin (SAM) to 14 anatomical head models using a novel definition for the mobile phone positioning. *Phys. Med. Biol.*, 50: 3423.

King WP & South GS (1981) *Antennas in Matter: Fundamental Theory & Application*. Cambridge, MA: MIT, p. 787.

Kumar S, Kesari KK, & Behari J (2011) Influence of microwave exposure on fertility of male rats. *Am. Soc. Reprod. Med. Fert. Steril.*, 95(4) :1500.

Kuster N & Schönborn F (2000) Recommended minimal requirements & development guidelines for exposure setups of bio-experiments addressing the health risk concern of wireless communications. *Bioelectromagnetics*, 21: 508.

Kuster N, Torres VB, Nikoloski N, Frauscher M, & Kainz W (2006) Methodology of detailed dosimetry & treatment of uncertainty & variations for in vivo studies. *Bioelectromagnetics*, 27: 378.

Laakso I, Ilvonen S, & Uusitupa T (2007) Performance of convolutional PML absorbing boundary conditions in finite-difference time-domain SAR calculations. *Phys. Med. Biol.*, 52: 7183.

Lin JC (2002) Cellular mobile telephones & children. *IEEE Antennas Propag. Mag.*, 44(50): 142.
Livesay DE & Chen KM (1974) Electromagnetic field induced inside arbitrarily shaped biological bodies. *IEEE Trans.*, 22: 1273.
Lyama T, Ebara H, Tarusawa Y, Uebayashi S, Sekijima M, Najma T, & Miyakoshi J (2004) Large scale in vitro experimental system for 2 GHz exposure. *Bioelectromagnetics*, 25(8): 599.
Markov M (2017) *Dosimetry in Bioelectromagnetics*. Ed. Natik, MA: CRC Press (Taylor and Francis Group).
Morgan L, Kesari S, & Davis DL (2014) Why children absorb more microwave radiation than adults. The consequences. *J. Microsc. Ultrastruct.*, 2(4): 197.
Murbach M, Neufeld E, Samaras T, Corcoles J, Robb FJ, Kainz W, & Kuster N (2016) Pregnant women models analyzed for RF exposure and temperature increase in 3T RF shimmed birdcages. *Magn. Reson. Med.*, 77(5): 2048.
Nikoloski N, Fröhlich J, Samaras T, Schuderer J, & Kuster N (2005) Reevaluation & improved design of the TEM cell in vitro exposure unit for replication studies. *Bioelectromagnetics*, 26: 215.
Okano Y, Ito K, Ida I, & Takahashi M (2000) The SAR evaluation method by a combination of thermographic experiments & biological tissue-equivalent phantoms, In: Rosen, A. Vender Vorst, & Y. Kotsuka (Eds.), Special Issue on Medical Applications & Biological Effects of RF/Microwaves. *IEEE Trans. Microwave Theory Tech.*, 48((11) Pt. II): 2094.
Panagopoulos DJ, Karabarbounis A, & Margaritis LH (2002) Mechanism for action of electromagnetic fields on cells. *Biochem. Biophys. Res. Commun.*, 298(1): 95.
Panagopoulos DJ, Messini N, Karabarbounis A, Philippetis AL, & Margaritis LH (2000) A mechanism for action of oscillating electric fields on cells. *Biochem. Biophys. Res. Commun.*, 272: 634.
Paulraj R & Behari J (2004) Radiofrequency radiation effect on protein kinase C activity in rats' brain. *Mutat. Res.*, 545: 127.
Pickard WF, Straube WL, & Moros EG (2000) Experimental & numerical determination of SAR distributions within culture flasks in a dielectric loaded radial transmission line. *IEEE Trans. Biomed. Eng.*, 47: 202.
Ray S & Behari J (1986) Microwave absorption in lossy liquids. *Phys. Med. Biol.*, 31(9): 1031.
Ray S & Behari J (1987) In vivo dielectric measurement of biological tissues in the frequency range 0.4–1.3 GHz. *Bioelectricity*, 6(1): 71.
Rodriguez V, d'Abreu G, & Liu K (2009) Measurements of the power handling of RF absorber materials: creation of a medium power absorber by mechanical means.*31st Annual Antenna Measurement Techniques Association Symposium (AMTA)*, Salt Lake City, UT.
Stuchly MA (1978) *Health Aspects of Radiofrequency & Microwave Radiation Exposure, Part 2*. Ottawa: Department of National Health & Welfare.
Stuchly MA & Stuchly SS (1980) Coaxial line reflection methods for measuring dielectric properties of biological substances at radio and microwave frequencies: A review. *IEEE Trans. Instrum. Meas.*, IM-29: 176.
Stuchly SS, Rzepecka MA, & Iskander MF (1974) Permittivity measurements at microwave frequencies using lumped elements. *IEEE Trans. Instrum. Meas.*, IM-23: 56.

Samaras T, Christ A, & Kuster N (2006) Effects of geometry discretization aspects on the numerical solution of the bioheat transfer equation with the FDTD technique. *Phys. Med. Biol.*, 51(11): N221.

Schönborn F, Pokovic K, Burkhardt M, & Kuster N (2001) Basis for optimization of in vitro exposure apparatus for health hazard evaluations of mobile communications. *Bioelectromagnetics*, 22: 547.

Schönborn F, Pokovic K, Wobus AM, & Kuster N (2000) Design, optimization, realization, & analysis of an in vitro system for the exposure of embryonic stem cells at 1.71GHz. *Bioelectromagnetics*, 21: 372.

Schuderer J & Kuster N (2003) Effect of the meniscus at the solid/liquid interface on the SAR distribution in Petri dishes & flasks. *Bioelectromagnetics*, 24: 103.

Stang A, Anastassiou G, Ahrens W, Bromen K, Bornfeld N, & Jöckel K-H (2001) The possible role of radiofrequency radiation in the development of uveal melanoma. *Epidemiology*, 12: 7.

Stratton JA (1941) *Electromagnetic Theory*. New York: McGraw-Hill.

Stuchly MA & Stuchly SS (1986) Experimental radio & microwave dosimetry. In *Handbook of Biological Effects of Electromagnetic Fields* (Polk C & Postow E eds.). Boca Raton, FL: CRC Press, p. 239.

Togashi T, Nagaoka T, Kikuchi S, Saito K, Watanabe S, Takahashi K, & Ito K (2008) FDTD calculations of specific absorption rate in fetus caused by electromagnetic waves from mobile radio terminal using pregnant women model. *IEEE Trans.*, 56(2): 554.

Vander Vorst A (1994) *Electromagnetisme. Champs et Circuits*. Brussels: De Boeck.

Wake K, Mukoyama A, Watanabe S, Yamanaka Y, Uno T, & Taki M (2007) An exposure system for long-term & large-scale animal bioassay of 105-GHz digital cellular phones. *IEEE Trans. Microwave Theory Tech.*, 55(2): 343.

Waker A & Lindborg L (2017) *Microdosimetry: Experimental Methods and Applications*. UK: CRC Press.

Wang J, Fujita M, Fujiwara O, Wake K, & Watanabe S (2006a) Uncertainty evaluation of an in vivo near-field exposure setup for testing biological effects of cellular phones. *IEEE Trans. EMC*, 48: 545.

Wang J, Fujiwara O, Kodera S, & Watanabe S (2006) FDTD calculation of whole-body average SAR in adult & child models for frequencies from 30 MHz to 3 GHz. *Phys. Med. Biol.*, 51: 4119.

Wang J, Saito T, & Fujiwara O (2004) Uncertainty evaluation of dosimetry due to plastic holder for restraining small animal in in vivo near field exposure setup. *IEEE Trans. EMC*, 46: 263.

Yee KS (1966) Numerical solution of initial boundary value problems involving Maxwell's equations in isotropic media. *IEEE Trans. Antenna Propag.*, 14(3): 302.

Young JL (1995) Propagation in linear dispersive media: Finite difference time-domain methodologies. *IEEE Trans. Antennas Propag.*, 43(4): 422.

Zhao H, Crozier S, & Feng L (2002) A high definition finite difference time domain method. *Magn. Reson. Med.*, 48: 1037.

Zhao JX (2005) Numerical dosimetry for cells under millimeter-wave irradiation using Petri dish exposure setups. *Phys. Med. Biol.*, 50: 3405.

Zhao JX & Wei Z (2005) Numerical modeling & dosimetry of the 35mm Petri dish under 46 GHz millimeter wave exposure. *Bioelectromagnetics*, 26: 481.

4

Biological Correlates of Microwave Field Exposure: Stress

4.1 Introduction

During the last five decades or so, there has been a growing concern on the effects of electromagnetic radiations on biological systems. This is because of electronic devices for communication, the air surveillance system, industry, diagnostic and therapeutic purposes in medicine—largely emitting microwaves/radiofrequency waves. In view of this, the importance of electromagnetic radiation pervading the environment has now significantly increased. This has added to the list of another pollutant in the environment (electro-pollution) after air, water, soil, noise. These effects can be further classified into two: thermal and nonthermal, though the line of demarcation between the two is not sharply defined. While the former leads to an increase in body temperature, the latter does not. Due to these exogenous fields of low intensity, nonthermal effects are attributed to the induced electromagnetic fields (Figure 4.1).

While the issue is still being debated, devices emitting these radiations have found their use in everyday life. While the thermal effects of microwaves are not commonly observed, nonthermal effects, if undetected, may have negative effects on human health. It is understood that emissions from RF-EMF to which humans are exposed (far-field exposures) are well below the safe levels.

In a survey, it was reported that around 4% of people claim that to some degree they are sensitive to RF-EMF (Eltiti et al. 2007). The biological effects also depend upon the intermittency of the exposure and the effects could be accumulative and may include membrane interactions that affect the ion fluxes, the modulation of neuronal impulse activity, and possibly induced arrhythmia in isolated hearts. The behavioral effects and those on reproductive pattern are also possible at low level of microwave exposure. There are important biomedical considerations associated with long-term exposure to any environmental factor capable of tissue interactions. These include effects specifically attributable to wave type, duration, frequency of recurrent exposure, interactions with regard to single or simultaneous

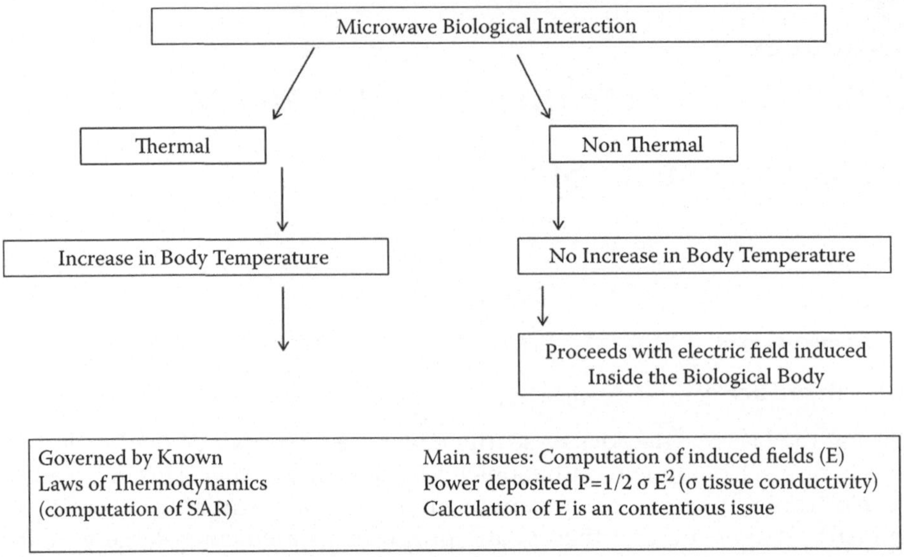

FIGURE 4.1
The boundary line between thermal and nonthermal effects is thin and not well defined.

exposure to multiple factors, and age at the onset of exposure and may also include considerations of ethnicity. While considering the biological effects and phenomena involved, it is realized that it is not only the external field but also the field within the tissue and the body that are also important. In this chapter an effort will be made to concentrate on nonthermal effects. From a biophysical point of view the mechanism is nonthermal if the interaction of the electric and magnetic vectors of the RF fields leads to specific effects other than caused due to heating (Glaser 2005). Foster and Glaser (2007) have noted that cells possess various temperature-sensitive molecules that can activate cellular responses to small changes in temperature (may be less than 0.1°C). Glaser (2005) further noted that subtle temperature effects may occur following low-level RF exposure that would be a part of the normal cellular responses encountered in everyday life and may not be of significance from health point of view. Energy of RF photon at 1 GHz is 4.10^{-5} eV ≪ thermal energy of molecules at room temperature (3.10^{-2} eV) and much lower than the energy of a chemical bond (~1 eV) and threshold of ionization (~10 eV). This line of reasoning has been prevalent since long and suggests that RF/MW exposure would not be able to cause direct damage to biological molecules through chemical bond disintegration.

While the mechanism of action has been a subject of debate, its biomedical effects have often been realized, and in conformity with this, several governments have imposed restrictions on the power level of these radiated fields. The biologists and the physicians have carried out a clinical exercise and have proposed a set of maximum values of the radiated fields, at various frequencies, extending from RF to well above the microwave frequencies. The paramount concerns are the biomedical fallout and the health of the people who are subjected to such exposures.

To date, heating of the tissue is the only biological effect agreed on and regulated by the SAR standard. However, a big part of the scientific community suggests that even at low intensity, man-made EMF interferes with human biological system, though the mechanism of such interaction is not yet fully understood. This includes interaction with immune function and metabolism giving rise to various illnesses and health problems and also brain cancer. The aspects will be discussed presently.

4.2 Radiofrequency Exposure and Health: Nonthermal, Microthermal, and Isothermal Effects

It may be pointed out that the possibilities of either nonthermal or microthermal effects on human body are the matter of continuing concern. In this, the first concern is to distinguish between thermal and nonthermal effects relating to biophysical phenomena.

The exposure to nonthermal microwave EMF-generated by mobile phones affects the expression of many proteins. This effect on transcription and protein stability can be mediated by the mitogen-activated protein kinase (MAPK) cascades, which serve as central signaling pathways and govern essentially all stimulated cellular processes. Indeed, long-term exposure of cells to mobile phone irradiation results in the activation of p38 using a 915 MHz field, switching modulation frequencies from 55 to 65 Hz at coherence times of 10s or longer produced full enhancement. These microwave coherence effects are similar to those observed in ELF fields (Litovitz et al. 1993).

There is also controversy about the possibility of nonthermal or microthermal effects. Accepting the idea that RFs may cause nonthermal effects or microwave exposure implies that such an exposure could be of a low or very low level. On the other hand, not all biological related effects are necessarily pathogenic. This underlies the whole question about how to establish guidelines for limiting electromagnetic field (EMF) exposure and more importantly to understand the mode of EMF biointeraction (e.g., with neurons/bone cells). The question is one of accepting or rejecting nonthermal effects.

Investigating the possibility of isothermal effects does not preclude the attention to be paid to "nonthermal" effects, which should probably better be termed microthermal effects (Vander Vorst et al. 1992). The question is:

can extremely weak EM exposure have biological significance and how is this possible? To answer this, one then has to consider the microwave trigger action.

(a) Microwaves as a Trigger

In principle when radiation falls upon a biological body, it transfers energy to the system, hence producing biological effects. In the RF/MW region the effects are frequency dependent and are largely governed by dielectric loss. It can be assumed that this loss is proportional to the intensity of the radiation. Microthermal effects, on the other hand, occur in certain frequency regions only and usually exhibit saturation at very low intensity. As a consequence, thermal effects might be drowned by microthermal effects. This is particularly to be expected when the signal of the considered effect in the nonthermal region is opposite to that of the thermal ones. One may find a link between frequency-dependent biological effects of resonance type to absorption bands in certain biomolecules. Frohlich (1980) has demonstrated, however, that such resonances are properties of the whole system and may depend on the biological activity.

It is important to realize that, in some instances, biosystems can exhibit properties similar to those of the most refined electronic instruments, achieving this in a way that is not well understood. For instance, at low intensities, the human visual system has a sensitivity that is close to the theoretical limit. Comparing the energy of a light quantum with that of a nerve impulse, there is a gain of more than 10^6. Clearly the light quantum acts as a trigger for a nerve impulse, the energy of which is provided by the biological system.

Control of activities represents another important set of in vivo biological properties. For instance, the uncontrolled proliferation cell leads to cancer. Of particular interest among materials are enzymes, which through their catalytic action regulate most biological chemical processes. Also is the maintenance of the electric potential difference across biological membranes, with a thickness of about 10 nm.

It is a general feature of active biological systems that energy is always available, through metabolic processes, and that this causes nonlinear changes in molecules or large subsystems. Hence, from the point of view of physics, there are nonlinear effects that changes with time and are maintained through constant energy supply. It is dangerous, therefore, to extrapolate from properties of biological molecules obtained by extracting them from the living system to their behavior in vivo, although in some cases this is possible. Still, from the point of view of physics, biological systems are relatively stable from a microscopic point of view: the thermal vibrations of single atoms are practically the same as in a corresponding nonbiological system. In some respect, however, involving relatively few degrees of freedom, they are very far from the thermal equilibrium, and these degrees of freedom dominate the overall behavior of the rest. They may be described in terms of collective properties or organizations that do not exist in individual particle physics. These collective properties evolve as a consequence of supply of energy (metabolism) and usually represent extreme nonlinear displacements.

Two physical models have been presented by Frohlich (1980). An essential feature in both cases is the basic importance of the nonlinear characteristics in conjunction with a supply of energy. One is quasi-static, showing that, under very general conditions, metastable states with very high electric polarization exist. The second is dynamic in terms of coherent excitation of electric vibrations may be excited by random metabolic energy. This leads to long-range selective forces that supplement short-range forces, including those leading to standard chemical processes. The selectively of the long-range forces depends on the frequency of the oscillating systems, which in turn depends on their structure.

At all levels of mammalian biological organization when subjected to an environmental impact elicits a complex array of nervous, endocrine, neurohumoral, and motor reaction to adjust body fluid balance, energy metabolism, and behavior to the needs, thus reprogramming itself to ensure its survival in an altered environment. The neuroendocrine system, a complex of hormone-secreting glands, and the central nervous system function as a chemical regulatory system in mammals to control and regulate metabolism and growth and to protect the body from endogenous and exogenous impacts.

4.3 Physics of the Problem

The biological bodies are inhomogeneous, having tissue-specific dielectric properties and the complexity of the shape; they make the computations of the induced field difficult. The fields induced inside the body act differently depending upon the frequency. The biological effects produced are dependent upon, but are not limited to, the following parameters:

- The location of the field with respect to the surroundings, e.g., if there are metallic objects around or if the person is grounded or not otherwise.
- Polarization of the incident wave with respect to the orientation of the human body (Figure 4.2).
- The portion of the human body exposed, if it is partial or full exposure and the electrical properties of the tissue undergoing exposure.

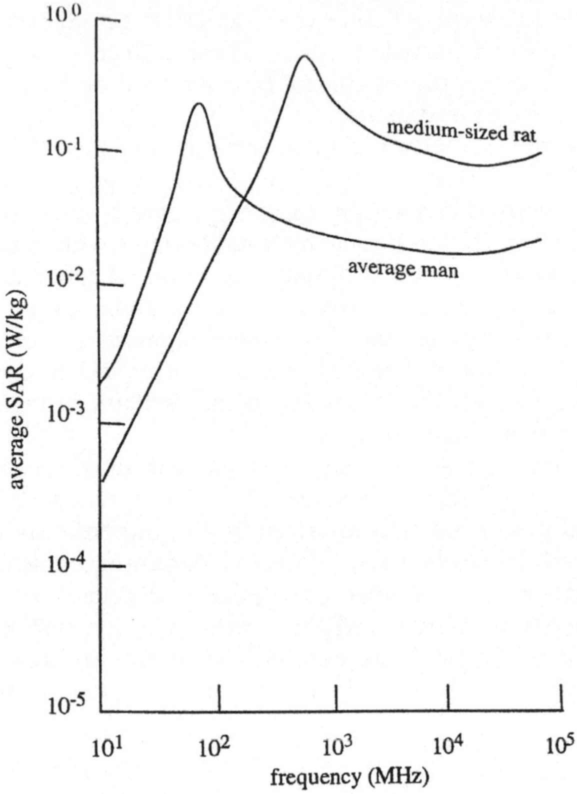

FIGURE 4.2
SAR for E polarization for an average man and for a medium-sized rat. For length of the object between A and B, the peak position is between the two. The resonance of the absorption is dependent upon its length.

In free space propagation of electromagnetic field, the power density is given by

$$\text{Power density} = E^2/1200\,\Pi\ \text{mW/cm}^2$$

where, E is the electric field strength.

Figure 4.2 illustrates how the average body SAR is size and frequency dependent (e.g., Gandhi 1979). The absorption characteristics for a prolate spheroidal model representing man, 175 cm long, oriented parallel to an incident electric field (maximum absorption). It shows that the average SAR, for man model, exposed to radiation at frequencies from 10 to 10,000 MHz, first increases as the square of the frequency, reaching a peak of

2W/kg at about 70 or 80 MHz and then gradually approaches an asymptotic value of approximately 0.16 W/kg. In the upright position, the grounded body has longitudinal resonance around 35 MHz (Gandhi 1975). This configuration may be obtained in a far-field exposure. However, near-field patterns of energy absorption, as in the case of user of cellular phone near the head, will be dominated by regional peaks determined by proximity of the transmitting antenna to specific body parts and their relative orientation.

It therefore follows from biophysical considerations, that each body has characteristic resonant frequency depending upon the length of the long axis. Correspondingly, for the same level of incident exposure, the average value of SAR is dependent upon the length of the body, the degree of decoupling decreases the average value of SAR by more than an order of magnitude. The absorbed RF energy can be converted into other form of energy and can cause interference with the functioning of the biological systems. A significant portion of this energy is converted into heat (absorption). However, the effects are frequency dependent. At frequencies well below 100 KHz, the induced fields can even stimulate nervous tissue.

4.4 Head as a Recipient of Electromagnetic Energy

In living systems, the electromagnetic signals are in existence in every physiological process, from EEG, EMG, protein folding, and nervous system function, and any other human activity, and can be perturbed through mobile communications frequencies. If we expose a living system to a weak external signal, it will interact and may interfere with normal physiological functioning, even though a direct frequency coupling may not be there (Parker & Winters 1992). It is this aspect of EMF-biological interaction that has aroused interest in past decades.

The electromagnetic waves falling on the biological objects may not necessarily penetrate through the entire body, but may be limited to a distance determined by the skin depth. The depth to which microwaves can penetrate inside the tissue depends on the electric and magnetic properties of the tissue and on frequency of the microwaves in question. In general, at a given frequency, the lower the water contents of the tissue, the greater the wave penetration and vice versa. Since the values of the reliable dielectric data are now available, the assessment of biointeraction mechanism can be better understood and quantified.

Out of all the organs, head is the targeted recipient of electromagnetic energy from many wireless systems (e.g., mobile phones), and the signal generated is transmitted to other organ and parts of the body. This interaction mode is, therefore, investigated for its physical and biological properties.

For a given incident field flux, the heating potential in the hot spot decreases rapidly with increasing head radius. Thus, in man, the expected temperature rise would be lower at this 1.0 GHz field frequency than seen in the 10 cm model. There are strong differentials in convective capacities between cerebral gray and white matter, attributable to substantially higher densities of blood vessel capillary beds in central cortical gray matter (Ranck 1964). For the human head, simulated as a sphere 15.0 cm in diameter with three layers representing brain, fat and skin, at 2.45 GHz (or higher frequency) field is rapidly absorbed at the surface of the head.

4.5 Quantification

As mentioned in Chapter 1, the dosimetry is spread over three frequency ranges: Low frequencies, Radiofrequency, and microwave frequencies. At low frequencies (<100 KHz), many biological effects are quantitated in terms of current density in tissue and this parameter is most often used as a dosimetric quantity. At higher frequencies, many (but not all) interactions are due to the rate of energy deposition per unit mass. This is why the SAR is used as the dosimetric measure at these frequencies. It is expressed as Watts per kilogram. The SAR is thus the absorbed power by the absorbing mass. The most obvious approach towards dosimetric analysis is to experimentally determine the SAR distribution in phantoms simulating animal and human bodies as well in real cadavers.

Even with these limitations, the SAR concept has proven to be a simple and useful concept in quantifying the interactions of RF/microwave radiation with living systems, enabling comparison of experimentally observed biological effects for various species under various exposure conditions. This provides (as of now) the only means, (howsoever imperfect), of extrapolating the animal data into potential hazards to humans exposed to RF radiation and facilitating, planning and effectively executing the therapeutic hyperthermic treatment (Stuchly & Stuchly 1996).

The SAR is defined as the time derivative of the incremental energy dW absorbed by or (dissipated in an incremental mass dm contained in a volume element dV of a given density ρ) (Sinclair 1981; WHO 1993). Correspondingly one has to resort to temperature measurement. The SAR is proportional to the temperature increase, when the effects of thermal conduction, convection and radiation are negligible in the time interval Δt.

$$\mathrm{SAR} = \left(\frac{d}{dt}\right)\left(\frac{dW}{dm}\right) = \left(\frac{d}{dt}\right)\left(\frac{dw}{\rho(dv)}\right) = C\frac{\Delta T}{\Delta t} \tag{4.1}$$

The same can also be evaluated, using the Poynting vector theorem for sinusoidal varying electromagnetic fields:

$$\text{SAR} = \sigma(\text{Ei})^2/\rho. \tag{4.2}$$

Where, $|\text{Ei}|^2$ is the peak value of the internal electric field (in volts per meter), σ is the conductivity and ρ is the density of the biological body in question. SAR is also dependent on the wave type, i.e., square, sine or triangular. The power of the square is larger than the other two. The average SAR is defined as the ratio of the total power absorbed in the exposed body to the mass in which it is absorbed, which is not necessarily that of the total body. The local SAR refers to the value within a defined unit volume or unit mass, which can be arbitrarily chosen.

To understand experiments on microwave exposure and their relationship to safety (and subsequent hazard), we can see Figure 4.3, where biological effects are shown relating to central nervous system and reproduction pattern in males is shown, with these being central to any effect on biosystems. The effects are shown to be frequency and SAR dependent. This offers difficulties in laying down criteria for safe exposure (Behari 2009a). Theoretically (Osepchuk & Petersen 2003) have plotted log–log coordinates of power (/SAR) on the ordinate and time on abscissa. They have shown that it is possible to show the demarcation between safety and limits of hazard. They have mentioned that to heat a sample for a long time (constant SAR), while heating a sample period for a short time (whereby no heat is lost from the system), the threshold curve is a line of constant specific absorption (SA). The intersection of the two lines determine the applicable thermal time constant and associated "average time" in setting exposure standards. However in vivo experiments for a short duration does not offer a reliable picture, while in vitro data are beset with short fall is simulating a realistic scenario.

As evident by equations (4.1 & 4.2), both approaches (temperature/field) have some common requirements. Any measurable field disturbance caused by the intrusion of the probe must be avoided. A further requirement is that any signal, picked by any part of the probe, other than the signal itself should be sufficiently suppressed. Further the spatial resolution should be better than the smallest spatial dimension of any local field maxima or minima, in order to enable accurate assessment of the SAR distribution. Determination of the SAR distribution requires measurements in the tissue volume of interest. In larger volumes with greatly nonuniform distributions, SAR varies from place to place, nessiciating measurements in several places and hence the location and the characteristics of the sensor must be accurately known.

From the animal experimentation (in the developing stage), as the animal age increases (and also the weight), the SAR value changes and dosimetric estimation demands a reset (Figure 4.4) (Behari 2009a).

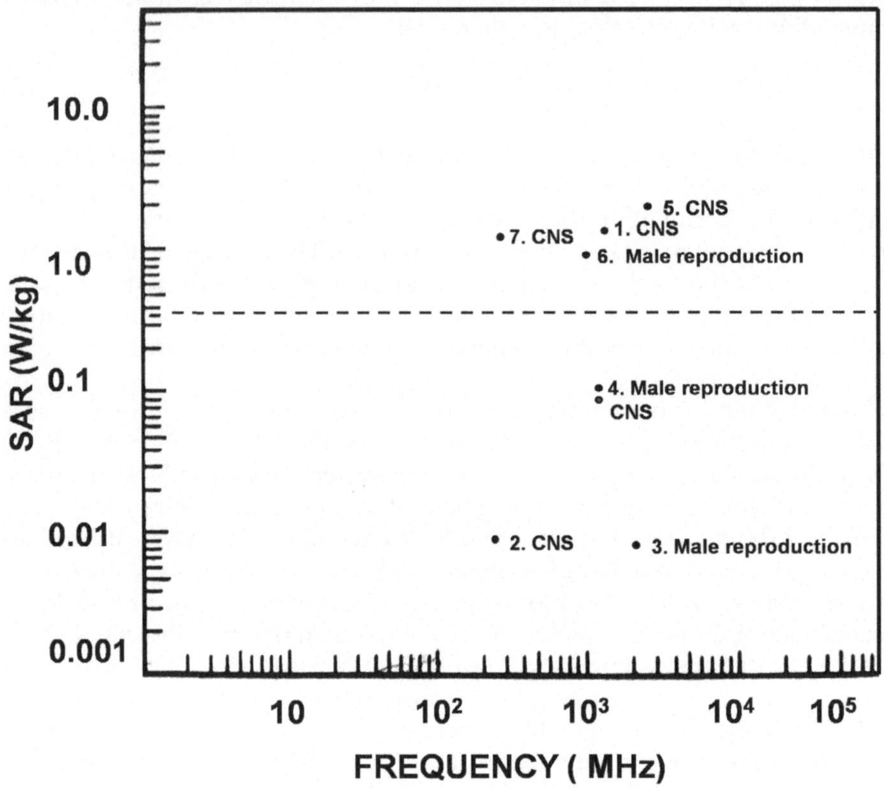

FIGURE 4.3
Occurrence of various biological effects as a function of frequency and SAR values.1: DNA strand break (Paulraj & Behari 2006), 2: cholinergic system (Kunjilwar & Behari 1993), 3: sperm count (Kumar et al. 2011), 4: male reproduction (Kesari et al. 2011), 5: CNS (Paulraj & Behari 2004), 6: cell phone, male fertility (Kesari et al. 2011), and 7: PKC (Paulraj & Behari 2004).

The concept of SAR is not sufficient when one is looking for biological effects based, depending on parameters other than absorption. This raises question about using these parameters for evaluating effects that may be of some other type. The possibility of nonthermal effects is thus a controversial one and therefore the problem of dosimetry becomes more pronounced. SAR may be a valid quantitative measure of interaction other than absorptive ones when the mechanism is dependent on the intensity of E field, except however when direction of the E field is of importance with respect to the biological structure (L/λ value). Similarly, the SAR concept may not be sufficient for the interactions directly through the E field. Further it is always a matter of uncertainty between perceived field strength and the actual RF exposure with

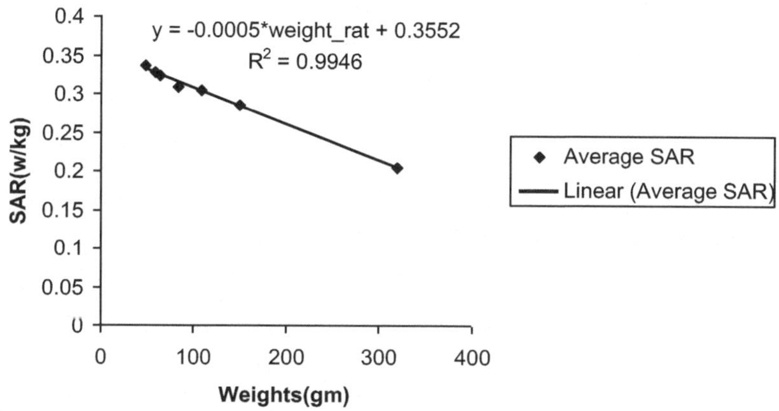

FIGURE 4.4
The linear regression model of the SAR as a function of weight of the rat.

respect to the biological object over a period of time. SAR may also depend upon the mobile phone used: i.e., GSM 900 or GSM 1800 MHz type (Panagopoulous et al. (2007)).

The extrapolation of results from animal experiments (mostly so) to humans is used in a reduced form, termed as frequency scaling. The approach essentially enables us to use results in one model experiment and the results predicted to another biological object, differing only by a scale factor. The frequency-scaling principle can be applied to determine the equivalence between the exposure of a man of height l_m and an animal of a length l_a, with both human and animal having the same orientation with respect to the exposure field. This is obtained by using the relationship:

$$f_m l_m = f_a l_a \tag{4.3}$$

where, f_m and f_a are the frequencies at which man and animal are exposed, respectively (Durney & Christensen 2000). It may be mentioned that the SAR distribution in the two cases will be similar in the two bodies (may not be the same). However, this relation is valid for low losses medium, which is not always the case for biologic structures.

4.6 Biological Effects

Potential biological effects due to nonthermal radiation effects may be classified under the following head:

(1) Low-intensity levels of RF radiation,
(2) Chronic versus acute exposure and,
(3) Pulsed RF radiation is reported to be more bioactive than constant wave RF radiation.

Human body is a complex system than what a simple thermal model would assume to be. It is sensitive to extreme periodic stimuli. Any pulsed modulation pattern supplies the energy and information to the biological system. However, the mode of this interaction remains unknown. This concept has been exploited in soft tissue and also in bone fracture healing (Behari 2009b). This is evident from the results, where the data are definitely emerging from the nonthermal effects. The features of biological effects of microwaves below thermal level are well described by several authors (Devyiatkov et al. 1994; Betskii et al. 1998; Behari 2009a).

(a) Investigations on Nonthermal Effects Can Be Divided into Two Heads

(1) In Vitro: altered cell responses and (2) In Vivo: results of chronic exposures on animals. The data available on biological effects of low-level electromagnetic field exposure are immense, though at times contradictory. These effects related to chronic exposure may not always produce adverse health impact. There is an element of uncertainty across various frequency bands and also on whether the target under investigation is brain, muscle tissue, or a total or a part body exposure.

Much experimental evidence of nonthermal influences of microwave radiation on living systems is now available—relating both to in vitro and in vivo studies—and was reviewed extensively (Bioinitiative 2012). From the use of microwave wireless technologies, the following nonthermal biological effects have been reported:

(1) Changes in the electrical activity in the human brain (Von Kltzng 1995);
(2) Increase in DNA single- and double-strand breaks from RF exposure to 2.45 GHz (Lai & Singh 1996; Paulraj & Behari 2004; Diem et al. 2005);
(3) Increased lymphoma rates (2-fold) in transgenic mice exposed twice a day for 30 minutes of cell phone (GSM) signals over 18 months (Repacholi et al. 1997);
(4) Permeability of the blood-brain barrier shows an increase in rats (Persson et al. 1997);
(5) Production of heat shock proteins and cancer risk (French et al. 2001);
(6) Higher risk of melanoma (Stang et al. 2001);

Other reported effects (Scientific and Technological Options Assessment Stoa 2001) include the following:

(a) Observation of an increase in resting blood pressure during exposure,
(b) Increased permeability of the erythrocyte membrane,
(c) Increase of chromosome aberrations and micronuclei in human blood lymphocytes,
(d) Synergistic effects with cancer-promoting drugs and certain psychoactive drugs,
(e) Depression of chicken immune systems,
(f) Increase in chick embryo mortality,
(g) Effects on brain dopamine/opiate electrochemistry,
(h) Neurogenetic effects and micronuclei formation in peritoneal macrophage.

4.7 Some Basic Systems That Have Been Targeted for Investigation Are as Follows:

(a) Immune System and RF

It is important to consider immunological system that relates to chronic and long-term exposure to EMF.

Vinogradov and Dumanski (1974) exposed white rats to EMF (2450 MHz, 50 μW/cm^2) for five hours/day for 14 days. These authors reported alterations in the structure and/or expression of tissue antigens using the method of anaphylaxis with desensitization. They used 25 rats, out of these 20 were microwave exposed. Sera from rats in remaining five (controls) were examined for the content of antibodies. Phagocytosis was determined in normal and exposed groups. The authors concluded that RF exposure could induce expression of antigens not normally expressed in brain tissues (and blood proteins) and/or alter antigen structure of normally expressed antigens. These changes are characterized by the changes of antigenic structure of tissues. The authors further reported that exposure to these fields (7h/day for 30 days, 50 μW/cm^2) induced auto antibodies reacting with brain tissue antigens in Guinea pigs, white Wistar rats, and rabbits. Autoimmune reactions were identified using the complement-binding reaction (CBR) and plaque-forming cell techniques that revealed the presence of antigen-specific antibodies and antigen-specific antibody-producing cells, respectively. Moreover, leukocytes from EMF (ultrahigh-frequency [UHF])-exposed Guinea pigs showed a reduced serum-mediated phagocytic activity. The results show the dependence in the formation of circulating antibodies against the brain. The antibody titer in Guinea pigs increased in time after the exposure and reached a maximum in 2 weeks after exposure. The authors concluded that chronic exposure to RF at a power density (PD) of 50 μW/cm^2 resulted in the formation of brain antigens in the animals. The highest titers of complement binding were observed 10–14 days after exposure. This indicates a similar time-dependent trend suggesting that the action was consistent. The authors investigated the cellular auto-immune reaction by determining the number of spot-forming cells, synthesizing antibodies against its own erythrocytes in the blood. The study was conducted on Guinea and white rats that were exposed for one month to EMF (UHF) fields at a power density of 50 μ/cm^2. In the same exposure set up, these authors investigated adverse properties of blood serum after UHF exposure based on the determination of changes in the phagocytic capacity of the cells. Guinea pigs were exposed for a period of 30 days and the measurement was performed before the exposure and two and four weeks after exposure. The effect was found to be maximum after two weeks of exposure and remained so till four weeks. These authors concluded that long-term RF exposure at this low intensity (50 μW/cm^2) results in auto-allergic reactions.

Shandala et al. (1983) exposed CBA mice and Wistar rats to 2375 MHz (7h/day). When mice were exposed to 0.1 or 10 mW/cm^2, increased spontaneous and mitogen-stimulated (PHA, phytohemagglutinin) cell proliferation, which persisted for 30 days after the last exposure. When rats were exposed for 3 months to 1 or 5μ/Wcm^2 or for 1 month at 10, 50, 500 μ/Wcm^2, there was a decrease in proliferative response to PHA, still evident 3 months after exposure. No effects were observed with 10 and 50 μ/Wcm^2 in rats. The authors have concluded that RF exposure–induced changes in T-cell immunity.

Vinogradov and Naumenko (1986) exposed Wistar rats to 2375 MHz fields at 50 or 500 μW/cm^2 for 30 days (7 h/day) and confirmed that exposure to 500 μW/cm^2 induced anti-brain antibodies using complement-binding and basophiles degranulation assays, and increased plaque-forming cells, suggesting RF exposure altered brain tissues rendering them immunogenic. The authors also reported an increased number of reticulo-endothelial plasma cells in bone marrow and spleen and a decreased number of small lymphocytes in bone marrow.

Vinogradov et al. (1987) exposed white Wistar rats for 30 days to (10, 50, 500 μW/cm^2, 2375 MHz) and a sham-exposed group used as controls. Induction of auto antibodies toward brain tissue antigens (brain extracts) was evaluated with the complement binding/fixation assay and pathological effects assessed by injecting auto-antibody-containing sera into pregnant animals. Electrophoresis patterns of sera immunoglobulin were also evaluated. Exposure to 50 and 500 μW/cm^2 induced auto antibodies to brain tissue antigens as revealed by indirect degranulation of basophiles and complement fixation assays. No effects were induced from exposure to 10 μW/cm^2. Exposure to 50 μW/cm^2 decreased cell proliferation. Sera from exposed (or sham-exposed) rats were injected into pregnant rats to verify whether the presence of the auto antibodies was pathological. Sera from rats exposed to 500 μW/cm^2 increased post-implantation loss and decreased the number, body weight and the length of newborns. Analysis of soft tissues from the fetus revealed the presence of hemorrhage in subcutaneous tissues, peritoneal cavity, liver, and brain. The authors also reported that exposure to 500 μW/cm^2 (but not 10 or 50 μW/cm^2) led to alterations in immunoglobulin electrophoresis, with the appearance of a new peak similar to that of class A antibodies, and concluded that it caused strong changes in physico-chemical and immunological properties of serum humoral factors. The authors concluded that such changes render proteins naturally produced in the body as immunologically "foreign" and stimulate autoimmune response.

In another experiment Vinogradov et al. (1991) exposed female Fisher rats to 2375 MHz (500 μW/cm^2), 7h/day for 15 days. Exposure effects were assessed by injecting lymph node cells from exposed or sham-exposed animals into normal recipient rats. The authors concluded that exposure reduced mitogen-stimulated cell proliferation (PHA and Con A) and induced auto-antibodies toward brain tissue antigens as shown by basophiles degranulation and plaque-forming cell assays.

(b) The Biology of Blood-Brain Barrier (BBB)

BBB is a protective barrier that prevents the flow of toxins into sensitive brain tissue. BBB serves as a regulatory system that optimizes the fluid environment of the brain's intracellular compartment (Pardridge 1991). The intact BBB protects the brain from damage, whereas the dysfunctioning BBB allows influx of normally excluded hydrophilic molecules into the brain tissue. Due to penetration of electromagnetic radiations, it is speculated that these radiations causes significant alteration in the BBB functionality (Lin 2001). It is a selectively permeable, hydrophobic barrier that is readily crossed by small, lipid-soluble molecules.

The BBB is anatomic/physiological complex associated with the cerebral vascular system. It is composed of a network of astrocytic pseudopodia which envelops the tight junctions of the vascular endothelium. It functions as a differential filter that permits the selective passage of biological substances from blood to brain. For instance, amino acids, anesthetics, and glucose may gain access to brain cells. The barrier is also highly permeable to ions such as sodium, potassium and chloride. On the other hand, carbohydrates, large molecules (proteins) and most microorganisms, water soluble chemicals and antibiotics are excluded from brain tissues by the BBB. Opening of the BBB may subject the CNS to assault from extraneous microorganisms. The BBB protects the mammalian brain from potentially harmful compounds in the blood. It is thus a natural defense system that maintains the physicochemical environment of the brain within certain narrow limits that are essential for life.

In a functional BBB, the membrane properties control the bidirectional exchange between the general circulation and the CNS. Water, most lipid soluble molecules, oxygen and carbon dioxide can diffuse from the blood to the nerve cells. However, when the barrier is damaged, conditions such as tumors, infarcts or infections prevails, and the normally excluded molecules can pass through, possibly bringing toxic molecules out into the brain tissue. The selective permeability is also disrupted temporally in cases of epileptic seizures (Mihaly & Bozoky 1984). Increased permeability of the BBB is seen in cases of oxidative stress (Parathath et al. 2006), where BBB dysfunction and neurodegeneration are shown to be mediated through an excitotoxicity mechanism by the serine protease tissue plasminogen, with NO and $ONOO^-$ as downstream mediators.

The selective permeability has the disadvantage that agents and drugs that are effective in treating diseases in the other parts of the body may not be able to gain entry into the brain to combat infection. On the other hand, the ability to selectively open the BBB suggests the possibility of using microwave regional hyperthermia to facilitate chemotherapy for brain tumors and facilitate the delivery of anti cancer drugs such as methotrexate. This drug is often used for high-dose chemotherapy.

(c) Nervous System

Due to the proximity of mobile phone to the head, most research efforts have been concentrated on estimating potentially toxic effect of RF (if any) on central nervous system. This is largely because nervous systems in the body mainly control the integrating network. Under some conditions like when the handset operates at full transmitter power because of a long distance to the next base station, local SAR values in the brain are reported to be in the range of 1 W/kg or more (Huber et al. 2003). Its activities are divided into two parts: sensing and then responding. In the first category it serves two functions: sensing intrinsic and extrinsic (environmental) stimulus and interpreting and integrating these signals. In the second phase, it responds to external perturbations by initiating actions in the form of muscular contractions or glandular secretions. When, the nervous system or the brain is perturbed, by the exposure due to radiofrequency radiations, where changes take place, relating to morphological (Kim et al. 2017), electrophysiological, and chemical systems. These include transient minor effects on the electroencephalogram (EEG), on sleep structure, and on cognitive processes in human subjects (Mann et al. 1998; Landgrebe et al. 2008). A significant change in these can lead to a change in overall behavior.

It is further reported that different areas of the brain have different sensitivities to radiofrequency radiations (Lai et al. 1984; Ray & Behari 1987). Exposure of brain to mobile phone may lead to an increase in temperature to the extent of 0.1°C (Van Leeuwen et al. 1999; Wainwright 2000), after taking into consideration the high blood perfusion rate. This is in contrast to skin blood perfusion that gets significantly elevated after exposure to mobile phone frequencies (Monfrecola et al. 2003).

(d) Electrophysiology

Effect on brain exposure to various modulation frequencies has been studied by various workers (Hinrikus et al. 2008). A variety of abnormalities have been identified (other than epileptic), which are included in the power spectrum (distribution of power over all the frequencies present). Several authors (Sun et al. 2006; Rojas et al. 2008) have reported altered gamma wave activity, and others showing reduction of spectral power across all bands (Tierney et al. 2012), while other workers showed increased high-frequency oscillations (Orekhova et al. 2007). Abnormalities in coherence and synchronization between various parts of the brain have been found (Muller 2008; Wass 2011), comparable to abnormal functional connectivity measured by fMRI (Just et al. 2004) and measuring with the use of electroencephalogram (EEG) or magnetoencephalogram (MEG) with higher temporal resolution (Isler et al. 2010). Several studies have identified an increased randomness in EEGs of people with autism (Catarino et al. 2011), as well as an increase in power but a reduction in coherence (Isler et al. 2010; Mathewson et al. 2012). Also Roschke and Mann (1997) did not notice any difference in the awake EEGs of subjects exposed to radiation emitted by cellular phones.

EMF/RFR also has impacts at levels of brain function at various frequencies and durations of exposure; it has been noted to impact alpha and beta rhythms (Hinrikus et al. 2008), to increase randomness (Marino & Carrubba 2009; Marino 2012), to alter power, to modulate interhemispheric synchronization (Vecchio et al. 2007), to alter electrical activity in brain slices (Tattersall et al. 2001), and to alter the patterns of coordination (spectral power coherence) across the major power bands (Houtala et al. 2008).

(e) Electrohypersensitivity (EHS)

In this case, the patient is not able to detect the presence or absence of EMF exposure (McCarty et al. 2011). Sandstrom et al. (2003) presented evidence that heart rate variability is impaired in people with electrical hypersensitivity and showed an imbalance of the autonomic nervous system. They reported a relatively "flat" representation of hourly recorded spectral power of the HF component of heart rate variability (HRV).

Landgrebe et al. (2007, 2008) reported that electrosensitive patients showed reduced intracortical facilitation as compared to two control groups. The EHS group of patients showed altered central nervous system function. These authors also reported that EHS patients, but not controls, demonstrated significant cognitive and neurobiological alterations pointing to a higher genuine individual vulnerability of electromagnetic hypersensitive patients.

Johansson et al. (2010) studied symptoms and stress in people with mobile phone-related effects and electromagnetic hypersensitivity. They reported that, there is support for difference between people with symptoms related to specific EMF sources and people with general electrohypersensitivity. The symptoms are anxiety, depression, somatization, exhaustion, and stress. The EHS group reported more neurasthenic symptoms.

In a study conducted by McCarty et al. (2011), with the fields either or not on the subject, experienced and reported temporal pain, feeling of unease, skipped heart beats, muscle twitches, and/or strong headache when the pulsed field (100 ms duration at 10 Hz) was on, but no or mild symptoms when it was off. Symptoms from continuous fields were less severe than with pulsed fields. The differences between field on and sham exposure were significant ($p < 0.05$). They concluded that electromagnetic hypersensitivity is a neurological syndrome, and statistically reliable somatic reactions would be provoked in the patient by exposure to 60Hz electric fields at 300 V/m. The authors conclude that EMF hypersensitivity can occur as a bonafide environmentally inducible neurological syndrome. Marino (2012) showed the link between EMF exposure and somatic responses ($p < 0.005$) and inferred that EHS is a nonlinear phenomena.

Aldad et al. (2012) exposed mice in utero to cellular telephones, with resultant aberrant miniature excitatory postsynaptic currents, dose responsive impaired glutamatergic synaptic transmission onto layer V pyramidal neurons of the prefrontal cortex. They showed that cell phone radiation significantly altered fetal brain development and produced ADHD (attention-deficit hyperactivity disorder)-like behavior in the offspring of pregnant mice. Exposed mice had a dose-dependent impaired glutamatergic synaptic transmission onto Layer V pyramidal neurons of the prefrontal cortex. The authors conclude the behavioral changes were the result of altered neuronal developmental programming in utero. Offspring mice were hyperactive and impaired memory function and behavior problems, much like the human children (Divan et al. 2008). They found that children born of mothers who used cell phones during pregnancy develop more behavioral problems by the time they have reached school age than children whose mothers did not use cell phones during pregnancy. Children whose mothers used cell phones during pregnancy had 25% more emotional problems, 35% more hyperactivity, 49% more conduct problems, and 34% more peer problems. They showed that cell phone radiation significantly altered fetal brain development and produced ADHD-like behavior in the offspring of pregnant mice. Exposed mice had a dose-dependent impaired glutamatergic synaptic transmission onto Layer V pyramidal neurons of the prefrontal cortex. In another experiment Lahijani et al. (2009) exposed pre- incubated chicken embryos to 50 Hz EMFs, and concluded that cell damage to elevated free radical-induced cell membrane disruptions.

Another study (Fragopoulou et al. 2009) reported altered development of the cranial bones of the mouse fetus from low intensity (0.6 to 0.9W/kg) in utero 900 MHz cell phone radiation. The authors have concluded that even modest exposure (e.g., 6 minutes daily for 21 days) is sufficient to interfere with the normal mouse developmental process. Another study by (Fragopoulou et al. 2010) report that brain astrocytes development followed by proteomic studies is adversely affected by DECT (Digital Electrical cordless telecommunication) and mobile phone radiation (Fragopoulou et al. 2012) and found that whole body exposure with GSM 900 MHz affects spatial memory in mice.

Andrianome et al. (2017) assessed the level of various salivary and urinary markers of patients with electromagnetic hypersensitivity (EHS) and compared them with those of a healthy control group. They analyzed samples from 30 EHS individuals and a matched control group of 25 individuals (non-EHS) aged between 22 and 66 years. The authors reported that sAA (saliva aphaamylase) was found to be significantly higher ($p < 0.005$) in the EHS group. uNeopterin (urine neopterin) and sAA analysis showed a significant difference based on the duration of EHS. Higher levels of sAA in EHS participants may suggest that the sympathetic adrenal medullar system is activated. However, most of the analyzed markers of the immune system, sympathetic activity and circadian rhythm did not vary significantly in the EHS group. There is a trend to the higher levels of some variables in subgroups according to the EHS duration.

Another related parameter is one of "microwave syndrome". This was highlighted several decades ago in Eastern Europe, related to a number of manifestations, such as headache, perspiration, emotional instability, irritability, tiredness, somnolence, sexual problems, loss of memory, concentration and decision difficulties, insomnia, and depressive hypochondriac tendencies. The evaluation is difficult because of the absence of a control group and well-established dosimetric data. Some workers support the idea that the RF sickness syndrome as a possible medical entity (Johnson 1998), due to modulated microwaves.

(f) Sensory Processing

At the symptomatic level issues with sensory processing are highly prevalent in autism spectrum disorders (ASDs). Phenomenology can include hypersensitivity to external stimuli, hypersensitivity to internal sensations and difficulty localizing sensation including pain and difficulty in processing more and more than one sensory channel at one time (Sacco et al. 2010; Robeldo et al. 2012). There is now an electrophysiological evidence of abnormalities at early (brainstem) stages of sensory processing, as well as in later stages of processing that occur in the cortex. Some studies have shown lower and some longer latencies of response to an auditory stimulus. Domain perception where the performance of people with ASDs is superior to that of neurotypical individuals have been identified (Marco et al. 2011). It is also possible that the mechanism is not neural—they may also be modulated by glial, metabolic, immune, perfusional, and other physiological processes and physical properties as well. Yet although there is some consideration of the pathophysiology-sensory function interaction (Kern et al. 2010), it has basically not been cleared in studies of ASDs with experimental designs integrating pathophysiological and electrophysiology. Kenet (2011) demonstrated environmental vulnerability of sensory processing in the brain by the exposure of rat dams to noncoplanar polychlorinated biphenyls (PCBs), during gestation and for three subsequent weeks of nursing. These authors reported that though the hearing sensitivity and brainstem development auditory responses of pups were normal, exposures resulted in the abnormal development of the primary auditory cortex (A1). A1 was irregularly shaped and marked by internal nonresponsive zones, its topographic organization was grossly abnormal or reversed in about half of the exposed pups, the balance of neuronal inhibition to excitation for A1 neurons was disturbed, and the critical period plasticity that underlies normal postnatal auditory system development was significantly altered. These findings demonstrate that development exposure to this class of environmental containment alters critical development. These findings are also important for RFR exposure.

(g) Physiological Effects on Brain Due to RF

By exposing mouse for a long duration, Repacholi et al. (1997) showed an elevated risk of developing lymphoma in a transgenic strain. Use of phone in driving stimulator leads to negative reaction time. Evidence for a direct memory effect on brain slices from the hippocampus of rat showed changes in long-term potentiation when exposed to 915 MHz (Scott et al. 1998). Mild et al. (1998), looking for a subjective response, suggested increased headache or sensation of warmness when using mobile phones. Braune et al. (1998) reported blood pressure increase (5–10 mm Hg) induced by exposure to the right side of the head. However, Barker et al. (2007) in a double-blind study reported no effect of GSM and TETRA (Terrestrial Trunked Radio) signals on blood pressure and related physiological parameters.

Some essential points can be summarized as below:

> Since nerve cells do not divide and are not likely to become cancerous, more likely consequences of DNA damage in nerve cells are changes in functions and cell death, which could either lead to or accelerate the development of neurodegenerative diseases. The effect of microwave radiation on DNA would be more significant on neurons than on other cell types, because nerve cells have a low capability to repair.

(ii) EMF-induced DNA damage could be blocked by treating the rats with antioxidants, including melatonin, immediately before and after exposure (Lai & Singh 1995, 1996). Melatonin is a hormone secreted from the brain's pineal gland. As a potent antioxidant, it effectively eliminates free radicals inside cells.

DNA damage leads to increased mutation rate could be linked to gene mutations. Gene is a section of DNA containing the information needed to make a particular protein or enzyme. There is also a section that can turn the gene on or off in response to outside signals. The growth of an organism from a fertilized fertilized egg involves a hugely complex pattern of switching genes on and off that regulates growth, cell division and differentiation into specific tissues. DNA damage causing unregulated growth to form tumors may not be immediate and may take years before it is fully replicated.

(h) Brain Function and EMF Effects: Fundamentals

Another important parameter is to measure neurotransmitter in various parts of brain (Zhou et al. 2012). Neurons transmit information across the synapses using a range of neurotransmitters. Calcium plays an essential role in this because a small amount of calcium must enter the neuron every time before it can release its neurotransmitters. If the electromagnetic field causes extra calcium to leak inside the cell (neuron), it would increase the background level and may trigger an early release of neurotransmitter. It has been shown that the excitation of acupuncture points by microwaves (0.2–3 GHz) may produce an efficient analgesic effect, as shown by the corresponding increase in the pain threshold (Teng et al. 1989).

Calcium in control of brain function has been found to be influenced by a range of modulating frequency. A statistically significant increase in net $^{45}Ca^{2+}$ transport was observed for modulating frequencies of 6–16 Hz followed by a fall in the frequency range of 20–35Hz (Bawin et al. 1978). The nonlinear effect of modulated waves on chicken cerebral tissue has been demonstrated with $^{45}Ca^{+2}$. The animals were exposed to 0.8 mW/cm^2 at 147 MHz, amplitude modulated by a sinusoidal signal (0.5–35 Hz). The existence of frequency windows has been confirmed (Blackman et al. 1979) for an incident power flux of 1 mW/cm^2. There was a positive response when the modulation lay between 6 and 12 Hz and there was little response at 0.5 and 20 Hz. A power window was also shown to exist at constant frequency: when the chicken cerebral tissue was submitted to a 450 MHz carrier wave modulated at 16 Hz. There was a significant increase in power levels of 0.1 and 1 mW/cm^2, while no effect was observed for power levels of 0.05 and 5 mW/cm^2. Similar results in terms of a low RF frequency and power windows were reported by Kunjilwar and Behari (1993). They exposed rats to 112 MHz, amplitude modulated at 16 Hz (power 1 mW/cm^2 SAR 0.01 W/kg) and reported changes in acetylcholinase estrase activity and Na^+/K^+phosphatase activity (Behari et al. 1998). They observed no significant changes when CW was changed to 73.5 MHz and 36.75 MHz and at the modulating frequency of 76 Hz. The limits of frequency and power window are 6–20 Hz and 0.1–1 mW/cm^2, respectively, in agreement with the work of Gandhi (1982). The author pointed out that the carrier frequency was less than 1 GHz, but itself has little effect, while the modulating frequencies are the controlling parameters. For avian brain tissue under AM wave, conductivity at modulation of 16 Hz was 1.2 times that of 3 Hz (Albert et al. 1987). For human brain, conductivity also increases as FM modulation increases from 9 to 16 Hz (Blackman et al. 1979).

Bawin and Adey (1976) have found that exposing brain tissue to weak VHF radio signals modulated at 16 Hz released calcium ions bound to the surface of cells. Blackman et al. (1979) concluded that weak fields were often more effective than strong ones, extra energy coming in is dissipated as heat. Without these ions, cell membranes are weakened and are more likely to tear under the stresses and strains imposed by the moving cell contents. Although the resulting holes are normally self-healing, these will increase leakage, while open and this than explains the bulk of the known biological effects of weak electromagnetic fields. Leaks in the membrane surroundings lysosomes can release digestive enzymes, including DNAase (an enzyme that destroys DNA).

In investigations carried out by Cetkin et al. (2017) a total of 32 male Wistar albino rats were randomly divided into three groups: control, sham and mobile phone speech (exposed, 2h/day) and stand by (12 h/day) groups. The speech and stand by groups were subjected to the exposed EMF for a total of 10 weeks. They reported no statistically significant difference between the serum iron and ferritin values of the rats in the speech and stand by groups than the control and sham groups ($p > 0.05$). The unsaturated iron binding capacity and total iron capacity values of the rats in the speech and stand by groups were significantly lower in comparison to the control group ($p < 0.01$). They found that exposure to EMF created by mobile phones affected unsaturated iron-binding capacity and total iron-binding capacity negatively.

(i) Effect on Brain DNA

Human DNA is about 2m long, and the molecule is greatly compacted so that it fits into nuclei of cells that are microns in diameter. The DNAmolecule in the nucleus conducts electricity (Hall et al. 1996) and is organized in a symmetrical pattern. It has two key characteristics of fractal antennas when interacting with EMF (Blank & Goodman 2011). DNA has a unique coiled coil structure where two strands of DNA are bound together by hydrogen bond between pair of nucleotide bases (one on each strand) and they long form a long twisted ribbon with delocalized π electrons that form continuous planar clouds on both surfaces of the ribbon.

The rate of conduction is influenced by the structure of DNA at the microscopic level. Changes such as the hairpin turns and mismatched bases can lead to the disruption of the ordered double helical structure in the rate of electron flow (Arkin et al. 1996; Hall et al. 1996; Giese & Vierling 2002). Electron motion can lead to local charging and the oxidative damage.

The result is a structure with two continuous paths that can conduct an electron current along the DNA. The coiled coil structure of DNA in the nucleus makes the molecule react like a fractal antenna for the electromagnetic field in general and RF field in particular. Fractal design is desirable for antenna because it minimizes the overall size, while reacting to a wide range of electromagnetic frequencies. However, these characteristics also become undesirable in DNA because it provides possibility of a wide range of frequencies present in the environment to interact with the DNA. The continuous cloud of delocalized electrons along both faces of the contour formed by the base pairs provides a conducting path for responding to EMF and makes it more vulnerable to damage. The chemical changes that result from electron transfer reactions are associated with molecular damage in DNA.

There have been reports regarding the effects on DNA damage in cells (C3H10T) exposed to radiofrequency radiations(Li et al. 2001) at high SARs of 3–5 W/kg, but no effect at the SAR value of 1.2 W/kg (Lagroye et al. 2004). DNA/DNA hybridization under controlled microwave (MW) power and temperature conditions were studied by Edwards et al. (2009). These authors demonstrated that microwaves (MW) affected double-stranded DNA well below their thermal melting temperature (may be nonthermal phenomena) and independent of the length of the DNAs. They suggested specific interaction of microwaves with DNA under MW heating. Dragan and Geddes (2014) showed that low-power microwave radiation accelerates both the formation of the anchor-DNA scaffold on the silver island film-surface and anchor/probe DNA hybridization. Thermotolerance, the ability to tolerate higher temperatures as a result of repeated exposure to high temperature, was originally demonstrated at the molecular level in connection with heat shock. Repeated exposure to increased temperature results in a decreased heat shock response. A similar mechanism applies when the cellular stress response is stimulated by EMF, since repeated EMF stimuli result in lower production of stress proteins. This could very well be a mechanism by which repeated exposure to EMF can result in less protection and more damage to molecules like DNA. The lower protection causes exposed individuals to an increased risk of mutation and initiation of cancer. Paulraj and Behari (2006) and Malyapa et al. (1998) also reported DNA strand break due to low-level microwave exposure.

Impact of EMF/RFR on cells in the brain is documented by some of the studies that have examined brain tissue after the exposure. Some aspects appearing after such exposures include dark neurons (neuronal damage), neuronal firing rate (Bolshakov & Alekseev 1992), and upregulation of genes related to cell death pathways in both neurons and astrocytes (Zhao et al. 2007). Astrocytic changes include increased GFAP and increased glial activity (Brillaud et al. 2007; Ammari et al. 2010). It has been observed that there is a marked protein downregulation of the nerve growth factor glial maturation factor beta (GMF) which is considered as an intracellular signal transduction regulator in astrocytes. This could have significant impact on neuronal-glial interaction as well as brain cell differentiation and tumor development. Diminution of Purkinje cell number and density has also been observed (Ragabetli et al. 2010). Promotion of pro-inflammatory responses in EMF-stimulated microglial cells has also been reported (Yang et al. 2010). It has been further identified that astrocyte abnormalities include altered expression of astrocyte markers GFAP abnormalities including elevation, antibodies, and altered signaling (Fatemi et al. 2008).

(j) DNA Damage and Cancer

Stress proteins are essential for cell protection. They help defend cells against damaging forces like increase in temperature and reductions in oxygen supply that could be life threatening. Body generates stress proteins to strengthen cellular resistance to the effects of EM radiation. However stress protein synthesis in reality is only an emergency measure and is designed to be an effective short-term measure. The response to repeated stimuli diminishes and this could be dangerous for health. This stems from the fact that two strands of DNA to come apart for the protein code to be read and for synthesis to proceed.

Based on epidemiological studies there is a consistent pattern of increased risk for glioma and acoustic neuroma associated with the use of mobile phones and cordless phones. No consistent pattern of an increased risk is seen for meningioma. Supportive evidence also come from anatomical localization of the tumor to the most exposed area of the brain, cumulative exposure in hours and latency time that add to biological relevance of an increased risk. In addition, calculations based on estimated absorbed dose give strength to the findings of (Hardell et al. 2011).

(i) Mechanisms in Cancer Development and Repair Models

Clinical evidence points to the significance of DNA repair mechanisms in tumor prevention and tumor initiation. Even the most trivial metabolic intervention, such as consumption of coffee, is known to produce numerous but transient breaks in nuclear DNA that are normally completely repaired in a matter of hours.

Defects in cloned DNA repair genes have been associated with a predisposition to some cancer and other disorders (Taylor et al. 1994). Moreover, free radicals of the oxygen and nitrogen species may act as complete carcinogens, the outcome depending on interactions between DNA damage, antioxidant levels, and DNA repair systems (Wiseman et al. 1995). Studies of breast cancer cases in one generation offer a model in which possible interaction between DNA repair proficiency and exposure to ionizing radiation in childhood (Helzlsourer et al. 1996) supports the hypothesis that a deficiency in repair of X-irradiation DNA damage may increase susceptibility to breast cancer.

Cancer development is a multi-stage process which is characterized a cumulative action of multiple events occurring in a single cell. This can be described by three stages: initiation, promotion, and progression. ROS can act in all these stages of carcinogenesis (Klaunig & Kamendulis 2004). The three stages model of carcinogenesis is shown in Figure 4.5a, b. Initiation involves a non-lethal mutation in DNA that produces an

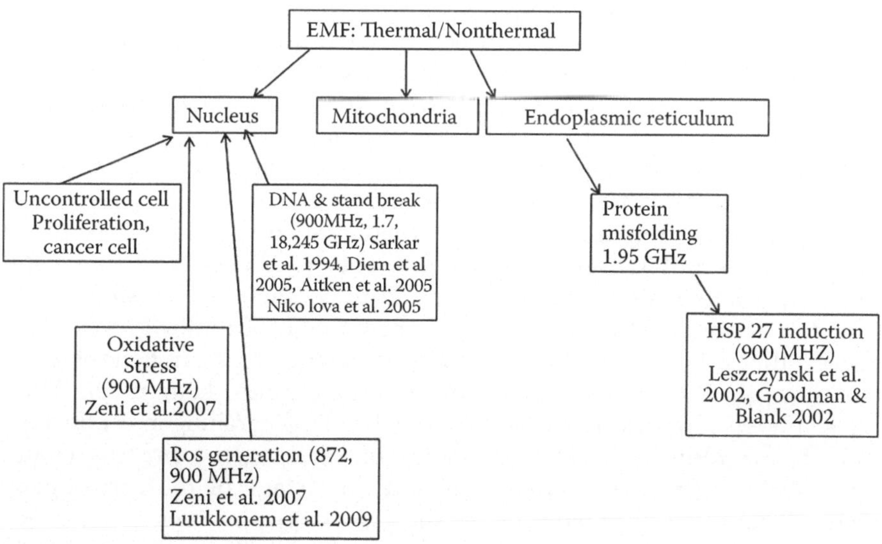

FIGURE 4.5a
Effect of electromagnetic field at the cellular level.

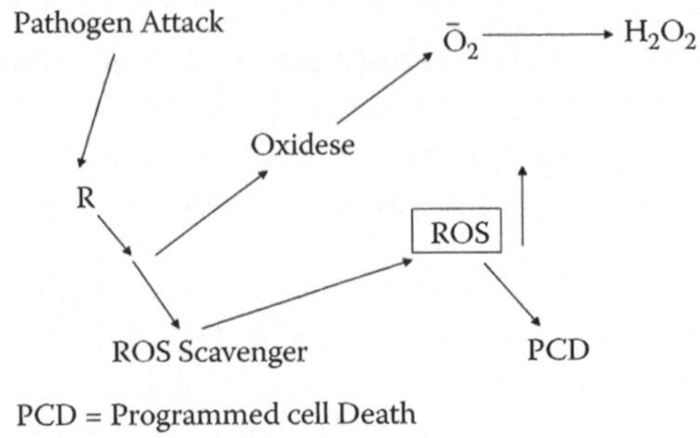

FIGURE 4.5b
Pathogen attack leading to ROS production.

altered cell followed by at least one round of DNA synthesis to fix the damage (e.g., 8-OH-G) produced during the initiation. If dividing cells are damaged for some reason, they are able to interrupt temporarily their cell cycle at stage G1, S, or G2, repair the damage, and resume division (Loft & Poulsen 1996). Oxidative DNA damage can occur via action of ROS, e.g., hydroxyl radicals, formed through the Fenton-type mechanism, along with other species. The process of initiation further proceeds through oxidative stress-induced Ca (II) changes leading to increase in intracellular free calcium as a result of its release from intracellular Ca (II) stores and through the influx of extracellular Ca (II) (Dreher & Junod 1996). The promotion stage is characterized by the clonal expansion of initiated cells by the induction of cell proliferation and/or inhibition of programmed cell death (apoptosis). This process results in the formation of an identifiable focal lesion. This stage dose-dependency requires the continuous presence of the tumors promotion stimulus and is a reversible process. Many tumors promoters have a strong inhibiting effect on cellular antioxidant defense systems such as SOD, catalase, glutathione, etc. While a high level of oxidative stress is cytotoxic to the cell and halts proliferation by inducing apoptosis or even necrosis. A low level of oxidative stress can in fact stimulate the cell division in the promotion stage and thus stimulate the promotion of tumor growth. This suggests that production of ROS during this stage of carcinogenesis is the main line of ROS-related tumor promotion (Figure 4.5a, b, c). Three stages model of carcinogenesis and the level of carcinogenic effect vs. level of free radicals at various stages of carcinogenic process (Valko et al. 2006). Progression is the third and final stage of the carcinogenic process (Klaunig & Kamendulis 2004). This stage involves cellular and molecular changes that occur from the preneoplastic to the neoplastic state. This stage is irreversible and is characterized by accumulation of additional genetic damage, leading to the transition of the cell from

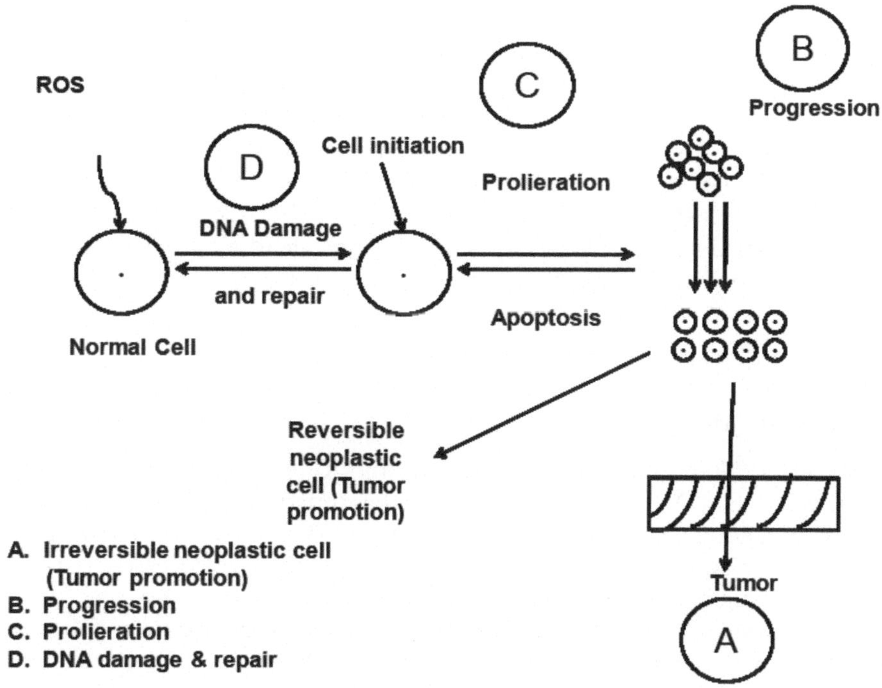

FIGURE 4.5c
Three-stage model of carcinogenesis.

benign to malignant. This stage is characterized by genetic instability and disruption of chromosome integrity. An important step in the growth of any tumor beyond a few millimeters is the generation of new blood supplies that feed the malignant cells (Carmeliet 2000). Angiogenesis is a multi-step process, involving degradation of the endothelial cell basement membrane, endothelial cell migration to the perivascular stroma and capillary sprouting. Previously, the tumor suppressor p53 was understood to regulate the process of angiogenesis through the activation of genes that inhibit neovascularization and the repression of genes that promote vessel growth. The effect of reactive oxygen and nitrogen species is balanced by the antioxidant action of non-enzymatic antioxidants, as well as by antioxidant enzymes. Such antioxidant defenses are extremely important as they represent the direct removal of free radicals (pro-oxidants), thus providing maximal protection for biological sites. Vitamin C (ascorbic acid) is a very important, and powerful, antioxidant that works in aqueous environments of the body, such as is present in the lungs and in the lens of the eye. Its primary antioxidant partners are Vitamin E and the carotenoids, as well as working along with the antioxidant enzymes. Genotoxic agents are usually chemicals that directly damage DNA, which in turn leads to mutation and/or clastogenic changes. A second category of carcinogenic compounds (non-genotoxic) function through non-DNA or indirect-DNA reaction mechanisms is the free radical generation) leading to carcinogenesis (progression) is shown in Figure 4.5a, b, c. This stage involves cellular and molecular changes that occur from the preneoplastic to the neoplastic state. This stage is irreversible and is characterized by accumulation of additional genetic damage, leading to the transition of the cell from benign to malignant.

(k) Role of Calcium and Effect of EMF Exposure

(i) Effects on Metabolism

Lerchl et al. (2008) have shown that chronic RF exposure (383 MHz, 900 MHz, and 1800 MHz) leads to frequency-dependent increase of body weight in Djungarian hamsters at moderate SAR values. These authors have concluded that this is indicative of metabolic processes may be affected by such exposures. It is possible that molecular processes involved with the brain energy metabolism of the rat may be perturbed by the radiation in the microwave frequency region. It has been reported that there are divalent iron atoms and two divalent copper atoms in the molecules of the respiratory chain (Lehninger 1965). Each of these is essential to the function of the respiratory at the molecular level. Charged particles in an electric field undergo translational motion if not otherwise constrained. Such a group of particles would possibly respond to the oscillating electric field having wide range starting from radiofrequency oscillation to the highest value that is limited by natural process to react (Sanders et al. 1984). Nicotinamide adenine dinucleotide (NADH), biochemical assay for adenosine triphosphate (ATP), and creatine phosphate (CP) are key compounds in brain energy metabolism. ATP is a key compound in energy metabolism because it is the carrier of energy to the processes in living cells. NADH oxidized produces ATP in the mitochondria, while brain ATP concentration is maintained at the expense of CP. When demand for ATP is higher than the mitochondrial production capacity, CP is rapidly converted to ATP to sustain its level and significant decrease in CP levels is observed prior to any decrease in ATP. The changes in these compounds are frequency dependent.

Another effect on metabolism of electromagnetic radiation is the leakage of free calcium ions, either through the cell's external membranes or those surrounding internal "calcium stores". This can have dramatic effects on many aspects of metabolism and explains results on stimulation of growth, an increased risk of cancer; symptoms suffered by electrosensitive humans besides several others. Calcium concentrations inside the cell control the rate of many metabolic processes, e.g., the activity of many enzyme systems and the expression of genes. Ca^{2+} ions use special channels to cross the membrane along the concentration gradient. The concentration of calcium ions in the cytosol is normally about a thousand times lower than that outside by metabolically driven ion pumps in its membranes. It is suggested that electromagnetic field stimulation increases membrane leakiness, causing release of unregulated amounts of extra calcium. The actual effects depend on the programmed state of cell at that instant of time, e.g., growth (rate), repair rate after injury or rate of healing be enhanced. On the other hand if there are mutant precancerous cell present, it may also lead to tumor promotion.

(ii) Calcium Release from Cell Membranes

Ca^{+2} are able to bind without causing deformations to either membrane proteins or to soluble proteins of cytoplasm or organelles. They have several ion bonding sites and by changing their configuration as a function of the occupied site, they are capable of exciting a specific target enzyme. Ca^{++} ion has been identified in relaying electrochemical messages to the cell surface thus become the most critical target of microwave exposure (Albert et al. 1987). It is known that Ca^{2+} signaling has extreme sensitivity for coherent excitation by very low-field energies within specific amplitude and frequency windows (Gartzke & Lange 2002). This causes a large electrostatic force generated at the cell surface. The level of the lowest level of exposure could be (0.00015 W/kg, 0.08 μW/cm^2) at 16 Hz modulated, (CW 240 MHz) signal (Schwartz et al. 1990). The mechanism of action of gonadotropin releasing hormone (GnRH) on the anterior pituitary gonadotropin reveals that Ca^{2+} functions as a second messenger in the GnRH-activated signal transduction cascade (Jennes et al. 1995; Haisenleder et al. 2001; Liu et al. 2003).

These ions are known to form bond without causing deformation to either membrane proteins or to soluble proteins of cytoplasm or organelles. Ca^{+2} ions use special channels to cross the membrane along the concentration gradient. These voltage gated channels are normally closed in excitable cells, but they open in response to action potential. This has always remained a question if the cell membrane (calcium ion channel) is directly involved in the electromagnetic field interactions (Liburdy 1992). This is important because the receptor sites and ion channels are located in the cell membrane and are first involved in the signal transduction processes. Also the alterations in the calcium fluxes are propagated down the signal transduction cascade to alter events such as gene activation. Further, changes in calcium ion second messenger are linked to induction of c-myc mRNA, a mid stage signal transduction marker, which in turn travel down the signal transduction cascade to alter gene activation events and cell proliferation.

(I) Electromagnetic Field Exposure and Enzyme Activation Ornithine Decarboxylase (ODC)

ODC is an enzyme essential for cell growth and DNA synthesis. It is rate limiting enzyme in the synthesis of polyamines. Polyamines (putrescine, spermidine, spermine, cadaverine) are long-chain molecules that are positively charged (polycationic). They have the highest charge/mass ratio of any biomolecule. High ODC activity occurs in the unregulated growth of tumor cells, as in the malignancy of prostate cancer (Figure 4.5a).

RF exposure has been shown to induce activity of enzyme ODC, levels of which are often elevated during cell growth and tumor promotion. The exposure of mouse fibroblasts to amplitude modulated microwaves at an SAR of 3 W/kg increased ODC activity (Penafiel et al. 1997), but to a much lower level than treatment with a chemical promoter. Litovitz et al. (1993) have examined the modulation frequency dependence of ODC activity in cultured cells (fibroblast), determining the minimal duration that a single ELF modulation frequency must be sustained (coherence time) in order to elicit an ODC response. Using a 915 MHz field, switching modulation frequencies from 55 to 65 Hz at coherence time of 1 s or less abolished enhancement of ODC responses, while coherence times of 10s or longer produced full enhancement. These microwave coherence effects and pulsed effects are similar to those observed in ELF fields.

In an investigation on murine L929 cell, ODC was activated by AM wave at 845 MHz, though it was not affected by FM at the same frequency (Penafiel et al. 1997). ODC synthesizes polyamines, which promotesthe permeability of superoxide dismutase across animal cell membrane (Podulso & Curran 1996).

(i) Protein Kinase C Activity

PKC plays a key role in a variety of pathologic states including oncogenesis (Nishizuka 1986; Harvey & French 2000) and in mediating cellular responses to extracellular stimuli involved in proliferation, differentiation, apoptosis and exocytotic release in a number of non-neuronal cells (Ohkusu et al. 1986). Several lines of evidence suggest that PKC modulates ion conductance by phosphorylating membrane proteins such as channels, pumps, and ion exchange proteins, besides its role in extrusion of Ca^{2+} immediately after its mobilization into cytosol. The enzyme has also been implicated in phosphorylation of several neuronal proteins, which are thought to regulate neurotransmitter release and long-term potentiation in memory formation (Suzuk 1994).

The activation of this enzyme is thought to be biochemically dependent on Ca^{2+}. Tumor promoting phorbol esters such as 12, O-tetradecanoyl phorbol-13-acetate (TPA) have a structure very similar to diacylglycerol and activate protein kinase C directly, both in vitro and in vivo (Castagna et al. 1982). It has been variously reported that protein kinase C is the receptor of tumor promoters (Parker et al. 1984). Tumor promoters such as phorbol esters increase the affinity of the enzyme for Ca^{2+}, resulting in its full activation at physiological Ca^{2+} concentration. TPA has a specific membrane receptor in the cell membrane (Hunter et al. 1984). In order to stimulate cell proliferation in cells; growth factor and PKC are needed to induce the signal pathways. Byus et al. (1984) reported a decrease in the activity of this enzyme following exposure of human lymphocytes for a period of 15–30 min to 450 MHz amplitude modulated at 16 Hz. Paulraj and Behari (2004) also reported that the activity of this enzyme is affected due to RF exposure.

Gökçek-Saraç et al. (2017) demonstrated molecular effects of acute and chronic exposure to both 900 MHz and 2100 MHz radiofrequency electromagnetic radiation (RF-EMR) on the hippocampal level/activity of some of the enzymes—including PKA, CaMKIIα, CREB, and p44/42 MAPK—from N-methyl-D-aspartate receptor (NMDAR) related signaling pathways. For this purpose rats were divided into following groups: Sham rats, rats exposed to 900 MHz and 2100 MHz RF-EMR for 2 h/day for acute (1 week) or chronic (10 weeks), respectively. The Western Blotting and activity measurement assays were used to assess the activity of the selected enzymes. The obtained results revealed that the hippocampal activity of selected enzymes was significantly higher in chronic groups as compared to acute groups at both 900 MHz and 2100 MHz exposure. In addition, hippocampal activity of selected enzymes was significantly higher at 2100 MHz RF-EMR than 900 MHz RF-EMR in both acute and chronic groups.

The authors concluded that both exposure duration (1 week versus 10 weeks) and different carrier frequencies (900 MHz versus 2100 MHz) had different effects on protein expression of hippocampus in Wistar rats, which may lead to further investigation on strategy for protection against RF-EMR exposure. Panagopoulous et al. (2007) working with Drosophila reported that between GSM (global system for mobile telecommunication) 900 MHz and DCS (digital cellular system) 1800 MHz, the former is more bioactive than the latter and attributed this to the higher field intensity of the GSM system.

(m) Genotoxic Effects

The microwave photon energy of RF radiation (10^{-3}–10^{-6} eV) is much less than the energy required to break the chemical bonds (hydrogen bands ~0.5 ev) and therefore it is was believed that these radiations do not cause any damage to hydrogen bonded structures and hence to DNA. Stronati et al. (2006) have used several standard *in vitro* tests for chromosomal and DNA damage in Go human lymphocytes exposed *in vitro* to a combination of x-rays and RFR. They have examined if a 24-h continuous exposure to a 935 MHz GSM basic signal (SAR of 1 or 2 W/Kg) is genotoxic *per se* or whether, it can influence the genotoxicity of the well-established clastogenic agent; x-radiation. Within the experimental parameters of the study in all instances no effect from the RFR signal was observed. However, it is possible that certain cell (Leal et al. 2000) and cellular constituents are altered by exposure to EMF, such as free radicals.

Free radicals (reactive oxygen species: ROS) have turned out to be a key parameter producing DNA damage. These are able to interact with DNA or other cellular components and are involved in cell regulatory processes. This phenomenon extends over a broad range of microwave portion of nonionizing electromagnetic radiations as reported earlier (Behari 2009a). Some of the characteristics of resonant behavior of microwave radiations are (Binhi 2002):

(I) The resonance response of biological systems to nonthermal (<1 mW/cm^2), the resonant line width being 10^{-2}–10^{-3} of peak frequency.

(II) The resonant behavior of system response as a function of modulation frequency of the microwave carrier.

(III) A weak dependence of the effect on the radiation intensity, often beyond a threshold power.

(IV) Physiological windows of the effect and sensitivity of spectra to the type of biological system and its physiological state.

From the above it is obvious that with the rapid use of high-frequency electromagnetic fields like mobile phones has in it an inherent global concerns about the negative health effects of its use, and possibility of an adaptive response is the ability of a cell or tissue to better resist stress damage by prior exposure to a lesser amount of stress. This study aimed to assess whether radiofrequency radiation can induce adaptive response by changing the antioxidant balance.

In order to assess RF-induced adaptive response in tissues, the level of GSH and the activity of GR were evaluated in liver. 50 rats were divided into 5 groups. Three groups were pre-exposed to 915 MHz RF radiation, 4 hours per day for one week at different powers, as low, medium and high. 24 hours after the last exposure to radiation, they were exposed to 4 Gy sublethal dose of gamma radiation and then sacrificed after 5 hours. Their livers were removed, washed and were kept at –80°C until used.

The results showed that pre-exposure to 915 MHz radiofrequency radiation with specific power could induce adaptive response in liver by inducing changes in the activity and level of antioxidant enzymes. It was concluded that pre-exposure to microwave radiation could increase the level of GSH and the activity of GR enzyme, although these increases were seen just in low power group, and the GR activity was indicated in medium power group. This increase protects tissue from oxidative damage induced by sublethal dose of gamma radiation.

This rearrangement of DNA has been further tested for both CW and pulsed microwave fields, using a fluorescence microscopy technique capable of detecting 1 break per 2×10^{10} daltons of DNA (Lai & Singh 1995). Immediately after a 2h exposure to pulsed microwaves (2.45 GHz, pulse width 2 μs, pulse repetition frequency 500/s), no effects were noted, but a dose rate-dependent increase in DNA single-strand breaks (0.6 vs. 1.2 W/kg whole body SAR) was found in rat brain cells at 4h post-exposure. By contrast, in rats exposed to 2.45 GHz CW fields for 2h (SAR 1.2 W/kg), increased single-strand breaks immediately, as well as at 4h post-exposure.

(n) The Effect of EMR on Cell Cycle Regulatory Factors in the Nucleus

There are key molecules that control the transition of the cell cycle from G2 to M phase. Histone kinase is an essential molecule that exerts its effect through phosphorylation and dephosphorylation of histones. During metaphase of both meiosis and mitosis, histones in the condensed chromatin are heavily phosphorylated and then dephosphorylation takes place after the anaphase and separation of the chromosomes. Histone kinase has a Cdc2 catalytic subunit which must bind with cyclin B to form a maturation promoting factor (MAP) (Gautier & Maller 1991). MAP promotes the entrance into mitosis from the G2 phase by phosphorylating multiple proteins, including histones. In highly proliferative cells such as sperm, the decreased activity of histone kinase is associated with defective progression in cell cycle and defective spermatogenesis. Kesari et al. (2011) have shown a statistically significant decrease in mean activity of histone kinase in sperm of rats post EMR radiation (SAR 0.9 W/kg), as compared to the control. This decline may also indicate a decrease in G2/M phase transition activity and decrease rate of proliferation.

(o) Fertility Pattern

In a bid to understand the effect of EMF exposure on humans, it is first to target the central nervous system and consequently their subsequent effect on reproductive system (Figure 4.7a, b). The information is then transferred by chemical messenger to other system. In pursuance of this a number of efforts have been made since about last four decades to investigate this aspect. This has been broadly divided into two parts: one concerning extremely low frequency (ELF) electromagnetic fields (EMFs) and second radiofrequency and microwave fields. The biological ELF effects are often found an overlap with RF modulated signals for ease to transfer information to the bio systems.

Sage et al. (2007) reported that personal and occupational use of personal digital assistants (PDAs or palm held wireless units) produce high intensity bursts of ELF-EMF exposure in persons that carry a PDA close to the body (i.e., in a pocket or in a belt); or held to the head for cell phone conversations. ELF-EMF emissions of 10μT were recorded on PDAs during normal office use over a 24 h test period. Results of ELF-EMF measurements show that transmit and receive functions produce rapid, short duration ELF-EMF spikes in the 2-10μT range, each lasting several seconds to over a minute, depending on the down load size. Switching the PDAs produced continuously elevated ELF-EMF pulses of over 90 μT on two units. Thus the user who wears the PDA may be receiving high-intensity ELF-EMF pulses throughout the day and night.

Any agent which effects the sperm motility or morphology (Ozguner et al. 2005; Forgacs et al. 2006) has potentiality of having a negative impact on male fertility. Since a good amount of data have accumulated indicating adverse effect of microwave radiations on sperms, there has also been a debate, if exposure to radio-frequency electromagnetic fields is associated with an elevated risk on reproduction. Radio waves from mobile phones may have their effect at the process of spermatogenesis. According to one study, lifestyle can decrease semen quality (Kilgalton & Simmons 2005) and prolonged use of cell phones has negative effects on sperm motility characteristics (Fejes et al. 2005). It has been shown that sperm DNA damage is not repaired, because of chromatin structure (Singh & Stephenes 1998).

Reactive oxygen species (ROS) such as superoxide anions (O^-), hydroxyl radicals (OH^-) and hydrogen peroxide (H_2O_2) may influence the structural integrity and function of sperm, such as motility, capacitation, and sperm-oocyte fusion (Griveau et al. 1995; Figure 4.5b). Spermatozoa are particularly vulnerable to oxidative stress because their plasma membrane is rich in polyunsaturated fatty acids (PUFAS) and membrane bound NADPH oxidase. ROS has been shown to correlate with reduced male fertility (Iwasaki & Gagon 1992), cause perioxidative damage to the sperm plasma membrane (Hughes et al. 1996), and induce both DNA strand breakages and oxidative base damage in human sperm (Kodama et al. 1997). A decrease in total antioxidant capacity of seminal plasma has been correlated with a reduction in sperm quality, such as concentration, motility and morphology (Smith et al. 1996).

The issue that biologic effects of RF radiations are genotoxic is still not fully resolved, though some of the available results indicate such a possibility. Some in vitro data show effects that are negative while others show these are positive, at field levels close to the guidelines levels for safe exposure.

(i) Effect on Sperm and Fertility

Several group of workers have replicated studies showing adverse effects on sperm quality, motility and pathology in men who use a cell phone, PDA (personal digital assistant) or pager on their belt or in a pocket (Aitkin et al. 2005; Wdowiak et al. 2007; Agarwal et al. 2009), with similar data on male rats (Kesari & Behari 2008; Kesari et al. 2011). Other studies conclude that usage of cell phone radiation, or storage of a mobile phone close to the testes of human males affect sperm counts, motility, viability and structure (Erogul et al. 2006; Yan et al. 2007; Agarwal et al. 2008). Animal studies have demonstrated oxidative and DNA damage, pathological changes in testes of animals, decreased sperm mobility and viability, and other measures of deleterious damage to the male germ line (Yan et al. 2007; Otitoloju et al. 2010; Salama et al. 2010). Agarwal et al. (2009) reported that cell phone radiations may lead to oxidative stress in human semen. These authors concluded that the cell phone kept in a trouser pocket in talk mode may negatively effect spermatozoa and impair male fertility. Avendano et al. (2012) provided evidence that a 4-hour exposure to WI-FI at exceedingly low levels (0.5–1.0 $\mu W/cm^2$) near a lap top computer caused decreased sperm viability and DNA fragmentation in human sperm samples. These authors have pointed out that exposure of human spermatozoa to a wireless internet-connected laptop decreased motility and induced DNA fragmentation by a nonthermal effect. They further speculated that keeping a laptop connected wirelessly to the internet on the lap near the testes may result in decreased male fertility. De Luliis et al. (2009) reported that RF-EMR in both the power density and frequency range of mobile phones enhances mitochondrial reactive oxygen species generation by human spermatozoa, decreasing the motility and vitality of these cells and leading to DNA fragmentation. They further mentioned that their findings have clear implications for the safety of extensive mobile phone use by males of reproductive age, potentially affecting both their fertility and the health and the well being of the offspring. This is based on damage from a 6-h exposure to 1800 MHz cell phone radiation in human sperm cells, causing reduced sperm motility and viability and also causing a significant increase in reactive oxygen species. The effects were worse with more exposure. Otitoloju et al. (2010) described sperm head abnormalities in mice exposed for six months to base-station level RF/MW at 70 to 100×10^{-9} W/cm^2: 39%–46% of exposed mice had damaged sperm, while only 2% of controls. The major abnormalities were knobbed hook, pin-head and banana shaped sperm head. The sperm head abnormalities were found to be dose dependent. These studies provide an indication that use of cell phone use is injurious to health. This further support the notion that much lower exposure levels associated with mobile phone base station (cell tower) RFR levels are deleterious, when over a over a period of time.

(p) Fetal Development Studies

Effect on the developing fetus from in-utero exposure to cell phone radiation has been observed in both human and animal studies since 2006. Divan et al. (2008) found that children born of mothers who used cell phones during pregnancy develop more behavioral problems by their reaching school age than children whose mother did not use cell phone during pregnancy. Children whose mother used cell phone during pregnancy had 25% more emotional problems, 35% more hyperactivity, 49% more conduct problems, and 34% more peer problems.

Sources of fetal and neonatal exposures of concern include cell phone radiation (both paternal use of wireless devices worn on the body and maternal use of wireless phones during pregnancy). Exposure to whole body RFR from base stations and WI-FI, use of wireless lap tops, use of incubators for newborns with excessively high ELF-EMF levels resulting in altered heart rate variability and reduced melatonin levels in newborns, fetal exposure to MRI of the pregnant mother, and greater susceptibility and asthma in the child where there have been maternal exposures to ELF-EMF.

Animal studies were conducted by Jensh et al. (1982) radiated pregnant Wistar albino rats at a power density level of 10 mW/cm^2, at a frequency of 915 MHz (average SAR 3.57 W/kg). The animals were exposed for 6 h/day from day 1 to day 21of gestation. No significant teratogenic signs were observed regarding the resorption rate, malformation rate, mean litter size, fetal weight and number of live and dead fetuses. The experiment was extended to include embryonic and postnatal development of offspring. The authors reported no significant morphologic changes.

In another study Berman et al. (1992) exposed (970 MHz, 22 h/day) pregnant rats (1st to 19th day). The SAR varied from 0.07, 2.4, and 4.8 W/kg. The embryo motility, fetal weight, skeletal ossification, as well as maternal fertility were evaluated. The exposure due to (4.8 W/kg) of these caused reduced (~ 12%). fetal body weight versus the control. All the other examined parameters were not significantly different. Klug et al. (1997) exposed rat embryos (9.5 days old) for up to 36 h at 900 MHz. The modulation frequency was fixed at 215 Hz and the SAR values were calculated as 0.2, 1, and 5 W/kg. The biomarkers chosen were crown-rump length, number of somites as well as embryonic malformation parameters of the embryos.

Grigoryev (2003) exposed chicken embryos to EMF from GSM Mobile phone during the embryonic development. The embryo mortality rate in the incubation period increased to 75% versus 16% in control group.

Ingole and Ghosh (2006) studied the developmental effects on the avian kidney of radiation from a cell phone handset (900 MHz frequency, power of 2W and SAR of 0.37 W/kg). The authors reported morphological alterations on the epithelium of the renal tubules as well as the renal corpuscles and chicken embryos. Margas and Xenos (1997) reported RF induced changes in the prenatal development of mice. A progressive decrease in the number of newborns per dam was observed, which ended in irreversible infertility. The prenatal development of the newborns, however, evaluated by the crown-rump length, the body weight, and the number of the lumbar, sacral, and coccygeal vertebrae, was improved.

On the other hand Kumlin et al. (2007) have reported no effect. They studied the development of the nervous system of Wistar rats due to exposure of 900 MHz radiation (2 h/day, 5 days per week).

It can be inferred that that in totality the effects is adverse, though the quantum of effect may be varying.

4.8 Non-Genotoxic Effects

Several studies reported the effect of RF fields on cell cycle kinetics, but in the majority of the investigations no effects were detected (Higashikubo et al. 2001; Pickard et al. 2001; Zeni et al. 2003; Miyakoshi et al. 2005; Lantow et al. 2006c). Alteration in cell proliferation was described only in a few reports (Pacini et al. 2002; Capri et al. 2004, 2004a).

Apoptosis is an important mechanism of protection against cancer. Several reports have reported that RF field effects on human peripheral blood mononuclear cells (Capri et al. 2004), lymphoblastoid cells (Marinelli et al. 2004), epidermis cancer cells (Caraglia et al. 2005), human Mono Mac 6 cells (Lantow et al. 2006c) and in Molts4 cells (Hook et al. 2004). No difference in apoptosis induction was detected between sham exposed and RF field exposed cells. On the other hand, Marinelli et al. (2004) have reported better survival rate of T lymphoblastoid leukemia cells exposed to 900 MHz non-modulated RF fields. Caraglia et al. (2005) found apoptosis induction in human epidermoid cancer cells after exposure to 1.95 GHz fields. Nikolova et al. (2005) described modulation in gene regulation after RF field exposure at a SAR of 1.5 W/kg in p53-deficient embryonic stem cells. Proteomic analyses of human endothelial cell lines showed RF fields induced changes in this expression and phosphorylation state of numerous proteins including the hsp27. However, these authors reported no effects of RF fields on cell cycle, cell proliferation, cell differentiation, apoptosis induction, DNA synthesis and immune cell functionality.

Analysis on whole genome cDNA arrays show alterations in gene expression after various RF exposure conditions using different cell types, but no consistent RF-signature such as stress response could be identified (Remondini et al. 2006).

Heat shock proteins act primarily as molecular chaperones to eliminate unfolded proteins, which can also appear from cellular stress. This stress response can be induced by many different external factors, including temperature, chemicals, oxidative stress, heavy metals, ionizing and non-ionizing radiation and ultrafine carbon black particles. Hsp70 has been shown to interfere with post mitochondrial events to prevent free radical mediated apoptosis (Gotoh et al. 2001). An increased expression level of

Hsp70 can thus offer protection against stress. Heat shock proteins are also involved in oncogenic processes (Inoue et al. 1999; Jolly & Morimoto 2000; French et al. 2001). Some investigators have described increased heat shock protein level after RF exposure (Kwee et al. 2001; Leszczynski et al. 2002; De Polimeri et al. 2003). However, these results are controversial, because there are negative findings also (Cotgreave 2005). It may be that data on Hsp70 awaits further confirmation, at different frequencies, wave forms and power levels.

4.9 Effect on Hearing

Particular interest has also been expressed, in the biological effects of pulsed-modulated RF and microwaves on ear. Human ear can perceive pulse modulated radiation between 200 MHz and 6.5 GHz as a buzzing or clicking noise, depending on modulation characteristics. The effect is attributed to the thermoelastic expansion of the brain tissue, following the small ($\ll$ 1°C) but rapid increase in temperature on the absorption of the incident energy, generating a sound wave in the head that is detected by the hair cells (cochlea) (Sienkiewicz et al. 2005). However, its clinical potential is yet to be fully utilized.

4.10 Weak NonthermalInteractions

It is quite often a matter of concern as to under the mechanism of weak nonthermal mechanism by which biological system could react to low intensity microwave fields. It requires fields of the order of a few kV/cm to orient long biopolymers, and probably still higher fields to excite internal vibrations or produce submolecular orientation. External fields acting on biopolymers should be able to overcome strong local fields. Transmembrane potentials induced by nonthermal microwave fields are vanishingly small relative to potentials required for stimulation and compare with membrane noise. Field induced force effects are unlikely to be significant on a single molecular or cellular level, since the threshold field strengths necessary to overcome thermal disturbances are too high (Schwan 1977). Field force effects become more probable as the volume of the exposed particle increases. Transmembrane potentials becomes larger for a given in situ field strength as the cell size is increased. Finally molecules can become significantly reoriented by the field if $\mu E \geq kT$, (where μ is the dipole moment, E is the field strength, k is the Boltzmann constant, and T is the absolute temperature). Thus larger permanent or induced dipole moment is more likely to respond to weak fields. But these very factors tend to limit responses to low frequencies for these interaction mechanisms. The large dimensions necessary for biological responses to weak microwave fields might be achieved by cooperative reaction of a number of cells or macromolecules to the microwave stimulus, which increases the effective size of the structure and correspondingly reduces the threshold that is required for an effect. It has been suggested that such cooperativity might be induced in the counter ions loosely bound near membrane surfaces which contain a loose framework of charged polysaccharides (Frohlich 1973; Bawin & Adey 1976).

4.11 Mechanism of Energy Transfer and Amplification

(a) Macromolecular Resonance

The electromagnetic field effects in biology and their variability is suggestive of the possibility of occurrence of resonance effects. So far resonance conditions are characterized in terms of narrow "windows", of frequency and amplitude ranges only (Blackman et al. 1979).

There are two broad situations, when perturbations are very short and when large in comparison with the field period. In the former case, every collision is quite effective in interrupting the molecule's radiation absorption emission process. In a fluid with a large rate of collision a coalitional broadened relaxation type spectrum results. In the later case, collisions for long duration compared to the EMF period, the spectrum becomes resonant. The collision time in a macromolecular fluid is a function of temperature, and therefore the EMF frequency determines the kind of spectrum (rotational or resonant). Water is a broad band attenuator of MW fields, which also shields other possible bimolecular absorption processes. Experiments suggest resonant absorption in growing cells at 41 GHz fields and in DNA at 11 GHz (Grundler et al. 1977; Azanza & Moral 1994). However the significance of these resonance frequencies in biological systems is yet to be established.

The nonthermal, pulsed microwave effects are connected with the transfer of information from irradiating field to the alive organism, through the latter's ability to identify certain frequency of radiation, with its ability to absorb energy from the field (Hyland 2001). The intensity of radiation needed for this recognition is many orders of magnitude below that, currently associated with nonthermal effect.

(b) Stochastic Resonance

Fields millions of times weaker than the membrane potential gradient of 10^7V/m modulate cell processes to surface stimulating molecules. This may underline the ability of biological systems to amplify small signals by extracting energy from the noise in the system (Bezrukov & Vodyanoy 1995). Viewed in this manner; it is possible to imagine an information processing system in which the presence of an on-going noise activity enhances information handling capacity. Low level effects are attributed to the direct interaction between neuron membranes and the local electric fields. A power level of 0.1 mW/cm^2 and 1 mW/cm^2 corresponds to free space values of 61V/m and 194 V/m respectively. This field is negligible as compared to static transmembrane potential of ~ 90 mV (~10^7 V/m) across a membrane of thickness of 4 nm. However, this is larger than the field due to slow brain wave (1 V/m) or from terrestrial field (10^{-3}–10^{-6} V/m) (Figure 4.6).

(c) Cell Surface Glycoproteins as a Possible Site for EM Field Interactions

Cells in tissue are separated by narrow fluid channels, typically not more than 150 A° wide, acting as windows on the electrochemical world surrounding each cell. These channels are preferred pathways for intrinsic and environmental electromagnetic field in tissue, since they offer much lower electrical impedance than cell membranes. Functional measures of brain electrical impedance are thus an index of conductance in this extracellular space and have been correlated with brain tissue physiological states in health and disease (Adey et al. 1963, 1965; Porter et al. 1965). These intercellular channels are also the site of electrochemical sensors that protrude as protein strands from within the cell membrane. They form a strongly negatively charged glycocalyx on the cell surface. They act as specific receptors for hormones, antibodies, neurotransmitter molecules, certain chemical cancer promoters and may be EMF signal. Their amplified signal to the cell interior elicits enzymatic responses regulating metabolism, messenger functions and cell growth. McConnell (1975) noted that intrusion of the phospholipid tails is constrained and they behave more rigidly.

It is now established that Cell Ca^{2+} signaling has extreme sensitivity for coherent excitation by very field energies within specific amplitude and frequency windows (Schwartz et al. 1990). Membranes are identified as sharply partitioning each cell from its neighbor, by reason of their high content of fat molecules (phospholipids). Its structure is identified as double layer of phospholipid molecules, the plasma membrane. The cell membrane is thus a physical and an electric barrier. Since generally accepted physiological findings have revealed sensitivities to induced tissue electric gradients from ELF environmental fields and from ELF-modulated fields. To explain the possibility of an extremely small signal to be effective it is postulated that power amplification mechanisms are operative in transductive coupling of these weak stimuli from fluid surrounding cells to the cell interior.

In search for a general mechanism of interaction of EM field with cells, Na^+ -K^+ ATPase, the "ion pump" enzyme in cell membrane has been

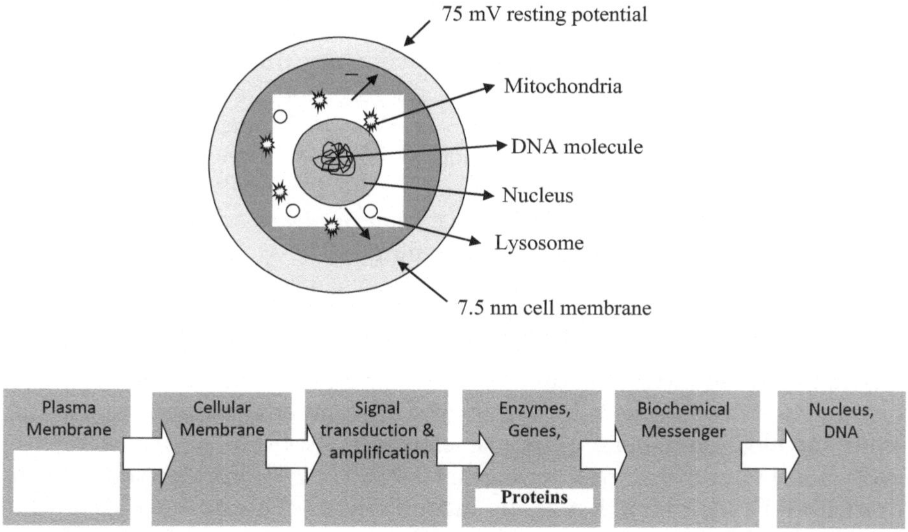

Co-operativism

+

Non linearity

+

Non-equilibrium thermodynamic Behaviour

↓

Amplifying effect of the Extremely Weak applied EMF

↓

Transmembrane coupling of the signal to the cytoplasm
(Solitonwaves may be responsible for such coupling)

FIGURE 4.6
An idealized excitable cell at rest in the human body.75mV across a thickness of 7.5 nm corresponds to an electric field of ten million Vm^{-1}.

studied by various groups (Blank 1992; Blank & Soo 1992; Behari et al. 1998). Changes in enzyme activity in either electric or magnetic fields show that the most important factor affecting signal transduction is the level of enzyme activation, the maximum biological (ATP-splitting) activity of the enzyme under a given set of conditions (i.e., ion concentration, temperature). Enzyme function involves communication between ATP-splitting catalytic sites and ion-binding sites in different parts of the molecule in a coordinated sequence and ion-binding sites in enzyme is essential and is probably brought about by charge movements during function. Such movements have been observed in the microsecond range. Ion fluxes via effects on ion pumps such as Na^+K^+ ATPase in human red blood cells exposed to RF and microwave radiation (Allis & Sinha-Robinson 1987; Christiansen 1989; Liu et al. 1990). These authors pointed out dependence of the optical properties on membrane excitation. Dark soliton propagation may be a means of transmembrane signaling.

(d) Stress Protein as a Fractal Antenna for RFR

EMF falling on to the biological target penetrates cell unattenuated and can directly interact with the cell nucleus and with other cell constituents. The ability of electromagnetic response elements (EMREs) to interact with EMF, after being transferred to another DNA chain, is further support for direct EMF-DNA interaction as the most likely mechanism for EMF initiation of the cellular stress response. The given structure makes DNA particularly vulnerable to EMF damage. It is possible for many EMF frequencies present in the environment causing this damage. The cellular response caused by the EMF-activated cellular stress response is an effective protective mechanism for cells exposed to a wide range of EMF frequencies. EMF stimulates stress proteins (impact on the cells). This amounts to stating that EMF efficiently harms cells at a billion times lower levels (nonthermal) than conventional heating (thermal effect).

In contrast to EMF, most biological agents are impeded by the membranes and require special mechanisms to enter the cell interior (Friedman et al. 2007). These authors have demonstrated that, in these scenarios, the initial step in transmitting extracellular information from the plasma membrane to the nucleus of the cell occurs when NADH oxidase rapidly generates reactive oxygen species (ROS). These ROS stimulate matrix metalloproteinases that allow them to cleave and release heparin binding epidermal growth factor. This secreted factor activates the epidermal growth receptor, which in turn activates the extracellular signal regulated kinase cascade. The ERK cascade is one of the four mitogen-activated protein kinase (MAPK) signaling cascades that regulate transcriptional activity in response to extracellular stimuli.

4.12 Biomarkers of Tumor Promotion

Animal studies have demonstrated that microwaves and radiofrequency fields can be called co-carcinogenic since they increase chemically induced skin cancer (Szmigielski et al. 1982). Cellular studies have verified that these carcinogenic effects are mediated by DNA since relatively weak fields increase DNA synthesis (Liboff et al. 1984) and can modulate DNA repair (Meltz et al. 1987). Some studies have also demonstrated that electric fields could break or nick DNA strands (Tamiya et al. 1988), and the change in secondary structure (conformation) of DNA, phenomena associated with cancer (Kitchin et al. 1989). It may be mentioned that these field emissions are largely at low EM field strengths.

Intracellular processes occurring under the influence of power line magnetic field related to free radicals and signal transmission may determine its biological effects. An uncontrolled oxygen radical release (oxidative stress), may cause protein oxidation, enzyme inactivation and lipid peroxidation, within the cellular membranes, causing structural and functional abnormalities. Superoxide dismutase (SOD) plays a key role in the system protecting the body from destructive free-radical activity. A decrease in SOD and Glutathione peroxidase activity while an increase in catalase (CAT) activity has been reported in powerline frequency generated magnetic field (Kula et al. 2002) and in radiofrequency field exposure alike (Kumar et al. 2011). It is possible that magnetic fields interact with the free radicals formed, rather than inducing them.

It can be concluded that there are various indicators of tumor promotion, due to electromagnetic field exposure. Following are some, but not limited to these:

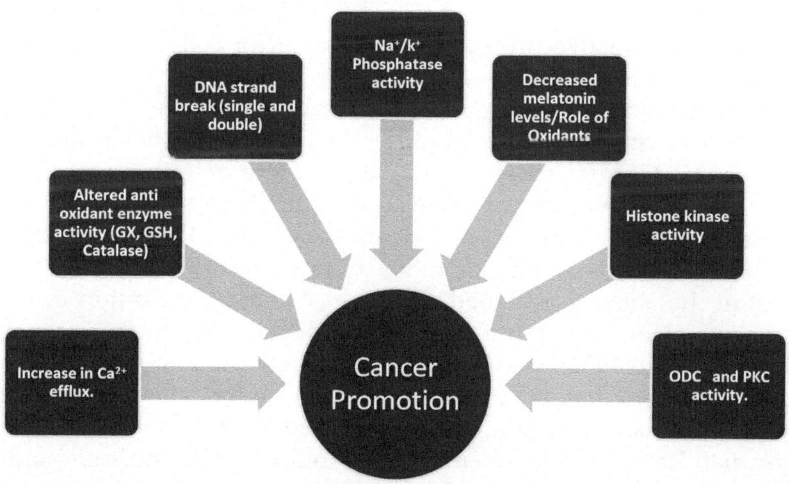

Cancer promotion (Stress Development/RF/MW Syndrome)/Effecting central nervous system and other parameters. Cancers are believed to be the long term result of the errors in DNA that occur during the normal functioning of cells. Living cells are continually growing (making protein) and errors in synthesis occur. The error rate is very small but finite, so the vast majority of errors are repaired but some still remains. When the error rate is too high, the cell activates apoptosis and destroys itself. When small number of errors remains they lead to mutation, some of which affect its function. Tumor may lead to tumor suppressor gene or a DNA repair gene and enables creation of oncogene, which accelerates the development of cancer. Although damage can occur during protein synthesis and cell division, as well as upon exposure to oxidizing chemicals, the probability of developing cancer is increased as a result of damage to DNA structure caused by exposure to EMF (Verschaeve 2008, 2014). The interconnection between stress and brain connectivity (or coherence) in ASDs is brought about by Narayanan et al. (2010). They tested the impact of the beta blocker propranolol on brain functional connectivity measured using functional MRI. An increase in functional connectivity was noted from propranolol-but not from nadolol which has the same vascular effects but does not cross the BBB. Propranolol decreases the burden of norepinephrine, thereby reducing the impact of stress systems on brain processing, and this creates an improvement in the signal to noise ratio of brain signals (Wallenstein & Hasselmo 1997), allowing it to utilize and coordinate more remote parts of its networks. This suggests that stressors such as EMF/RFR, act by adding non-biologically meaningful noise to the system, might have the opposite effects, degrading coherent integration.

Combined effect of one or all of these parameters causes the development of stress, which is the end result. The EMF-activated cellular stress response is an effective protective mechanism for cells exposed to a wide range of EMF frequencies.

Proteins are important components of cells and make about 50% of the dry weight of most cells. Many different types of proteins are classified according to their functions, and stress proteins are now considered recognized as a new class of proteins with function related to cell protection. Cellular stress proteins are synthesized when cells come in contact with stimuli that cause damage to macromolecules (Kultz 2005).

Most of the above mentioned effects are having their origin in nonthermal effects. However these effects are dependent upon a number of physical and biological parameters, which also become relevant in determining the criteria for safe exposure. A unifying formulation for a possible biological mechanism to account for very weak EMF bioeffects other than cancer may lie with field interactions of pulsed RFR and ELF-modulated RFR as disrupters of synchronized neural activity. Electrical rhythms in our brain can be influenced by external signals. This is consistent with established weak field effect on coupled biological oscillators in living tissues. Biological system of heart, brain and gut are dependent on the cooperative actions of cells that function according to principles of nonlinear, coupled biological oscillations for synchrony (Strogatz 2003; Buzsaki

2006). The key to synchronization is the joint actions of the cells that cooperate electrically linking population of biological oscillators that couple together in large arrays and synchronize spontaneously. Synchronous biological oscillations in cells (pacemaker cells) can be disrupted by artificial, exogenous environmental signals, resulting in desynchronization of neural activity that regulates critical functions in the brain, gut and heart and circadian rhythms governing sleep and hormone cycles (Strogatz 1987). The brain contains a population of oscillators with distributed natural frequencies, which pull one another into synchrony. Rhythms can be altered with wide variety of agents and that these perturbations must seriously alter brain performance (Buzsaki 2006).

Organisms are continually driven by internal (generated by specialized cellular clocks within the organism) and external driving from the environment. The example of the former is the cardiac pacemaker located at the sinoatrial node in the mammalian hearts and the circadian clock residing at the suprachiasmatic nuclei in mammalian brains. These rhythms are composed of thousands of clock cells that are intrinsically diverse that nevertheless manage to function in a coherent oscillatory state. This is the case for the circadian oscillations exhibited by the suprachiasmatic nuclei, the period of which is determined by the individual neurons making the circadian clock (Strogatz 2003).

4.13 Oxidative Stress: Cell Signaling

Cell communicates with each other and responds to extracellular stimuli through cell signaling (signal transduction) is a well-established biological mechanism. Signal transduction is a process enabling information to be transmitted from the outside of a cell to various functional elements inside the cell. Signal transduction is triggered by extracellular signals (hormones, growth factors, cytokines and neurotransmitters). Signals sent to the transcription machinery are responsible for expression of certain genes that are normally transmitted to the cell nucleus by a class of proteins called transcription factors. Because ROS act as oxidants by nature, they influence the redox status and may, according to their concentration, cause either cell proliferation, or cause growth arrest or cell death or even necrosis (Sharma et al. 1999). The effects of ROS on cell proliferation occur exclusively at low or transient concentration of radicals. Low concentration of superoxide radical and hydrogen peroxide in fact stimulate proliferation and enhanced survival in a variety of cell types. ROS can thus play a very important physiological role as secondary messengers.

The hydroxyl radical is highly reactive and immediately removes electrons from any molecule in its path, turning that molecule into a free radical and thus propagating a chain reaction. However, hydrogen peroxide is actually more damaging to DNA than the hydroxyl radical, since the lower reactivity of hydrogen peroxide provides enough time for the molecule to travel into the nucleus of the cell, subsequently reacting with macromolecules such as DNA.

In leukocytes, physiological activation is associated with the onset of phagocytosis and leads to increased formation of reactive oxygen species (ROS). These cells exert a wide variety of functions including the regulation of the immune response (pro and anti inflammatory processes), scavenging of senescent cells, and phagocytosis of infected or malignant cells, wound healing, repair and detoxification. The generation of free radicals enhances important physiological processes, e.g., signal transduction processes of various membrane receptors and further immunological functions. An imbalance between excessive formation of reactive oxygen species and the limited antioxidant defense system may take place. However, several authors (Lantow et al. 2006a, 2006b) reported no increase in free radical level.

ROS are produced intracellularly through multiple mechanisms and depending on the cell and tissue types, the major sources being the regular producers of ROS: NADPH oxidase (NOX) complexes in cell membranes. One of these, i.e., mitochondria converts energy for the cell into a usable form, adenosine triphosphate (ATP). The process by which ATP is produced, called oxidative phosphorylation involves the transport of protons (hydrogen ions) across the inner mitochondrial membrane by means of the electron transport chain (Hall et al. 1996). If too much damage is done to mitochondria, a cell undergoes apoptosis (programmed cell death). The cellular stress response is a specific response of individual cells, and stress proteins are the chemical agents that also serve as markers of the magnitude of the external agent.

4.14 Multifold EMR Behavior

It is quite intriguing that the mode of EMF interaction with biological system is not simple but multifold. There is ample of evidence that low level electromagnetic fields causes DNA strand break in brain cells and sperm. An application of a low level pulsed electromagnetic field on induced fracture and induced osteoporosis in rats causes an accelerated healing in rat bones *(Behari 2009a) and in decelerating osteoporosis (Behari & Lochan 2003; Jayanand and Behari 2009a).*

Some other investigations (Prakash & Behari 2009a) reveals that synergistic effect of nanoparticles and pulsed electromagnetic can prevent the microgravity induced osteoporosis. This is evidenced by an increase in bone mineral content, bone mineral density and morphological changes. Results indicate that the extremely low frequency field components of the clinical PEMF signals are far more capable of stimulating bone remodeling activity than higher frequency components. This is because the pulsed signals carry multiplicity of messages to the biological systems as compared to continuous ones. This in contrast to other low level EMF effects

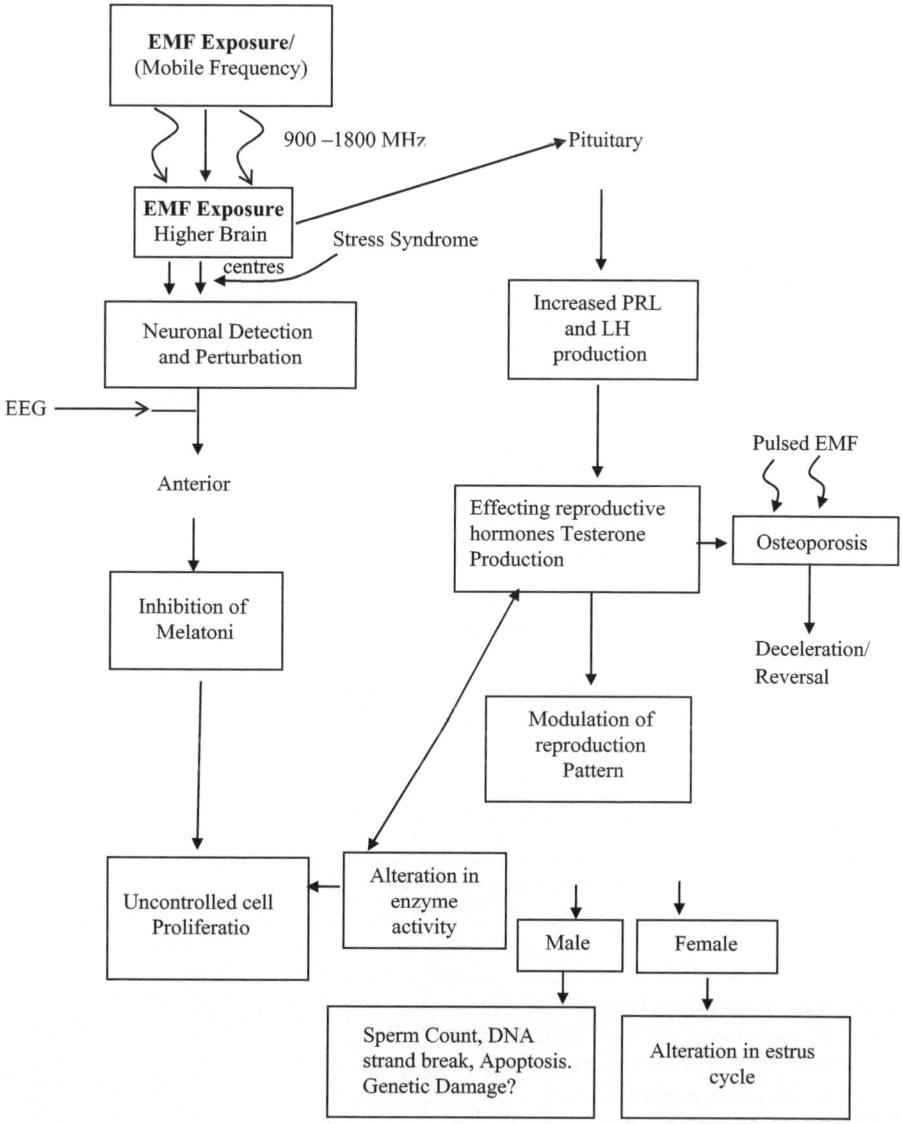

FIGURE 4.7a
Proposed model of EMF exposure, which influences brain cells and promotes the growth of initiated tumor cells, osteoporosis, and reproduction pattern.

which are often implicated in tumor promotion. In contrast to high power, the use of weak electromagnetic fields to study the sequences and energetic of events that couple humoral stimuli from surface receptor sites to the cell interior has identified cell membranes as a primary site of interaction with these low frequency fields in the pericellular fluid. A summary of mode of EMF-biointeraction is summarized in Figure 4.7 a,b.

Long-term biological consequences of repeated microwave irradiation depend on the parameters of irradiation. Experiments have shown that after repeated microwave exposure changes in cholinergic receptors also depend on the endogenous signals in the brain. The microwave effects could be blocked by pretreatment, with narcotic antagonist naltrexone before each session of daily exposure. It is apparent from these results that endogenous opioids may play a mediating role in some of the neurological effects of microwaves (Lai 1992). The microwave effects can be summarized as follows (1) microwaves enhanced morphine induced catalepsy in the rat (2) narcotic antagonist can block a transient increase in body temperature after microwave exposure; (3) the effect of acute

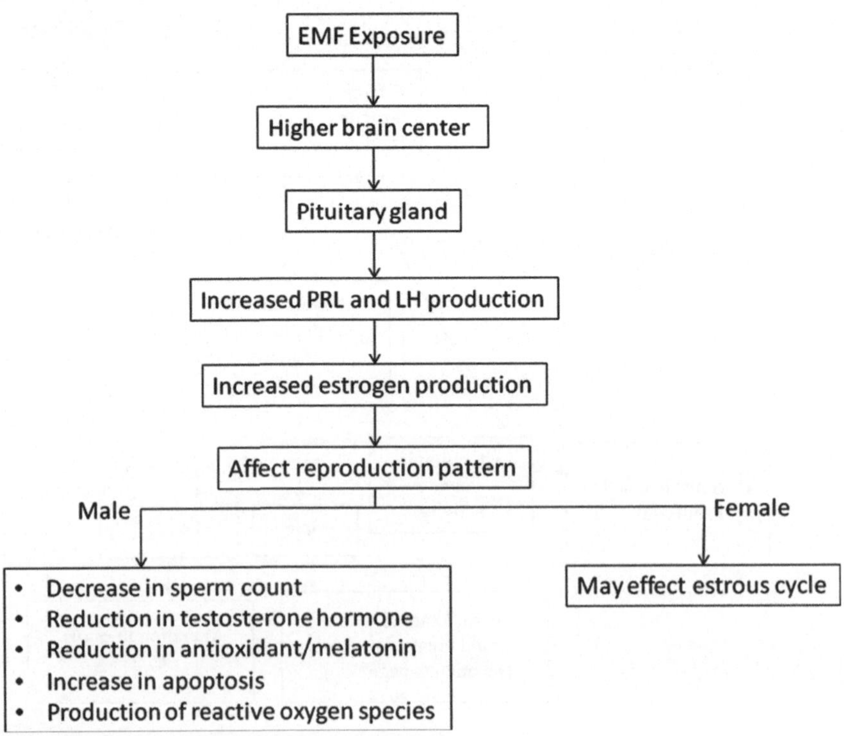

FIGURE 4.7b
Mode of EMF-CNS-reproduction axis exemplified.

microwave exposure on amphetamine-induced hyperthermia; (4) microwave induced changes in high affinity muscarinic cholinergic receptors in the brain after repeated sessions of microwave exposure can be blocked by pretreatment with narcotic antagonist before each session of microwave exposure; (5) the three major subtypes of opioid receptors, μ, δ and κ are involved in mediating the effect of microwaves in brain.

4.15 Stress

The pathophisiologic picture of stress has been characterized as the general adaptation syndrome which develops in three stages, the alarm reaction, the stage of resistance, and the stage of exhaustion (Sclye 1946). The cellular stress response was described by (Ritossa 1962), which accounts for the proteins initially being called heat shock proteins, generated by elevated temperature of the external environment. Several external physical and chemical environmental influences (e.g., pH and osmotic pressure changes) are capable of influencing this. Goodman et al. (1994, 1998) were the first to show that the response was stimulated by extremely low frequency EMF. In fact cells are far more sensitive to EMF than to thermal stimuli, the EMF energy being one billion times smaller than the thermal stimuli. These findings support the view that EMFs are potentially harmful to cells, and protective biological response to EMF occurs long before there is a significant change in temperature.

Buchner and Eger (2011) studied health impacts of exposures from new base station yielding exposure to EMF/RFR, saw a significant elevation of the stress hormones adrenaline and noradrenaline during the first six months with a concomitant drop in dopamine, with a failure to restore the prior levels after a year and a half. These impacts were felt by the young, the old and the chronically ill, but healthy adults. Bellieni et al. (2008) found that heart rate variability is adversely affected in infants hospitalized in isolettes where ELF-EMF levels are in the range 0.8 to 0.9 μT range. Infants suffer adverse changes in heart rate variability, similar to adults. This electromagnetic stress may have lifelong developmental impacts (Witter et al. 2009).

The stress proteins act as the chemical agents that also serve as markers. The cellular stress response is a protective reaction of individual cells to potentially harmful stimuli in the environment. The ability of EMF extends from extremely low frequency range (Goodman & Blank 1998; Blank 2012) to radiofrequency range (De Polimeri et al. 2003) and by amplitude modulated RF/microwave fields (Czyz et al. 2004; Paulraj & Behari 2011). The cellular stress response differs from the more familiar responses of entire organism to stresses that lead to secretion of cortisol and adrenalin and that result in the activation of various systems throughout the body.

The cellular stress response is a protective reaction of individual cells to potentially harmful stimuli in the environment. The different physical and chemical stimuli that can initiate this response cause the two strands of DNA to fall apart for amino acid code for protein synthesis to be read. Therefore, the observed stress protein synthesis is evidence reacted with DNA to start the process. Many different type of cells that respond to cells both in vivo and in vitro, include epithelial, endothelial and epidermal cells, cardiac, muscle cells, fibroblasts, yeast, E coli, developing chick eggs, and dipteran cells. The EMF does not produce stress response in all type of cells.

Microwave as Stressor

It has been suggested (Michaelson 1982) that microwaves of high power density can act as a stressor effecting regulatory and integrative homeokinetic activity resulting in an alteration of homeostasis. It is generally agreed (Lu et al. 1980) that threshold of 50 mW/cm^{2}exists for a 60 minutes exposure for 300 gm rats. It is shown that corticosterone (CS) increases within 15–30 minutes of the start of exposure and falls sharply within 15–30 minutes after termination of exposure (Guillet et al. 1975). Growing amount of Clinical observations and evidences support a significant role for stress in ASDs (Anderson & Colombo 2009; Ming et al. 2011; Anderson et al. 2013) with variability among individuals in the severity of the stress response but a tendency to have high tonic sympathetic arousal at baseline (Chang et al. 2012; Cheshire 2012). The impact of EMF/RFR exposure can also be greatly influenced by the stress system status of the individual.

Extending the above line of arguments to low level of microwave exposure would shed light on the mode of microwave interaction with humans. It has been suggested that a chronic exposure of low intensity pulsed microwave can be a source of stress. This has been investigated by giving low intensity, single and repeated exposure on benzodiazepine receptors in three areas of brain: cerebral cortex, hippocampus, and cerebellum (Lai 1992). The cerebral cortex and hippocampus are known to play significant role in stress responses and along with the cerebellum, contain high concentration of benzodiazepine receptors. The authors investigated the effects of single (45 minutes) and repeated (10 days daily dose of 45 minutes each session) of microwave exposure (2.45 GHz, 1 mW/cm^2, average whole body SAR 0.6 W/kg, pulse 500 ppm with pulse width 2ms) on the concentration and affinity of benzodiazepine in the cerebral cortex, hippocampus and cerebellum of the rat. The mechanism by which acute stress affects benzodiazepine receptors in the brain needs more investigation.

The similarity of the effects of microwaves and those of established sources of stress (nonspecific) led to the suggestion that microwave irradiator is a "stressor" (Salford et al. 1994). The effect (and magnitude) of absorption of electromagnetic energy on brain tissue and cell membrane depend on type of electromagnetic field (cw/modulation). These effects appear to be important at frequency and amplitude modulation below 300 Hz. Pre development of mice is also affected by RF induced changes (Margas & Xenos 1997). The effect of these extremely low frequencies is important to examine for those falling close to EEG frequencies, though their direct coupling may be unlikely (Takashima et al. 1984). It has been reported (Thuróczy et al. 1994) that whole body exposure at 30 mW/cm^2 (25 W/kg, SAR) of rats causes an increase in EEG activity (sum of EEG wave frequency bands) immediately at the first stage after exposure and also a slight increase in delta waves (0.5–4.0Hz) of the EEG spectrum.

At all levels of mammalian biological organization adverse environment elicits a complex array of nervous, endocrine, neurohumoral, and motor reactions to adjust body fluids balance, energy metabolism, and behavior, concomitantly with need to survive in a changed environment. The neuroendocrine system, a complex of hormone secreting glands, and the central nervous system function as a chemical regulatory system in mammals to control and regulate metabolism and growth and to protect the body from endogenous and exogenous alterations in homeostasis. The cellular stress response is activated by a mechanism that involves interaction of EMF with the DNA molecule. The reaction of DNA, and/or the stress proteins synthesized, could be used to develop new EMF safety standards (Blank & Goodman 2012). It may be mentioned that stress response does not occur in reaction to EMF in all type of cells, and that tissue cultured cells (as compared to natural cells) are less likely to show an effect of. The cellular stress response is quite widespread.

It is concluded that microwave induced corticosterone response observed in rats is dependent upon adrenocorticotropin secretion by the pituitary, i.e., the adrenal gland, is not directly stimulated by microwave exposure.

Studies of effect of EMF on characterized electron transfer reactions, involving cytochrome oxidase, ATP hydrolysis by Na, K-ATPase, and the redox reaction, have shown that (Blank 2012):

(1) Electron transfer rates are accelerated due to the exposure of EM fields.
(2) Effect of EMF varies inversely with the intrinsic reaction rate, and that EMF effects are only seen when intrinsic rate are low. This arises because of low energy components of EMF.
(3) Experimentally determined thresholds are low (~0.5 μT).
(4) Effects vary with frequency with different optima for reactions studied: the two enzymes showed broad frequency optima close to the reaction turnover members for NaK-ATPase (60 Hz) and cytochrome oxidase (800Hz), suggesting that EMF interacted optimally when in synchrony with the molecular kinetics. EMF interaction

with DNA in both ELF and RF ranges do not appear to involve electron transfer reactions with defined kinetics.

Variations in the rate of electron flow can lead to the accumulation of charge. The temporary build-up of charge at a site results in strong repulsive forces that can cause disruption of H bonds. A net charge can disrupt the structure of a complex molecule, such as occurs when the four protein chains of hemoglobin disaggregate in response to a gradual build up of charge in the hemoglobin tetramer (Blank & Soo 1998). For similar reasons, one would expect disaggregating forces at the DNA site where charge builds up.

The stress response has provided opportunity to investigate EMF interaction with DNA, and in particular, how this results in stimulating DNA to start the hypothesis of proteins. Because the DNA sequence is known for hsp 70, it is possible to study the effects of changes in the DNA sequence on protein synthesis. As a result of these experiments, it was possible to identify two distinct regions in the promoter region of the HSP 70 gene-an EMF sensitive region that was not sensitive to increased temperature, as well as a region sensitive only to temperature. These electromagnetic response elements (EMREs) are also found on the c-myc promoter which also reacts to EMF. This mechanism is based on direct interaction with specific segments of DNA and there is reason to believe that EMF can interact similarly with other segments of DNA.

The classic triad of alarm reaction (adrenocortical stimulation, thymicolymphatic hypotrophy and gastrointestinal ulcer) denotes the stereotyped response of the body to any demand that severely taxes the regulatory process. The alarm reaction also points the involvement of the hypothalamohypophyseal-adrenocortical (HHA) system and the autonomic control. It is well established that in both the sex of rats acute stress inhibits growth hormone (GH) secretion (Collu & Jequier 1976) and stimulates adrenocorticotrophic hormone (ACTH) (Matsuyama et al. 1971). The most important aspect of the stress-induced secretory pattern of these adenohypophyseal hormones is that it establishes the nonspecific character of the response. These stress induced hormonal changes are related to the intensity and duration of the stressing agent. However it is established that stress is caused by the microwave exposure and not due to any other environmental stress by seeking comparison with control/sham exposed animal data. The neuroendocrine data are consistent with the hypothesis that the adenohypophyseal responses are the integral result of CNS processing of multiple signals from many body locations, cells that no single localization of absorbed energy is pivotal to the onset of a response.

4.16 Health Implications and Possible Remediation

The increasing use of electromagnetic fields for a variety of purposes (domestic, occupational, and industrial) give rise to the problem of their health implications. The International Agency for Research on Cancer (IARC) has classified RF fields as "possibly carcinogenic to humans," This is also for emissions from exposure to the brain from RF fields from cell phone base stations (mounted on roofs or towers), which is less than 1/100th the exposure to the brain from mobile devices such as cell phones.

Some people are concerned about potential health effects, especially on the developing brains and bodies of children. However the reported data on this issue are conflicting: some concluding negative results, while other reporting just the reverse otherwise. Scientists continue to study the effects of long-term exposure to low levels of RF.

Various functional properties of DNA including DNA synthesis (Liboff et al. 1984) and repair (Meltz et al. 1987) are altered by EM fields. Direct effects on DNA may be mediated by its conformational state. Conformational states in turn are controlled by hydrogen bonds which hold together the folded secondary structure of biomolecules (Takano et al. 1999). Cellular phones speed up DNA rewinding, suggesting an increase in hydrogen bond formation. If cellular phones are found to have effect on hydrogen bonds, it will have implications in biology.

Some technologies have emerged utilizing a concept that one type of EM field can reverse or neutralize the biological effects produced by another type of EM field. Industry frequency magnetic fields are important because of the biophysical influence on the cell (Kula & Drozdz 1996; Kula et al. 2000; Kumar et al. 2011a).

One of the major molecular effects of magnetic fields is their influence on nuclear spins of paramagnetic molecules (Grissom 1995). This mechanism plays an important role when in the course of a chemical reaction the chemical bond is disrupted and two molecules with unpaired electrons are formed (a pair of radicals). Depending on their electron spin orientations, radical recombination or diffusion and formation of free radicals (e.g., oxygen radicals) may take place. DC field reverses neutralizes the effect of a Pulsed magnetic field on nitrites outgrowth in neuronal cellular studies (Blackman et al. 1979). Another related study has been the use of incoherent noise fields to undo neutralize magnetic field effects on ornithine decarboxylase induction (Farrell et al. 1998). In case of mobile frequencies exposures it has been demonstrated that it increased the number of fruit fly offspring, as well as some biochemical markers. It also increased the levels of transcription factors which are known to activate DNA synthesis. This effect can be reversed when a commercially available aluminum shield is added to the cellular phone. Syldona (2007) have demonstrated that cellular phone induced changes in DNA rewinding are completely reversed when an Aulterra Neutralizer is added to the cellular phone. This effect is seen 77% of the time, yielding a statistically significant result.

DNA rewinding has been utilized as a classical property for studying in vitro effects of cellular phone radiation. This hypothesis however contradicts other data suggesting that primary sight of EMF-biointeraction is the plasma membrane and/or the ions that bind to various protein receptors within the plasma conditions require a complex interaction between the EM fields from the cellular phone. In systems, where two EMFs interact, the strength and orientation between the two fields is critical in order to obtain resonance conditions.

The radiofrequency exposure causing increased DNA damage in cells is cumulative. Various evidences suggest that responses of the central nervous system to these radiations could lead to stress response (Lai et al. 1987; Lai 1992). Stress effects cumulate over time and involve first adoption and then an eventual breakdown of homeostatic processes when it persists. The results of major reports (Rubin et al. 2005; Seitz et al. 2005; WHO 2005) support these findings.

In leukocytes, physiological activation is associated with the onset of phagocytosis and leads to increased formation of reactive species (ROS). These cells exert a wide variety of functions including the regulation of the immune response (pro and anti inflammatory processes), scavenging of senescent cells, and phagocytosis of infected or malignant cells, wound healing, repair and detoxification. The generation of free radicals enhances important physiological processes, e.g., signal transduction processes of various membrane receptors and further immunological functions. An imbalance between excessive formation of reactive oxygen species and the limited antioxidant defense system may take place. However, several authors (Lantow et al. 2006a, 2006b) reported no increase in free radical level.

It is evident that there are lot of controversies regarding brain tumors associated with mobile phone users. Mobile phones generate electromagnetic radiation in two ways. First, from the antennae that are present around our towns and secondly from the telephones themselves. Present international standards permit GSM 900 mobile phones to transmit at a pulsed power of 2 W with an average output of 0.25 W. Mobile phones have been found to generate electromagnetic radiation well below the guidelines of the International Commission on Non Ionizing Radiation Protection (ICNIRP 1998).

Above data and discussions are suggestive of the fact that RF-EMF is bioactive and have a potential to cause health impacts. Bioeffects can occur in the first few minutes at levels associated with cell and cordless phone use. Bioeffects can also occur from just minutes after exposure to mobile phone masts (cell towers): Wi-Fi and wireless utility smart meters that produce whole body exposure. Chronic base station exposures can result in illness. This is because they interfere with normal body processes (disrupt homeostasis), prevent the body from healing damaged DNA, produce immune system imbalances, metabolic disruption and lower resistance to disease across multiple pathways. Normal body processes can eventually be disabled by external stresses (from systemwide electrophysiological interference) and lead to pervasive impairment of metabolic and reproductive functions.

There is a consistent pattern of increased risk for glioma and acoustic neuroma of wireless phones (mobile phones and cordless phones). An important aspect of this is that Bioeffects can occur at very low level of electromagnetic field exposure, provided proper widow sets are available.

4.17 The Non-linearity between Electromagnetic Exposure and Biological Effect

The biological/health effects from man-made EMFs/non-ionizing radiation, do not follow a linear dose-response (or cause-effect) relationship according to the experimental evidence. Experiments have shown that, the absorption of a larger amount of energy by the same mass of a given tissue and within the same time-interval, does not necessarily induce a larger biological effect. In other words, a more intense field or larger *SAR* does not necessarily relate to a larger biological response and correspondingly health effects. Viewed in this context it may be said that experimental data on energy dependency of biological effects by EMF present SAR formulation, very often do not adequately explains (a) the nonlinear character of EMF-induced bio effects due to the existence of amplitude, frequency and "exposure time windows" and (b) EMF-induced bio effects are significantly dependent on physical and chemical composition of the surrounding medium.

The non-linearity of biological effects of man-made EMFs, and especially RF/microwave fields modulated by Extremely Low Frequency (ELF) signals (0–300 Hz), where the largest effects do not correspond to the largest *SAR* or intensity values, has been reported (e.g., Blackman et al. 1979). Since then, it has also verified by various other studies (Goodman et al. 1994; Eberhardt et al. 2008; Panagopoulos et al. 2010a, 2010b). For example, in one of the studies regarding effect of GSM radiation on the permeability of the blood-brain barrier in rats, although other studies found no effect on the blood-brain barrier (Stam 2010). Some authors (Panagopoulos et al. 2010a) have reported that the strongest effect was produced by the lowest *SAR* values which corresponded to the weakest radiation intensity, may be because of the windows existing in the range of their investigations (frequency, intensity).

Moreover, in several studies, regions of increased bioactivity called "windows" were recorded, where the biological effects reach a maximum compared to the effects at smaller or larger values of a directly measurable physical parameter like the intensity (and thus *SAR*) or frequency of the radiation. The "windows" represent an unexplained phenomenon of the biological effects of EMFs, where increased bioactivity appears within certain values of a physical parameter of the field/radiation, but not for lower or higher values of this parameter (Blackman et al. 1979; Liboff et al. 1984). An intensity window on the biological effects of mobile telephony radiation was discovered where the effect on DNA damage was more intense around the value of 10 $\mu W/cm^2$ in terms of the microwave – carrier – radiation intensity than for intensities larger than 250 $\mu W/cm^2$. More specifically, the borders of this "window" were found to be located between 8 and 28 $\mu W/cm^2$ (Panagopoulos et al. 2010a; Panagopoulos & Margaritis 2010b). In such a case of non-linearity the dose-effect relationship cannot be predicted. Any inaccuracy in the intensity measurement, as for example it may occur within an antenna's reactive near field, would be further reflected in corresponding SAR estimation. More specifically, if the electric field intensity E varies significantly within an antenna's near field, the corresponding SAR value depending on E^2 (Equation 4.2) will include this variation plus the variation in the conductivity and density of the biological matter.

The reason for the non-linearity between electromagnetic exposure and biological effect may well be exactly the fact that the amount of absorbed energy or the rate of its absorption (*SAR*, field intensity) does not determine the biological effect. Indeed, the amount of absorbed energy during a certain time-interval (i.e., the rate of energy absorption) increases with increasing intensity or *SAR*. If the corresponding biological effect increased proportionally, there would be no "windows" or other non-linear effects in regards to intensity or *SAR*. Nevertheless such effects exist.

Finally, the non-linearity of several types of biological effects has been reported regardless of exposure to EMFs, and in response to a variety of external factors such as ionizing radiation, physiological, pharmacological, or chemical agents, environmental contaminants, etc., indicating that a non-linear response to environmental factors is associated with living subject.

From the scientific point of view, adverse human health effects of non-thermal radiation levels cannot be exactly quantified, and repeated with utmost reproducibility, or even excluded at this time. Only limited toxicological information is available (that too not in an isolated environment) in respect to the widespread use. The economical impact of the cellular phone systems in industrial nations is a sensitive factor. On one side, there is always a demand for scientific proof for human adverse health effects and dose response when establishing official guideline exposure threshold values. On the other side, insufficient limit of detection, lack of sufficient dosimetry and exposure control, and industry friendly research bias, is an impediment in risk assessment for long-term adverse health effects.

References

Adey WR, Kado J, Didio J et al. (1963) Impedances changes in cerebral tissue accompanying a learned discriminative performance in the cat. *Exptl. Neurol.*, 7: 259.

Adey WR, Kado RT & Walter DO (1965) Impedance charactersics of cortical & subcortical structures, evaluation of regional specificity in hypercapnea & hypothermia. *Exptl. Neurol.*, 11: 190.

Agarwal A, Deepinder F, Sharma RK, Ranga G & LiJ (2008) Effect of cell phone usage on semen analysis in men attending infertility clinic: anobservational study. *Fertil. Steril.*, 89(1): 124.

Agarwal A, Desai NR, Makker K, Varghese A, Mouradi R, Sabanegh E & Sharma R (2009) Effects of radiofrequency electromagnetic waves (RF-EMW) from cellular phones on human ejaculated semen: an in vitro pilot study. *Fertil. Steril.*, 92(4): 318.

Aitkin RJ, Bennetts LE, Sawyer D, Wilklendt AM & King BW (2005) Impact of radiofrequency electromagnetic radiation on DNA integrity in the male germline. *Int. J. Androl.*, 28(3): 171.

Albert EN, Slaby F & Roche J (1987) Effect of amplitude modulated 147 MHz radiofrequency radiation on calcium ion efflux from avian brain tissue. *Radiat. Res.*, 109(1): 19.

Aldad TS, Geliang G, Gao XB & Taylor HS (2012) Fetal radiofrequency radiation exposure from 800–1900 Mhz-rated cellular telephones affects neurodevelopment & behavior in mice. *Sci. Rep.*, 2: 312. doi:10.1038/srep00312

Allis JA & Sinha-Robinson BL (1987) Temperature specific inhibition of human red cell Na +/K – aTPase by 2,450 MHz microwave radiation. *Bioelectromagnetics*, 8: 203.

Ammari M, Gamez C, Lecomte A, Sakly M, Abdelmelek H & De Seze R (2010) GFAM expression in the rat brain following sub-chronic exposure to a 900 MHz electromagnetic signal. *Int. J. Radiat. Biol.*, 86(3): 367.

Anderson CJ & Colombo J (2009) Larger tonic pupil size in young children with autism spectrum disorder. *Dev. Psychobiol.*, 51(2): 207.

Anderson CJ, Colombo J & Unruh KE (2013) Pupil & salivary indicators of autonomic dysfunction in autism spectrum disorder. *Dev. Psychobiol.*, 55(5): 465.

Andrianome S, Hugueville L, de Seze R & Selmaoui B (2017) Increasing levels of saliva alpha amylase in electrohypersensitive (EHS) patients. *Int. J. Radiat. Biol.*, 93 (8): 841.

Arkin MR, Stemp EDA, Holmlin RE, Barton JK, Hoermann A, Olson EJC & Barbara PF (1996) Rates of DNA mediated electron transfer between metalointercalators. *Science*, 273: 475.

Avendano C, Mata A, Sanchez Sarmiento CA & Doncei GF (2012) Use of laptop computers connected to internet through WI-FI decreases human sperm motility & increases sperm DNA sperm fragmentation. *Fertil. Steril.*, 97(1): 39.

Azanza MA & Moral AD (1994) Cell membrane biochemistry & neurobiological approach to biomagnetism. *Prog. Neurobiol.*, 44: 517.

Barker AT, Jackson PR, Parry H, Coulton LA, Cook GC & Wood SM (2007) The effect of GSM & TETRA mobile handset signals on blood pressure, catechol level s & heart rate variability. *Bioelectromagnetics*, 28: 433.

Bawin AM & Adey WR (1976) Sensitivity of calciumbinding in cerebral tissue to weakenvironmental fields oscillating at low frequency. *Proc. Natl. Acad. Sci.*, 73: 1993.

Bawin S, Adey W & Sabbot I (1978) Ionic factors in release of 45 Ca2+ fro chicken cerebral tissues by electromagnetic fields. *Proc. Natl. Acad. Sci.*, 75(12): 6314.

Behari J (2009a) Biological correlates of low level electromagnetic field exposure. In: *General & Applied Toxicology*. (Ballantyne B, Mars TC & Syver T, eds., 3rd Edition), John Wiley & Sons Asia Pvt. Ltd., p. 1.

Behari J (2009b) *Biophysical Bone Behavior: Principals & Applications*. Singapore: John Wiley & Sons (Asia) Pvt. Ltd, p. 173.

Behari, J & Behari, J (2009) Changes in bone histology due to capacitive field stimulation of ovariectomized rat. *Indian J. Med. Res.*, 130: 720.

Behari J, Kunjilwar KK & Pyne S (1998) Interaction of low level modulated RF radiation with Na+ _ K= -ATpase. *Bioelectrochem. Bioener.*, 47: 247.

Behari J & Lochan R (2003) Effect of low level pulsed radiofrequency fields on induced osteoporosis in tat bone. *Indian J. Exp. Biol.*, 41: 587.

Bellieni CV, Acampa M, Maffei M, Maffei S, Perrone S, Pinto I, Stacchini N & Buonocore G (2008) Electromagnetic fields produced by incubators influence heart rate vaiability in newborns. *Arch. Dis. Child Fetal. Neonatal. Ed.*, 93(4): F298.

Berman E, Weil C, Philips PA, Carter HB & House DB (1992) Fetal & maternal effects of continual exposure of rats to 970 MHz circularly polarized microwaves. *Electromgn. Biol. Med.*, 11: 43.

Betskii O, Devyatkov N & Kislov V (1998) Low intensity millimetre waves in medicine & biology. *Biomed. Radioelektron*, 4: 13.

Bezrukov SM & Vodyanoy I (1995) Noise induced enhancement of signal transduction across voltage dependent ion channel. *Nature*, 378: 362.

Binhi VN (2002) *Magnetobiology*. San Diego, Tokyo: Academic Press, An Elsevier Science Imprint, p. 353.

Bioinitiative (2012) In: *A Rationale for Biologically – Based Exposure Standards for Low – Intensity Electromagnetic Radiation* (Cindy Sage and David O Carpenter, eds.). Bioinitiative Working Group. www.bioinitiative.org.

Blackman CF, Elder JA, Weil CM, Benane SG, Eichinger DC & House DE (1979) Induction of calcium-ion efflux from brain tissue by radiofrequency radiation: effects of modulation frequency & field strength. *Radio Sci.*, 14: 93.

Blank M (1992) Na + -K – ATPase function in alternating electric fields. *FASEB J*, 6: 2434.

Blank M (2012) The cellular stress response: EMF-DNA interaction. *Bioinitiative (Supplement)*, 2(7): 1.

Blank M & Goodman R (2011) DNA is a fractal antenna in electromagnetic fields (EMF). *Int. J. Radiat. Biol.*, 87: 409.

Blank M & Goodman R (2012) Electromagnetics & health: DNA-baseddosimetry. *Electromag. Biol. Med.*, 31: 243.

Blank M & Soo L (1992) Threshold for inhibition of Na K-ATPase by ELF alternating currents. *Bioelectromagnetics*, 13: 329.

Blank M & Soo L (1998) Frequency dependency of cytochrome oxidase activity in magnetic fields. *Bioelectrochem. Bioenerg.*, 46: 139.

Bolshakov MA & Alekseev SI (1992) Bursting responses of Lymnea neurons to microwave radiation. *Bioelectromagnetics*, 13(2): 119.

Braune S, Wrocklage C, Raczek J, Gailus T & Lucking CR (1998) Resisting blood pressure during exposure to radiofrequency electromagnetic field. *Lancet*, 351: 1857.

Brillaud E, Plotrowski A & de Seze R (2007) Effect of an acute 900 MHz GSM exposure onglia in the rat brain: a time dependent study. *Toxicology*, 238(1): 23.
Buchner K & Eger H (2011) Changes in clincally important neurotransmitters under the influence of modulated RF fields-a long –term study under real-life conditions (origional in German). *Umwelt-Medizin-Gesellschaft*, 24(1): 44.
Buzsaki G (2006) *Rhythms of the Rain*. New York: Oxford University Press.
Byus CV, Lundak RK, Fletcher RM et al. (1984) Alterations in protein kinase activity following exposure of cultured lymphocytes to modulated microwave elds. *Bioelectromagnetics*, 15: 34.
Capri M, Scarcella E, Bianchi E, Fumelli C, Mesirca P, Agostini C et al. (2004) 1800 MHz radiofrequency (mobile phones, different global system for mobile communication modulations) does not affect apoptosis & heat shock protein 70 level in peripheral blood mononuclear cells from young & old donors. *Int. J. Radiat. Biol.*, 80: 389.
Capri M, Scarcella E, Fumelli C, Bianchi E, Salvioli S, Mesirca P et al. (2004a) In vitro exposure of human lymphocytes to 900 MHz CW & GSM modulated radio-frequency: studies of proliferation, apoptosis & mitochondrial membrane potential. *Radiat. Res.*, 162: 211.
Caraglia M, Marra M, Mancinelli F, D'Ambrosio G, Massa R, Giordano A et al. (2005) Electromagnetic fields at mobile phone frequency induce apoptosis & inactivation of the multi-chaperone complex in human epidermoid cancer cells. *J. Cell Physiol.*, 204: 539.
Carmeliet P (2000) Mechanisms of angiogenesis & arteriogenesis. *Nat. Med.*, 6: 389.
Castagna M, Takai Y, Kaibuchi K et al. (1982) Direct activation of calcium activated phospholopid – dependent proteinkinase by tumor – promoting phorbol esters. *J. Biol. Chem.*, 257: 7487.
Catarino AO, Churches S, Baron-Cohen S, Andrade A & Ring H (2011) A typical EEG complexity in autism spectrum conditions: amultiscale entropy analysis. *Clin. Neurophysiol.*, 122(12): 2375.
Cetkin M, Demirel C, Kizlkan N, Aksoy N & Erbagci H (2017) Evaluation of the mobile phone electromagnetic radiation on serum iron parameters in rats. *Afr. Health Sci.*, 17(1): 186.
Chang MC, Parham LD, Blanche EI, Schell A, Chou CP, Dawson M & Clark F (2012) Autonomic & behavioural responses of children with autism to auditory stimuli. *Am. J. Occup. Ther.*, 66(5): 567.
Cheshire WP (2012) Highlights in clinical autonomic neuroscience: newinsights into autonomic dysfunction in autism. *Auton Neurosci.*, 171(1-2): 4.
Collu R & Jequier JC (1976) Pituitary response to auditory stress: effects of treatment with α-methyl-p-tyrosine. Usefulness of a factorial mix design for statistical analysis. *Can. J. Physiol. Pharmacol.*, 54: 596.
Cotgreave IA (2005) Biological stress responses to radio frequency electromagnetic radiation: are mobile phones really so (heat) shocking? *Arch. Biochem. Biophys.*, 435: 227.
Czyz Z, Zeng Q, Niolova T, Mester A, Schderer J, Kuster N & Wobus AM (2004) High frequency electromagnetic fields (GSM signals) affect ene suppressor p-53 deficient stem cells. *Bioelectromagnetics*, 25(4): 296.
De Luliis GN, Newey RJ, King BV & Aitken RJ (2009) Mobile phone radiation induces reactive oxygen species production & DNA damage in human spermatozoa in vitro. *PLOS One*. doi:10.1371/journal.pone.0006446

De Polimeri DI, Smith B, Dawe A, North K, Smith T, Archer DB, Duce IR, Jones D & Candido EP (2003) Microwave radiation can alter protein confirmation without bulk heating. *FEBS Lett.*, 543(1–3): 93.
Devyiatkov ND, Pletnev SD, Chernov ZS & Shchitkkov KG (1994) Effect of low energy pulses of EHF-and SHF-radiation of nanosecond duration of nanosecond duration with a high peak intensity on biological structures (mkalignant neoplasm). *Doklady Akademi Nauk*, 336(6): 826.
Diem E, Lerchal A & Wilhelm A (2005) Critical comments on DNA breakage by mobile phone electromagnetic fields. *Mutat. Res.*, 583: 18.
Divan HA, Kheifets L, Obel C & Olsen J (2008) Prenatal & postnatal exposure to cell phone use & behavioural problems in children. *Epidemiology*, 19: 523.
Dragan A & Geddes CD (2014) 5 color multiplexed microwave accelerated metal-enhanced flurosence detection & analysis of multiple DNA sequences from within from one sample well within a few seconds. *J. Fluores.*, 24(6): 1715.
Dreher D & Junod AF (1996) Role of oxygen free radicals in cancer development. *Eur. J. Cancer*, 32A: 30.
Durney HD & Christensen DA (2000) *Basic Introduction to Bioelectromagnetics*. Boca Raton, London, NY, Washington, DC: CRC Press, LLC, 2000 Corporate Blvd. p. 139.
Eberhardt JL, Persson BR, Brun AE, Salford LG & Malmgren LO (2008) Blood –brain barrier & nerve cell in rat brain damage 14 & 28 days after exposure to microwaves from GSM mobile phones. *Electromag. Biol. Med.*, 27(3): 215.
Edwards WF, Young DD & Deiters A (2009) Efect of microwave irradiation on DNA hybridization. *Org. Biomol. Chem.*, 7(12): 2506–2508. doi:10.1039/b903609a
Eltiti S, Wallace D, Zougkou K, Russo R, Joseph S, Rasor P et al. (2007) Development & evaluation of the electromagnetic hypersensitivity questionnaire. *Bioelectromagnetics*, 28: 137.
Erogul O, Oztas E, Yildirim I, Kir T, Aydur E, Komesli G, Irkilata HC, Irmak MK & Peker AF (2006) Effects of electromagnetic radiation from a cellular phone on human sperm motility in in vitro study. *Arch. Med. Res.*, 37: 840.
Farrell JM, Barber M, Krause D & Litovitz TA (1998) The superposition of a temporally incoherent magnetic field inhibits 60 Hz-induced changes in the ODC activity of developing chick embryos. *Bioelectromagnetics*, 19(1): 53.
Fatemi SH, Folsom TD, Reutiman TJ & Lee S (2008) Expression of astrocytic markers aquaporin 4 & connexion 43 is altered in brains of subjects with autism. *Synapse*, 62(7): 501.
Fejes I, Zavacki Z, Szollosi J, Koloszar Daru J, Kovacs L & Pal A (2005) Is there a relationship between cell phone use & semen quality? *Arch. Androl.*, 51: 385.
Forgacs Z, Somoy Z, Kubinyl G, Bakos J, Hudak A, Surjan A & Thurocczy G (2006) Efects of whole body 1800 MHz GSM-like microwave exposure on testicular steridogenesis & histology of mice. *Reprod. Toxicol.*, 22: 111.
Foster KR & Glaser R (2007) Thermal mechanism of inreraction of radiofrequency energy with biological exposure systems with relevance to exposure guidelines. *Health Phys.*, 92(6): 609.
Fragopoulou AF, Koussoulakes SL & Margaritis LH (2009) Cranial & postcranial skeletal variations induced in miouse embryos by mobile phone adiation. *Pathophysiology*, 17(3): 169.
Fragopoulou AF, Miltiadous Stamatak A, Stylianopoulou F, Koussoulakes SL & Margaritis LH (2010) Whole body exposure with GSM 900 MHz affects spatial memory in mice. *Pathophysiology*, 17(3): 179.

Fragopoulou AF, Samara A, Antonelou MH, Xanthopoulou A, Papadopoulou A, Vougas K, Koutsogiannopoulou E, Anastasiadou E, Stravopodis DJ, Tsangaris GT & Margaritis LH (2012) Brain proteome response following whole boy exposure of mice to mobile phone or wireless DECT base radiation. *Electromag. Biol. Med.*, 31(4): 250.

French PW, Penny R, Lauorence JA & McKenzie DR (2001) Mobile phones, heat shock proteins & cancer. *Differentiation*, 67: 93.

Friedman J, Kaus S, Hauptman Y, Schiff Y & Seger R (2007) Mechanism of short term ERK activation by electromagnetic field at mobile phone frequencies. *Biochemistry J.*, 405: 559.

Frohlich H (1980) The biological effects of microwaves & related questions. In: *Advances in Electronics & Electron Physics* (L Marton & C Marton, eds.). New York: Academic press, p. 85.

Gandhi OP (1975) Strong dependence of whole animal absorption on polarization & frequency of radiofrequency energy. *Ann. N. Y. Acad. Sci.*, 247: 532.

Gandhi OP (1979) Dosimetry-the absorption properties of man & experimental animals. *Bull. N. Y. Acad. Med.*, 55(11): 973.

Gandhi OP (1982) Electromagneticabsorption in an inhomogeneous model of man for realistic exposure conditions. *Bioelectromagnetics*, 3(1): 81.

Gandhi OP, Hagmann MJ & D'Andrea JA (2012) Part body and multibody effects and absorption of radiofrequency electromagnetic energy. *Radio Sci.*, 14(6S): 15–21.

Gartzke J & Lange K (2002) Cellular target of weak magnetic field: ionic conduction along actin filaments of microvilli. *Am. J. Physiol.*, 283: C1333.

Giese KC & Vierling E (2002) Changes in oligomerization are essential for the chaperone activity of a small heat shock protein in vivo and in vitro. *J. Biol. Chem.*, 277: 46310.

Glaser R (2005) Are thermoreceptors responsible for "non thermal" effects of R F fields? *Edition Wissenschaft FGF*, 21: 12.

Gökçek-Saraç Ç, Er H, Kencebay Manas C, Kantar Gök D, Özen Ş & Derin N (2017) Effects of acute & chronic exposure to both 900 MHz & 2100 MHz electromagnetic radiation on glutamate receptor signaling pathway. *Toxicology*, 238(1): 23.

Goodman R & Blank M (1998) Magnetic field induces expression of hsp70. *Cell Stress Chaperones*, 3: 79.

Goodman R, Blank M, Lin H, Khorkova O, Soo L, Weisbrot D & Henderson AS (1994) Increased levels of hsp70 transcripts are induced when cells are exposed to low frequency electromagnetic fields. *Bioelectrochem. Bioenerg.*, 33: 115.

Gotoh T, Terada K & Mori M (2001) Hsp 70-DnaJ chaperone pairs prevent nitric oxide-mediated apoptosis in RAW 264.7 macrophages. *Cell Death Differ.*, 8: 357.

Grigoryev Y (2003) Biological effects of mobile phone electromagnetic field on chick embryo (Risk assessment using the mortality rate). *Radiats Biol. Radioecol.*, 43: 541.

Grissom CB (1995) Magnetic field effects in biology: a survey of possible mechanisms with emphasis on radical – pair recombination. *Chem. Res.*, 3: 95.

Griveau JF, Dumont E, Renard P, Callegari JP & Le Lannou D (1995) Reactive oxygen species, lipid peroxidation & enzyme defence systems in human spermatozoa. *J. Reprod. Fertil.*, 103: 17.

Grundler WF, Keilmann F & Frohlich H (1977) Resonant growth rate response of yeast cell irradiated by weak microwaves. *Phys. Lett.*, 62(6): 463.

Guillet R, Lotz WG & Michaelson SM (1975) Time course of adrenal response in microwave exposed rats. In Proceedings of USNC? URSI, p. 316.

Haisenleder DJ, Workman LJ, Burger LL, Aylor KW, Dalkin AC & Marshall JC (2001) Gonadotropin subunit transcriptional responses to calcium signal in rat evidence for regulation by pulse frequency. *Biol. Reprod.*, 65: 1789.

Hall DB, Holmin RE & Barton JK (1996) Oxidative DNA damage through long range electron transfer. *Nature*, 382: 731.

Hardell L, Carlberg M & Hansson MK (2011) Pooled analysis of case-control studies on malignant brain tumours & the use of mobile & cordless phones including living & deceased subjects. *Int. J. Oncol.*, 38: 1465.

Harvey C & French PW (2000) Effects on protein kinase C & gene expression in a human mast cell line, HMC-1, following microwave exposure. *Cell Biol. Int.*, 23 (11): 739.

Helzlsourer KJ, Harris EL, Parshad R, Perry HR, Price FM & Sanford KK (1996) DNA repair proficiency: potential susceptibility factor for breast cancer. *J. Natl. Cancer Inst.*, 88: 754.

Higashikubo R, Ragouzis M, Moros EG, Straube WL & Roti Roti JL (2001) Radiofrequency electromagnetic fields do not alter the cell cycle progression of C3H 10T & U87MG cells. *Radiat. Res.*, 156: 786.

Hinrikus H, Bachman M, Lass J, Tomson R & Tuulik V (2008) Effect of 7, 14 & 21 Hz modulated 450MHz microwave radiation on human electroencephalographic rhythms. *Intl J. Radiat. Biol.*, 84(1): 69.

Hook GJ, Zhang P, Lagroye I, Li L, Higashikubo R, Moros EG et al. (2004) Measurement of DNA damage & apoptosis in Molt-4 cells after in vitro exposure to radiofrequency radiation. *Radiat. Res.*, 161: 193.

Houtala CD, Maganioti AE, Papageorgiou CC, Nanou ED, Kyprianou MA, Tsiafakis VG, Rabavilas AD & Capsalis CN (2008) The spectral power coherence of the EEG under different EMF conditions. *Neurosci. Lett.*, 441(2): 188.

Huber R, Schuderer J, Graf T et al. (2003) Radio frequency electromagnetic field exposure in human estimation of SAR distribution in the brain, effects on sleep & rate. *Bioelectromagnetics*, 24: 262.

Hughes CM, Lewis SE, Mckelvey-Martin VJ & Thompson W (1996) A comparison of baseline & induced DNA damage in human spermatozoa from fertile & infertile men, using a modified comet assay. *Mol. Hum. Reprod.*, 13: 1240.

Hunter T, Ling N & Cooper JA (1984) Protein kinase C phosphorylation of the EFF receptor at a theonine residue close to the cytoplasmic face of the plasma membrane. *Nature*, 311: 480.

Hyland GJ (2001) *The physiological Environmental Effects of Non Ionising Electromagnetic Radiation*. Brxelles: EU Parliament.

ICNIRP (1998) Guidelines for limiting exposure to time varying electric, magnetic, & electromagnetic fields (upto 300 GHZ). *Health Phys.*, 74: 494.

Ingole IV & Ghosh SK (2006) Cell phone radiation & developing tissues in chicken embryo-a light microscope study of kidneys. *J. Anat. Soc. India*, 55: 19.

Inoue Y, Sato Y, Nishimura M, Seguchi M, Zaitsu Y, Yamada K et al. (1999) Heat-induced drug resistance is associated with increased expression of Bcl-2 in HL60. *Anticancer Res.*, 19: 3989.

Isler JR, Martein KM, Grieve PG, Stark RI & Herber MR (2010) Reduced functional connectivity in visual evoked potentials in children with autism spectrum disorder. *Clin. Neurophysiol.*, 121(12): 2035.

Iwasaki A & Gagon C (1992) Formation of reactive oxygen species in spermatozoa of infertile patients. *Fertil. Steril.*, 57: 409.

Jennes L, Bramem B, Centersm A, Janovickm JA & Conn PM (1995) Regulation of hippocampal gonadotropin releasinghormone (GnRH) receptor mRNA & GnRH-stimulated inositolphosphate production by gonadal steroid hormones. *Mol. Brain Res.*, 33: 104.

Jensh RP, Vogel WH & Brent RI (1982) Postnatal functional analysis of prenatal exposure of rats to 915 MHz microwave radiation. *Int. J. Toxicol.*, 1: 73.

Johansson A, Nordin S, Heiden M & Sandsstrom M (2010) Symptoms, personality traits, & stress in people with mobile phone-related symptoms & electromagnetic hypersensitivity. *J. Psychosom. Res.*, 68(1): 37.

Johnson LAG (1998) Radiofrequency (RF) sickness in the linefield study: an effect of modulated study? *Arch. Environ. Health*, 53(3): 238.

Jolly C & Morimoto RI (2000) Role of the heatshock response & molecular chaperones in oncogenesis & cell death. *J. Natl. Cancer Inst.*, 92: 1564.

Just MA, Cherkassky VL, Keller TA & Minshew NJ (2004) Cortical activation & synchronization during sentence comprehension in high-functioning autism: evidence of underconnectivity. *Brain*, 127(8): 1811.

Kenet T (2011) Sensory functions in ASD. In: *The Neuropsychology of Autism* (Foun D ed.). New York: Oxford University Press.

Kern JK, Geier DA, Adams JB & Geier MR (2010) A biomarker of mercury body burden correlated with diagnostic domain specific clinical symptoms of austism spectrum disorder. *Biometals*. 23(6): 1043.

Kesari KK & Behari J (2008) Comparative study of 900MHz & 2.45 GHz radiation effect on reproductive system of male rats. In: *Recent Advances & Challenges in Reproductive Health Research* (Sharma RS, Rajanna A & Rajalakshmi M, eds.) Proceedings of theconference on "Recent Advances & Challenges in Reproductive Health Research" (Feb 19–21, 2007). New Delhi: ICMR Publication, p. 363.

Kesari KK, Kumar S & Behari J (2011) Effects of radiofrequency electromagnetic wave exposure from cellular phones on the reproductive pattern in male Wistar rats. *Appl. Biochem. Biotechnol.*, 164(4): 546.

Kilgalton SJ & Simmons LW (2005) Image content influences men's semen quality. *Biol. Lett.*, 1: 385.

Kim JH, Yu DH, Huh YH, Lee EH, Kim HG & Kim HR (2017) Long term exposure to 835 MHz RF-EMF induces hyperactivity, autophagy & demyyelination in the cortical neurons of mice. *Sci. Rep.*, 20(7): 41129. doi:10.1038/step41129

Kitchin KT, Brown JL & Lijinsky W (1989) Biochemical studies of six nitrogen-containing heterocycles in rat tissues. *Biochem. Pharmacol.*, 38(16): 2733.

Klaunig JE & Kamendulis LM (2004) The role of oxidative stress in carcinogenesis. *Ann. Rev. Pharmacol. Toxicol.*, 44: 239.

Klug S, Hestcher M, Giles S, Kohlsman S & Kramer K (1997) The lack of effects of nonthermal RF electromagnetic fields on the development of rat embryos grown in culture. *Life Sci.*, 61: 789.

Kodama H, Yamaguchi R, FukadaJ, Kasai H & Tanaka T (1997) Increased oxidative deoxyribonucleic acid damage in the spermatozoa of infertile male patients. *Fertil. Steril.*, 68: 519.

Kula B & Drozdz M (1996) A study of magnetic field effects on fibroblast cultures. Part 2. The evaluation of effects of static and extremely low frequency (ELF) magnetic fields on free radical processes in fibroblasts cultures. *Bioelectrochem. Bioenerg.*, 39: 27.

Kula B, Sobczak A & Kuska R (2002) Effects of electromagnetic field on free radical processes in steelworkers' part I: magnetic field influence on the antioxidant activity in red blood cells & plasma. *J. Occup. Health*, 44: 226.

Kula B, Sobczak K & Kuska R (2000) Effects of static& ELF magnetic fields on free – radical processes inrat liver& kidney. *Electrro-Magnetobiol.*, 19: 99.

Kultz D (2005) Molecular & evolutionary basis of the cellular stress response. *Ann. Rev. Physiol.*, 67: 225.

Kumar S, Kesari KK & Behari J (2011) The influence of microwave exposure on male fertility. *Fertil. Steril.*, 95(4): 1500.

Kumar S, Kesari KK & Behari J (2011a) The therapeutic effect of a pulsed electromagnetic field on the reproductive patterns of male wistar rats exposed to a 2.45 GHz microwave field. *Clinics*, 66(7): 1237. Print version ISSN 1802-5932.

Kumlin T, Liyonen H, Miettenen P, Iunoven A, van Groen T, Puranen L, Pitkaaho R, Juutilainen R & Tanila H (2007) Mobile phone radiation & the behavioural developing brain: morphological effects in juvenile rats. *Radiat. Res.*, 168: 471.

Kunjilwar KK & Behari J (1993) Efect of amplitude modulated radiofrequency radiation on cholinergic system of developing rats. *Brain Res.*, 61(1–2): 321.

Kwee S, Raskmark P & Velizarov S (2001) Changes in cellular proteins due to environmental nonionizing radiation. 1. Heat shock proteins. *Electro Magnetobiol.*, 20: 141.

Lagroye I, Anane R, Wettring BA, Moros EG, Straube WL & Laregina M (2004) Measurement of DNA damage after acute exposure to pulsed-wave 2450 MHz microwaves in rat brain cells by two alkaline comet assay methods. *Intl. J. Radiat. Biol.*, 80(1): 11.

Lahijani MS, Tehrani DM & Sabouri E (2009) Histopathological & ultrastructural studies on the effects of electromagnetic fields on the liver of preincubated white chicken embryo. *Electromag. Biol. Med.*, 28(4): 391.

Lai H (1992) Research on the neurological effects of nonionizing radiation at the University of Washington. *Bioelectromagnetics*, 13: 513.

Lai H, Horita A, Chou CK & Guy AW (1984) Low level microwave irradiation affects ethanol-induced hypothermia & ethanol consumption. *Bioelectromagnetics*, 5: 213.

Lai H, Horita A, Chou CK & Guy AW (1987) A review of microwave irradiation & actions of psychoactive drugs. *IEEE Eng. Med. Biol.*, 6(1): 31.

Lai H & Singh NP (1995) Acute low intensity microwave exposure increases DNA single strand breaks in rat brain cells. *Bioelectromagnetics*, 16: 207.

Lai H & Singh NP (1996) Single & double strand breaks in rat brain after exposure to radiofrequency electromagnetic radiation. *Int. J. Radiat. Biol.*, 69: 513.

Landgrebe M, Hauser S, Langguth B, Frick U, Hajak G & Eichhammer P (2007) Altered cortical excitiability in subjectively electrosensitive patients: results of a pilot study. *J. Psychsom Res.*, 62(3): 283.

Landgrebe M, Rick U, Hauser S, Langguth B, Rosner R, Hajak G & Eichhammer P (2008) Cognitive & neurobiological alterations in electromagnetic hypersensitive patients: results of a case controlled study. *Psychol. Med.*, 38(12): 1781.

Lantow M, Lupke M, Frahm J, Mattsson MO, Kuster N & Simkó M (2006a) ROS release & Hsp70 expression after exposure to 1800 MHz radiofrequency electromagnetic fields in primary human monocytes & lymphocytes. *Radiat. Environ. Biophys.*, 45: 55.

Lantow M, Schuderer J, Hartwig C & Simkó M (2006b) Free radicalrelease & Hsp70 expression in two human immune relevant cell lines after exposure to 1800 MHz radio frequency radiation. *Radiat. Res.*, 165: 88.

Lantow M, Viergutz T, Weiss DG & Simkó M (2006c) Comparative study of cell cycle kinetics & induction of apoptosis or necrosis after exposure to radiofrequency radiation in human Mono Mac 6 cells. *Radiat. Res.*, 166: 539.

Leal BZ, Szilagyi M, Prihoda TJ & Meltz ML (2000) Primary DNA damage in human blood lymphocytes exposed to 2450 MHz radiofrequency radiation. *Radiat. Res.*, 153: 479.

Lehninger AL (1965) *Components of the Respiratory Chain & Approaches to Its Reconstruction in the Mitochondrion*. New York: W A Benjamin.

Lerchl A, Kruger H, Niehaus M, Streckert JR, Bitz AK & Volkert H (2008) Effects of mobile phone electromagnetic fields at nonthermal SAR values on melatonin & body weight of Djungarian hamsters (Phodopus Sungorus). *J. Pineal. Res.*, 44: 267.

Leszczynski D, Joenväärä S, Reivinen J & Kuokka R (2002) Non-thermal activation of the hsp27/p38MAPK stress pathway by mobile phone radiation in human endothelial cells: molecular mechanism for cancer & blood-brain barrier-related effects. *Differentiation*, 2–3: 120.

Li L, Bisht KS, LaGroye I, Zhang P, Straube WL, Moros EG, Pickrd WE & Roti JL (2001) Measurement of DNA damage in mammalian cells exposed to radiofrequency fields at high SAR of 3-5 W/kg. *Radiat. Res.*, 156: 328.

Liboff AR, Williams T Jr, Strong DM & Wistar R Jr. (1984) Time-varying magnetic fields: effect on DNA synthesis. *Science*, 223(4638): 818.

Liburdy RP (1992) Calcium signalling in lymphocytes & ELF fields metric & a site of interaction involving the calcium ion channel. *FEBS Lett.*, 301: 53.

Lin JC (2001) The blood brain barrier, cancer, cell phones, & microwave radiation. *IEE Mag.*, 2(4): 26.

Litovitz T, Krause D, Penafiel M et al. (1993) The role of coherence time in the effect of microwaves on orthine decarboxylase activity. *Bioelectromagnetics*, 14: 395.

Liu DS, Astumian RD & Tsong TY (1990) Activation of Na+ & K+ pumping modes of Na +K –aTPase by an oscillating electric field. *J Biol. Chem.*, 265: 7260.

Liu F, Austin DA & Webster NJG (2003) Gonadotrophin releasing hormone desensitized LßT2 Gonadotrope cells are refractory to acute protein kinase C, Cyclic AMP,& Calcium-dependent signalling. *Endocrinology*, 142: 2284.

Loft S & Poulsen HE (1996) Cancer risk & oxidative DNA damage in man. *J. Mol. Med.*, 74: 297.

Lu ST, Lotz WG & Michaelson SM (1980) Advances in microwave-induced effects. Theconcept of stress. *Proc. IEEE*, 68(1): 73.

Malyapa RS, Ahern EW, Straube WL, Moris EG, Pickard WF & Roti Roti JL (1998) Measurement of DNA damage after exposure to 2450 MHz electromagnetic radiation. *Radiat. Res.*, 148: 608.

Mann K, Wagner P, Brunn G, Hassan F, Hiemke C & Roschke J (1998) Effect of pulsed high frequency electromagnetic fields on the nonendocrine system. *Neuroendocrinology*, 67: 139.

Marco EJ, Hinlley LB, Hill SS & Nagarajan SS (2011) Sensory processing in autism: a review of neurophysiologic findings. *Pediatr. Res.*, 69(5 Pt2): 48R.

Margas IN & Xenos TD (1997) RF radiation – induced changes in the prenatal development of mice. *Bioelectromagnetics*, 18(6): 455.

Marinelli F, La Sala D, Cicciotti G, Cattini L, Trimarchi C, Putti S et al. (2004) Exposure to 900 MHz electromagnetic field induces an unbalance between pro-apoptotic & pro-survival signals in T-lymphoblastoid leukaemia CCRF-CEM cells. *J. Cell Physiol.*, 198: 324.

Marino A (2012) Response to letter to the editor concerning 'Electromagnetic Hypersensitivity'. *Int. J. Neurosci.* 122(7):402 (on Line), 1–2.

Marino AA & Carrubba S (2009) The effects of mobile-phone electromagnetic fields onbrain electrical activity: acritical analysis of the literature. *Electromagn. Biol. Med.*, 28(3): 250.

Mathewson KJ, Jetha MK, Drmic IE, Bryson SE, Goldberg JO & Schmidt LA (2012) Regional EEG Alpha power, coherence, and behavioural symptomatology in austim spectrum disorder. *Clin. Neurophysiol.*, 123(9): 1798. doi:10.1016/j.clinph.2012.02.061

Matsuyama S, Ogasa Q & Yokoki H (1971) Quantitative study of spermatogenesis in androgen treated hypophysectomised rats. *Natl. Inst. Health Q. (Tokyo)*, 11: 46.

McCarty DE, Carrubba S, Chesson AL, Frilot C, Gonzalez-Toledo E & Marino AA (2011) Electromagnetic hypersensitivity: evidence for a novel neurological syndrome. *Int. J. Neurosci.*, 121: 670.

McConnell HM (1975) Coupling between lateral & perpendicular motion in biological membranes. In *Functional Linkage in Biomolecular Systems* (Schmitt FO, Schneider DM & Crothers DM eds.). New York: Raven Press, p. 123.

Meltz ML, Walker KA & Erwin DN (1987) Radiofrequency (microwave) radiation exposure of mammalian cells during UV-induced DNA repair synthesis. *Radiat. Res.*, 110(2): 255.

Michaelson SM (1982) Health implications of exposure to radiofrequency/microwave energies. *Bri. J. Idust. Med*, 39: 105.

Mihaly A & Bozoky B (1984) Immunohistochemichal localization of extravagated serum albulin in the hippocampus of human subjects with partial & generalized epilepsies & epileptiform convulsions. *Acta Neuropathol. (Berlin)*, 9: 540.

Mild KH, Oftedal G, Sandstrom M, Wilen J, Tynes T, Haugsdai B & Hauger E (1998) *Comparison of Systems Experienced by Users of Analogue & Digital Mobile Phones: A Swedish – Norwegian Epidemiological Study*. Sweeden: Report for the National Institute for Working life.

Ming X, Bain JM, Smith D, Brimacombe M, Gold von-Simson G & Axlrod FB (2011) Assessing autonomic dysfunction symptoms in children: a pilot study. *J. Child Neurol.*, 26(4): 420.

Miyakoshi J, Takemasa K, Takashima Y, Ding GR, Hirose H & Koyama S (2005) Effects of exposure to a 1950 MHz radio frequency field on expression of Hsp70 & Hsp27 in human glioma cells. *Bioelectromagnetics*, 26: 251.

Monfrecola G, Moa G & Procaccini EM (2003) Non-ionizing electromagnetic radiations, emitted by a cellular phone, modify cutaneous blood flow. *Dermatol.*, 207: 10.

Muller RA (2008) From loci to networks & back again: anomalies in the study of autism. *Ann. N. Y. Acad. Sci.*, 1145: 300.

Narayanan A, White CA, Saklayen S, Scaduto MJ, Carpenter AL, Abduljalil A, Schmalbrock P & Beversodorf Q (2010) Effect of propranolol on functional connectivity in autism spectrum disorder – a pilot study. *Brain Imaging Behav.*, 4(2): 189.

Nikolova T, Czyz J, Rolletschek A, Blyszczuk P, Fuchs J, Jovtchev G et al. (2005) Electromagnetic fields affect transcript levels of apoptosis-related genes in embryonic stem cell-derived neural progenitor cells. *FASEB J*, 19: 1686.

Nishizuka Y (1986) Studies & perspectives of protein kinase C. *Science*, 233: 305.

Ohkusu K, Isobe K, Hidaka H & Nakashima I (1986) Elucidation of the protein kinase C-dependent apoptosis pathway in distinct of T lymphocytes in MRL-lpr/pr mice. *Eur. J. Immunol.*, 25: 3180.

Orekhova EV, Stonganova TA, Nygren G, Tsetlin M, Posikera IN, Gillberg C & Elam M (2007) Excess of high frequency electroencephalogram oscillations in boys with austism. *Biol Psychiatry*, 62(9): 1022.

Osepchuk JM & Petersen RC (2003) Historical review of RF exposure standards & the international committee on Electromagnetic safety (ICES). *Bioelectromagnetics Suppl.*, 6: S7.

Otitoloju AA, Obe IA, Adewale OA, Otubanjo OA & Osunkalu VO (2010) Preliminary study on the reduction of sperm head abnormalities in mice, Mus musculus, exposed to radiofrequency radiations from global system for mobile communication base stations. *Bull. Environ. Contamin. Toxicol.*, 84(1): 51.

Ozguner M, Koyu A, Cesur G, Ural M, Ozguner F, Gokcimen A & Delibas N (2005) Biological & morphological effects on the reproductive organ of rats after exposure to electromagnetic field. *Saudi Med. J.*, 26: 405.

Pacini S, Ruggiero M, Sardi I, Aterini S, Gulisano F & Gulisano M (2002) Exposure to global system for mobile communication (GSM) cellular phone radiofrequency alters gene expression, proliferation, &morphology of human skin fibroblasts. *Oncol. Res.*, 1: 19.

Panagopoulos DJ, Chavdoula ED & Margaritis LH (2010a) Bioeffets of mobile telephony radiation in relation to is intensity or distance from the antenna. *Int. J. Radiat. Biol.*, 86(5): 345.

Panagopoulos DJ & Margaritis LH (2010b) The identification of an intensity "window" on the bioeffects of mobile telephone radiation. *Int. J. Radiat. Biol.*, 6(5): 358.

Panagopoulous DJ, Chavdoula ED, Karabarbounis A & Margaritis LH (2007) Comparison of bioactivity between GSM 900 MHz & DCS 1800 MHz mobile telephoney radiation. *Electromag. Biol. Med.*, 26: 33.

Parathath SR, Parathath S & Tsirka SE (2006) Nitric oxide neurodegeneration & breakdown of the blood brain barrier in tPA-dependent excitotoxic injury in mice. *J. Cell Sci.*, 119(pt2): 339.

Pardridge WM (1991) Blood brain barrier biology & methodology. *J. Neurovirol.*, 5(6): 556.

Parker JE & Winters W (1992) Expression of gene specific RNA in cultured cells exposed to rotating 60 Hz magnetic fields. *Biochem. Cell Biol.*, 70: 237.

Parker PJ, Stabel S & Waterfield MD (1984) Purification to homogeneity of protein Kinase C from bovine brain-identity with the phorbol ester. *EMBO J*, 3(5): 953.

Paulraj R & Behari J (2004) Radio frequency radiation effects on protein kinase C activity in rats' brain. *Mutat. Res.*, 545: 127.

Paulraj R & Behari J (2006) Single strand and DNA breaks in rat brain cells exposed to microwave radiation. *Mutat. Res.*, 596: 76.

Paulraj R & Behari J (2011) Effect of low level microwave radiation on carcinogenesis in swiss Albino mice. *Mol. Cell Biochem.*, 348(1–2): 191.

Penafiel LM, Litovitz T, Krause D, Desta A & Mullins JM (1997) Role of modulation on the effect of microwaves on ornithidine decarboxylase activity in L929 cells. *Bioelectromagnetics*, 18: 132.

Persson BRR, Salford LG & Brun A (1997) Bood – brain barrier permeability in rats exposed to electromagnetic fields used in wireless communication. Wireless networks-special issue: exposure hazards & health prediction in personal communication services. *Wireless Netw.*, 3(6): 455.

Pickard WF, Bisht KS, Leal BZ, Meltz ML, Roti JL, Straube WL & Moros EEG (2001) Cytogenic studies in human blood lymphocyte exposed in vitro to radiofrequency radiation at a cellular frequency (835.62 MHz, FDMA). *Radat. Res.*, 155: 113.

Podulso JF & Curran GL (1996) Increased permeability of superoxide dismutase at the blood-nerve & blood-brain barriers with retained enzymatic activity after covalent modification with naturally occurring polyamine putrescine. *J. Neurochem.*, 67: 734.

Porter R, Adey WR & Kado RT (1965) Measurement of electrica impedance in the human brain: somepreliminary observations. *Neurology*, 14: 1002.

Prakash P & Behari J (2009a) Synergistic effect of hydroxyapatite nanoparticles & pulsed electromagnetic field to prevent osteoporosis in rat induced by stimulated microgravity. *Int. J. Nanomed.*, 4: 133.

Ragabetli MC, Aydinlioglu A, Koyun N, Ragbetli C, Bektas S & Ozdemir S (2010) The effect of mobile phone on the number of Purkinje cells: a stereological study. *Intl. J. Radiat. Biol.*, 86(7): 548.

Ranck JB (1964) Specific impedance of cerebral cortex during spreading depression & an analysis of neuronal & interstitial contributions. *Exp. Neurol.*, 9: 1.

Ray S & Behari J (1987) Dielectric dispersion in rat brain tissue. In: Proceedings of the First Asia-Pacific Microwave Conference. Microwave Technology & Applications, p. 496.

Remondini D, Nylund R, Reivinen J, Poulletier de Gannes F, Veyret B, Lagroye I, Haro E, Trillo MA, Capri M, Franceschi C et al. (2006) Gene expression changes in human cells after exposure to mobile phone microwaves. *Proteomics*, 6(17): 4745.

Repacholi MH, Basten A, Gebski V, Noonan D, Finni J & Harris AW (1997) Lymphomas in E-Pim1 transgenic mice exposed to pulsed 900 MHz electromagnetic fields. *Radiat. Res.*, 147: 631.

Ritossa FM (1962) A new puffing pattern induced by a temperature shock & DNP in Drosophilla. *Exp. Basel*, 18: 571.

Robeldo J, Donnellan AM & Strandt-Conroy K (2012) An exploration of sensory & movement differences from the perspective of individuals with autism. *Front Integr. Neurosci.*, 6: 107.

Rojas DC, Maharaih K, Teale P & Rogers SJ (2008) Reduced neural synchronization of gamma-band MEG oscillations in first-degree relatives of children with autism. *BMC Psychiatry*, 8: 66.

Roschke J & Mann K (1997) No short term effects of digital mobile radio telephone on the awake human electroencephalogram. *Bioelectromagnetics*, 18: 172.

Rubin GJ, Das Munshi J & Wessely S (2005) Electromagnetic hypersensitivity: a systematic review of provocation studies. *Psychosom. Med.*, 67: 224.

Sacco RP, Curatolo B, Manzi B, Militerni R, Bravaccio C, Frolli A, Lenti C, Saccani M, Elia M, Reichelt KL, Pascucci T, Pluglisi-Allegra S & Persico AM (2010) Principal pathogenetic components & biological endophenotypes in autism spectrum disorders. *Autism Res.*, 3(5): 237.

Sage C, Johansson O & Sage SA (2007) Personal digital assistant (PDA) cell phone units produce units elevated extremely low frequency electromagnetic field emissions. *Bioelectromagnetics*, 28: 386.

Salama N, Kishimoto T & Kanayama HO (2010) Effects of exposure to a mobile phone on testicular function & structure in adult rabbit. *Int. J. Androl.*, 33(1): 88.

Salford LG, Brun A, Sturesson F, Eberhart JL & Persson BR (1994) Permeability of the blood-brain barrier induced by 915 MHz electromagnetic radiation, continuous wave & modulated at 8, 16, 50 & 200 Hz. *Microscopy Res. Tech.*, 27: 535.

Sanders AP, Joines WT & Allis JW (1984) The differential effects of 200, 591 &2450 MHz radiation on rat brain energy metabolism. *Bioelectromagnetics*, 5: 419.

Sandstrom M, Lyskev E, Hornsten R, Hansson MK, Wiklund U, Rask P, Klucharev V, Stenberg B & Bierle P (2003) Holter ECG monitoring in patients with prcieved electrical hypersensitivity. *Int J Psychophysiol.*, 49(3): 227.

Schwan HP (1977) Field interactions with biological matter. *Ann. N. Y. Acad. Sci.*, 303: 198.

Schwartz JL, House DE & Mealing GA (1990) Exposure of frog hearts to CW or amplitude modulated VHF fields: selective efflux of calcium ions at 16Hz. *Bioelectromagnetics*, 11: 349.

Scientific & Technological Options Assessment Stoa (2001) The Physiological & Environmental Effects of Non-Ionising Electromagnetic Radiation. Working document for STOA.

Sclye H (1946) The general adaption syndrome & diseases of adaption. *J. Clin. Endocrinol. Metab.*, 6: 117.

Scott IR, Wood SJ & Tattersell JEH (1998) Effects of radiofrequency radiation on long term potentiation in rat hippocampus slices. In: Poceedings of Bioelectromagnetics Society 20th Annual Meeting, St. Petersburg, FL.

Seitz H, Stinner D, Eikmann TH, Herr C & Röösli M (2005) Electromagnetic hypersensitivity (EHS) & subjective health complaints associated with electromagnetic fields of mobile phone communication – a literature review published between 2000 & 2004. *Sci. Total Environ.*, 349: 45.

Shandala M, Vinogradov GI, Rundev MI & Rudakov SF (1983) Influence of microwave radiation on some parameters of cellular immunity in conditions of chronic exposure. *Radio-biology*, XXIII(4): 544(in Russian).

Sharma PK, Pasqalotto FF, Nelson DR, Thomas AJ Jr. & Agarwal A (1999) The reactive oxygen species-total antioxidant capacity score is a new measure of oxidative stress to predict male infertility. *Hum. Reprod.*, 14: 2801.

Sienkiewicz Z, Jones N & Bottomley A (2005) Neurobehavioural effects of electromagnetic fields. *Bioelectromagnetics*, Sl7: S116–S126.

Sinclair WK (1981) Radiation protection: the NCRP guidelines & some considerations for the future. *Yale J. Biol. Med.*, 54(6): 471.

Singh NP & Stephenes RE (1998) X-ray induced DNA double strand breaks in human sperm. *Mutagen.*, 13: 75.

Smith R, Vantman D, Ponce J, Escobar J & Lissi E (1996) Andrology: total antioxidant capacity of human seminal plasma. *Hum. Reprod.*, 11(8): 1665.

Stam R (2010) Electromagnetic fields & the blood brain barrier. *Brain Res. Rev.*, 65(1): 80.

Stang A, Anastassiou G, Ahvens W, Bromen K, Bornfeldn K & Jockel K-H (2001) The possible role of radiofrequency radiation in the development of uveal melanoma. *Epidemiology*, 12(1): 7.

Strogatz SH (1987) Human sleep & circadian rhythms: a simple model based on two coupled oscillators. *J Math Biol.*, 25: 327.

Strogatz SH (2003) *Non Linear Dynamics & Chaos. With Applications to Physics, Biology, Chemistry & Engineering*. Advanced Book Program. Perseus Books CRC Press.

Stronati L, Testa A, Moquet J, Edwards A, Correlli E, Villani P, Marino C, Fresgna AM, Appolloni M & Lloyd D (2006) 935 MHz cellular phone radiation. An vitro study of genotoxicity in human lymphocytes. *Intl. J. Radiat. Biol.*, 82: 339.

Stuchly MA & Stuchly SS (1996) Dielectricproperties of biological substances-tabulated. *J. Microwave Power*, 15(1): 19.

Sun LX, Yao K, He JL, Lu DQ, Wang KJ & Li HW (2006) DNA damage & repair induced by acute exposure of microwave from mobile phone on cultured human lens epithelial cells. *zhonghua yank e Za Zhi*, 42: 1084.

Suzuk T (1994) Protein kinase C involved in the expression of long term potentiation. *Int. J. Biochem.*, 26: 735.

Syldona M (2007) Reducing the in-vitro electromagnetic field effect of cellular phones on human DNA & the intensity of their emitted radiation. *Acupunct Electrother Res.*, 32(1–2): 1.

Szmigielski A, Pietraszek A, Janiak M, Wrembel J, Kalczek M & Szigielski S (1982) Acceleration of the development of benzopyrene induced cancer in mice by microwave radiation. *Arch Dermatol Res.*, 274: 303.

Takano S, Takahashi T, Ohishi H, Kono S, Kawakami S & Iwai S (1999) Radical surgery for Budd-Chiari syndrome. Direct excision & repair for obstruction of the vena cava (Budd-Chiari syndrome) under hepatic vascular exclusion using a centrifugal pump. *Eur. J. Surg.*, 165(7): 632.

Takashima S, Gabriel C, Shepard RJ & Grant EH (1984) Dielectric behaviour of DNA solution at radio frequency & microwave frequencies. *J. Biophys.*, 46: 29.

Tamiya T, Yamasaki M, Maeo Y, Yamashiro T, Ogoshi S & Fujimoto S (1988) Complement activation in cardiopulmonary bypass, with special reference to anaphylatoxin production in membrane &bubble oxygenators. *Ann. Thorac. Surg.*, 46(1): 47.

Tattersall JE, Scott IR, Wood SJ, Nettel JJ, Bevir MK, Wang Z, Somasiri NP & Chen X (2001) Effect of low intensity radiofrequency electromagnetic field on electrical activity in rat hippocamapal slice. *Brain Res.*, 904(1): 43.

Taylor AMR, McConville CM & Byrd PJ (1994) Cancer & DNA processing disorders. *Brit. Med. Bull.*, 50: 708.

Teng J, Vanhoenacker D & Vander Vorst A (1989) Biological effects of microwave in acupuncture. In: 19th European Microwave Conference, London, p. 918.

Thuróczy G, Kubinyi G, Bodó M, Bakos J & Szabó LD (1994) Simultaneous response of brain electrical activity (EEG) & cerebral circulation (REG) to microwave exposure in rats. *Rev Environ Health*, 10(2): 135.

Tierney AL, Gabard-Durman L, Vogel Farley V, Tagwe-Flusberg H & Nelson CA (2012) Developmental trajectories of resting EEG power: an endophenotype of autism spectrum disorder. *PLoS One*, 7(6): e39127.

Valko M, Leibfritz D, Moncol J, Cromin MTD, Mazur M & Tesler J (2006) Free radicals and antioxidant in normal physiological functions and human disease. *Int. J. Biochem. Cell Biol.*, 39: 44.

Van Leeuwen P, Lange S, Bettermann H, Grönemeyer D & Hatzmann W (1999) Fetal heart rate variability & complexity in the course of pregnancy. *Early Hum. Dev.*, 54: 259.

Vander Vorst A, Teng J & Vanhoenacker D (1992) The action of microwave electromagnetic fields on the nervous system. *Actes Journees. Int. Antennes, Niece*, 111.

Vecchio FC, Babiloni C, Ferreri F, Circio G, Fini R, Del Percio C & Rossini PM (2007) Mobile phone emission modulates interhemispheric functional coupling of EEG alpha rhythms. *Eur J Neurosci.*, 25(6): 1908.

Verschaeve L (2008) Genetic damage in subjects exposed to radiofrequency radiation. *Mutat. Res.* doi:10.1016/jmrrev.2008.11.002

Verschaeve L (2014) Environmental impact of radiofrequency fields from mobile phone base stations. *Crit. Rev. Environ. Sci. Technol.*, 44: 1313.

Vinogradov G, Andrienko LG & Naumenko GM (1991) Phemomenon of adaptive immunity under the effect of non-ionisung microwave radiation. *Radiobiology*, 31: 718(In Russian).

Vinogradov G, Naumenko G, Vinarskaya E & Gonchar N (1987) Biological significance of auto immune reaction of the organism after exposure to environmental factors. *Gigiena I Sanitaria*, 1: 55(in Russian).

Vinogradov GI & Dumanski YD (1974) On the sensitization action of ultrahigh frequency electromagnetic fields. *Gig Sanit*, 9: 31(in Rusian).

Vinogradov GI & Naumenko G (1986) Experimental modelling of autoimmune reactions as affected by non-ionizing microwave radiation. *Radiobiology*, XXVI(5): 705.

Von Kltzng L (1995) Low frequency pulsed electromagnetic field influence EEG of man. *Phys. Med. Biol.*, XI(2): 77.

Wainwright P (2000) Thermal effects of radiation from cellular telephones. *Phys. Med. Biol.*, 45: 2363.

Wallenstein GV & Hasselmo ME (1997) Gabaergic modulation of hippocampal population activity: sequence learning, place field development, & the phase precession effect. *J. Neurohysiol.*, 78: 393.

Wass S (2011) Distortions & disconnections: disrupted brain connectivity in autism. *Brain Cong.*, 75(1): 18.

Wdowiak A, Wdowiak L & Wiktor H (2007) Evaluation of the effect of using mobile phones on male fertility. *Ann. Aqric. Environ. Med.*, 14: 169.

WHO (World Health Organization) United Nations Environment Programme? World Health Organization/International Radiation Protection Association (1993) *Electromagnetic Fields (300 Hz-300 GHz)*. Geneva: WorldHealth Organization, Environmemtal Health Criteria, Vol 137, p. 494.

WHO (World Health Organization) (2005) *Electromagnetic Fields & Public Health. Electromagnetic Hypersensitivity. WHO Fact Sheet No 296*. Geneva: World Health Organization.

Wiseman H, Kaur H & Halliwell B (1995) DNA damage & cancer: measurement & mechanism. *Cancer Lett*, 93(1): 113.

Witter FR, Zimmerman AW, Reichmann JP & Connors SL (2009) In utero beta 2 adrenergic agonist exposure & adverse neurophysiologic & behavioural outcomes. *Am J Obstet Gynecol*, 201(6): 553.

Yan JG, Agresti M, Bruce T, Yan YH, Ganlund A & Matloub HS (2007) Effect of cellular phone emissions on sperm motility in rats. *Fertil. Sterli.*, 88(4): 957.

Yang X, He G, Hao Y, Chen C, Li Y, Wang Y & Zhang G (2010) The role of the JAK2-STAT3 pathway in pro-inflammatory responses of EMF-stimulated N9 microglial cells. *J. Neuroinflammation*, 7: 54.

Zeni O, Chiavoni AS, Sannino A, Antolini A, Forigo D, Bersani F et al. (2003) Lack of genotoxic effects (micronucleus induction) in human lymphocytes exposed in vitro to 900 MHz electromagnetic fields. *Radiat. Res.*, 160: 152.

Zhao TY, Zou SP & Knapp PE (2007) Exposure to cell phone radiation up regulates apoptosis genes in primary cultures of neurons & astrocytes. *Neurosci. Lett.*, 412: 34.

Zhou J, Gennatas ED, Kramer JH, Miller BL & Seeley WW (2012) Predicting regional neurodegeneration from the healthy brain functional connectome. *Neuro.*, 73(6): 1060.

5

Biological Responses of Mobile Phone Frequency Exposure

5.1 Introduction

A large number of individuals (>10^9 worldwide) are exposed to the radiofrequency (RF) signals from cellular phones and other personal communication services and the number is increasing exponentially. Cellular phones are defined as devices emitting radiofrequency electromagnetic waves (RF-EMW). These waves transmit signals from cellular phone to the base stations and antennas. Since mobile phones and other wireless gadgets are held close to the body and are used frequently, these devices are potentially the most dangerous sources of electromagnetic radiation that the average person possesses. The increasing scientific evidence of various health hazards on exposure of radiofrequency radiation (RFR) emitted from both the cell phones and base stations have caused significant media attention and public discussion in recent years. This has given rise to an increasing concern for any unknown effects that may be potentially detrimental to the human health. Antennas of modern mobile telephones are located close to the head and the radiations from base stations are distributed all over in areas around it. There is now an added worry if these radiations are carcinogenic or tumor promoter or have any other health implications. There is another concern, if the mechanism of interaction of RF fields with developing tissues of children and fetuses may be different from that of adults due to their smaller physical dimension size and variation in tissue electromagnetic properties.

Regionally, cancer incidence has distribution due to variations in age and gender besides many others. Global system for mobile communication (GSM) radiation does seem to affect a variety of brain functions (including neuroendocrine systems) and health problems reportedly happen to be neurological. It may be pointed out that mobile phone frequency has two components: one is the continuous wave (CW) and other in the low frequency range (8.3 Hz). The latter is close to delta and alpha range of brain wave frequencies, having similarity in the oscillatory behavior, and therefore a possibility of mutual interactions seems possible.

Salford et al. (2003) reported neuronal damage caused by nonthermal microwave (MW) exposure. The cortex as well as the hippocampus and the basal ganglia in the brains of exposed rats contain dark neurons.

The mobile system may be classified as analog (advanced mobile phone system—AMPS). On the other hand, digital cellular phones operate under various standards such as GSM and digital AMPS (DAMPS). All the systems developed for cellular phones transmit encoded, digitized information using some form of phase or frequency modulation (Penafiel et al. 1997). Two low-frequency waves of GSM at 8.3 and 217 Hz act on the composite pulsed GSM signal in which these frequencies are present. This signal carries no power when the user is not talking or receiving but when the user communicates the power of this electromagnetic field (EMF) reaches a maximum of 250 mW. This leads to raises a question regarding the negative effect on human health. In the present day technology, the specific absorption rate of mobile phone varies in the range 0.1–1.2 W/kg depending upon the manufacturing details. Based on this criterion, the field emission from these devices remains below the known safety limits.

The development of wireless (mobile) telephony has resulted in the transmission and propagation of microwaves modulated by very specific signals. Radio waves transmitted by mobile phones of the GSM type present a characteristic pattern that results from the particular time structure of such a signal (time division multiple access, TDMA). It is an electromagnetic signal with extremely low frequency (ELF) modulated pulsed microwave carrier. This is not the case for analog radio and television. One may say that digital cellular phones using the GSM system transmit information in bursts of microwaves. The presence of ELF components in the signal and the bursting activity of these waves have given rise to a new controversial question: Can this signal structure exert a negative influence on human head tissues and more specifically on the brain by way of inducing non-thermal effects? This stems from the fact that modulated or pulsed radio frequency radiations are more effective in producing biological effects. They may produce a different effect when compared with continuous wave radiation of the same or different frequency, as modulated signal carries multiplicity of messages. This finding is important because mobile telephonic radiation is modulated at low frequencies. Biological effects of extremely low frequency (<100 Hz) electric and magnetic fields are well established. Therefore, frequency, intensity, exposure duration, and the number of exposure episodes can affect the exposure to radio frequency radiations.

While mobile phones are handheld, wireless communication systems operate at several frequencies in the electromagnetic spectrum. In the United States, it operates at two frequencies: the old existing ones at 850 MHz and the newer personal communication services at 1900 MHz (Figure 5.1). European mobile phones operate at slightly different frequencies than these. In 2G system, frequencies used were 800–900 MHz, extending upto 1800 MHz in Europe and 1500 MHz in Japan. 2G phones mainly employed the TDMA

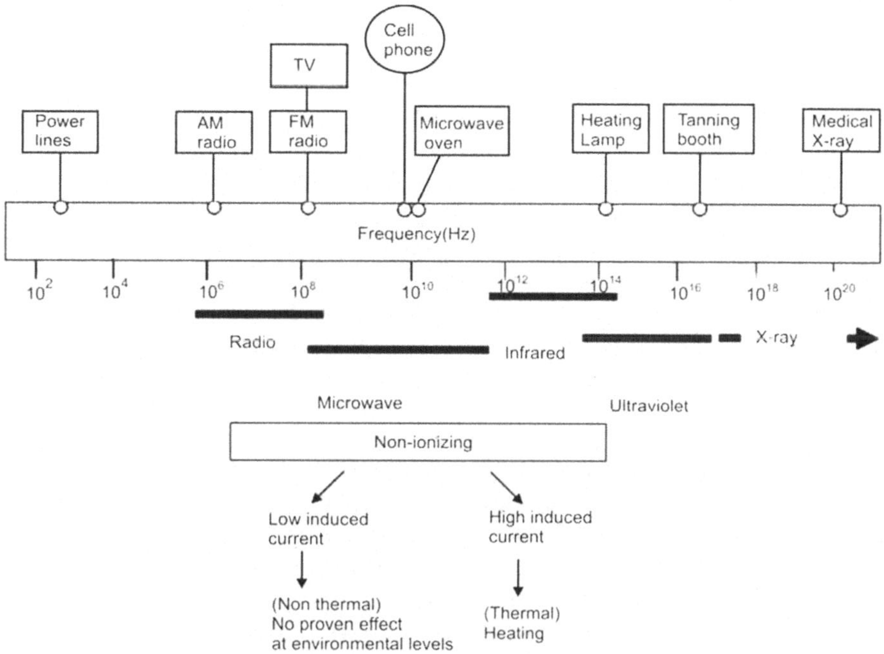

FIGURE 5.1
In terms of the electromagnetic spectrum, cell phones fall between microwave ovens and TV transmitters. Such radiation, through nonionizing, can induce biologically significant effects.

system, and the waveforms were pulsed ones. The characteristic for 3G is higher data rates, which may go as high as 384 kbits to 2 Mbits. The maximum power from a mobile 3G phone (2100 MHz) is 0.125 watts produced over 0.2 MHz. On the other hand, GSM phones (900 and 1800 MHz) have a maximum power of 1 watt. In recent years, 2G system is partially replaced by 3G and 4G (2300 MHz) system in India. In wireless communications ranging from 1G to 4G (400–2700 MHz), and possibility of 5G (6GHz), energy exposures that occur from these radiations are very broad and more so in view of the fact that mode of interaction is frequency dependent. This implies that the talk of one single number as criteria for safe exposure (like for ionizing radiation) is not possible. Before 1990 the range of microwave exposure was only limited to 0.800–3 GHz. However, the waveform of interest has been changing. An in vitro experimental investigation was conducted to verify if pure magnetic fields at 8.3 and 217 Hz could induce any effect on the spontaneous bioelectric activity of the neurons from the brain ganglia of the snail Helix aspersa (Azanza et al. 2002). Changes have been observed, as well as the reversibility of the effects induced under exposure to magnetic fields of low magnetic flux densities in the ranges of 0.37–6.68 and

0.6–3.6 mT for 8.3 and 217 Hz, respectively. Mobile phones generate magnetic pulses that peak at several tens of micro tesla, while biological effects are reported around 0.2 μT (Jokela et al. 2004; Sage et al. 2007; Manjhi et al. 2013). The results indicated that, in most cases, the neurons reacted to the lowest values of applied magnetic flux density, that is, 50 μT, and that some neurons would probably react to even a lower exposure level (Lederer et al. 2001). A second series of results demonstrated the ability of the neurons to recover their spontaneous activity, after it has been modified under exposure to 8.3 and 217 Hz sinusoidal applied magnetic flux density values between 0.6 and 6.68 mT. These results show the reversibility of the bioelectric-induced alterations on neurons under the specified experimental conditions. The investigations are important in view of obtaining practical conclusions about sensitivity threshold and reversibility for actual mobile phone ELF magnetic field exposure.

Mobile telecommunication equipment consists of a single unit with integrated microphone, ear piece, transreceiver, and antenna. Mobile phone operates at low power levels: 600 mW in case of analog, while 125 mW in case of digital phones. It is speculated that these may possibly cause exposure level limit close or above the prescribed limit, which has many uncertainties. Fields induced inside the head depends upon the position of the handset with respect to the head and the electric properties of the tissues. The problem is further compounded because different types of antennas cause different amount of field induced in the human head (Jansen & Rahmat-Samii 1995). The telephone antennas are modeled as a dipole or monopole on a metal box (Figure 5.2). These have led to (a) characterization of the performance of antenna of the cellular phones and to improve upon it at various distances of the antenna with respect to the head in various configurations and (b) to compute the RF energy deposition in various tissues and to calculate the specific absorption rate (SAR). This can be compared with the suggested standards (ANSI/IEEE C95.1 1992; Stuchly 1994).

Since mobile phones are used close to the head, the emitted radiations are absorbed by the brain (Ismail & Ibrahim 2002). A typical value of the distance between antenna and head is about 2 cm or less. Microwaves in the frequency range 800–1000 MHz can penetrate the cranium and nearly 40% of these can reach the deep brain (Kang et al. 2001; Klemn & Troester 2006; Barnett et al. 2007). The energy corresponding to these frequencies is insufficient to knock an electron from atoms in a living tissue and belong to the nonionizing part of the electromagnetic spectrum. A commonly occurring partial body exposure of humans to microwave radiation occurs with the use of cellular phones. Owing to the proximity of the phone antenna to the head, much effort has gone into determining the dosimetry profile of microwaves in the head in various possible configurations (Figures 5.3a and 5.3b). The geometry of holding a mobile phone suggests that the exposure will be principally to the side of the head for the

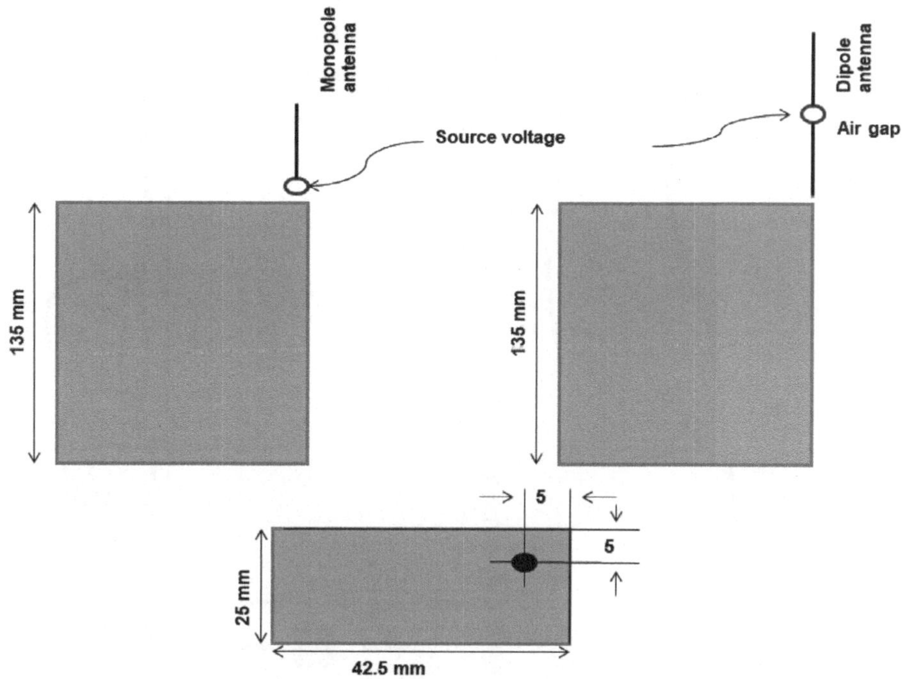

FIGURE 5.2
Portable radio models related to human health.

handheld use or to the other parts of the body closest to the phone during hands-free use. Accordingly, cell phone radiation intensity decreases as the distance from the cell phone increases, suggesting the possibility of showing variability of effects if the cell phone is only a short distance away. By contrast, the use of headsets connected to the cell phone may greatly reduce the absorbed cell phone radiation. Wearing an air-tube headset has been found to intensify radiation into the ear canal, the wire being a transmitter of radiation and serving as an antenna that can attract EMFs from the surroundings. Microwaves used by mobile cells are generated by an antenna and are carried by line of sight propagation to the transmitter. In between the path of this propagation, these low-intensity radiations fall on biological objects. Frey (1998) opined that headache was linked to microwave emissions from cellular phones. The body of research is controversial in several respects since the experimental results as of now are mostly understood in terms of thermal effects. However, the effects due to nonthermal effects are amply documented, though not fully understood. The accepted existence of nonthermal phenomena in biological systems is difficult to explain within the framework of known laws of physics.

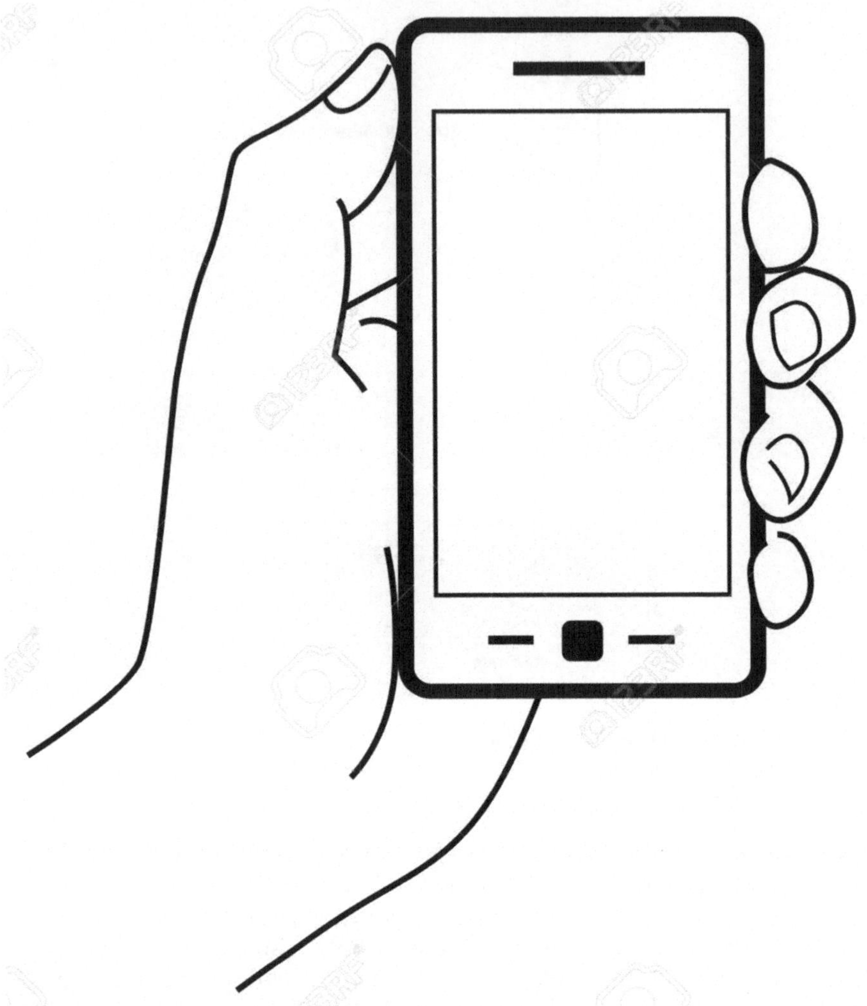

FIGURE 5.3a
A normal way of holding mobile phone.

In the frequency range of 40 MHz to 6 GHz, the electromagnetic field penetrates deep into the tissue, causing an increase in the random molecular motion. This is suggestive that while defining the exposure time and the volume of the tissue over which the temperature rise is measured needs to be defined. The tissue shape is often taken as cubic, largely for geometric and numerical convenience. In the process of electromagnetic (EM) propagation, radiation falling on the population and hence in the process the energy is intercepted by the human body (or any other biological object) and

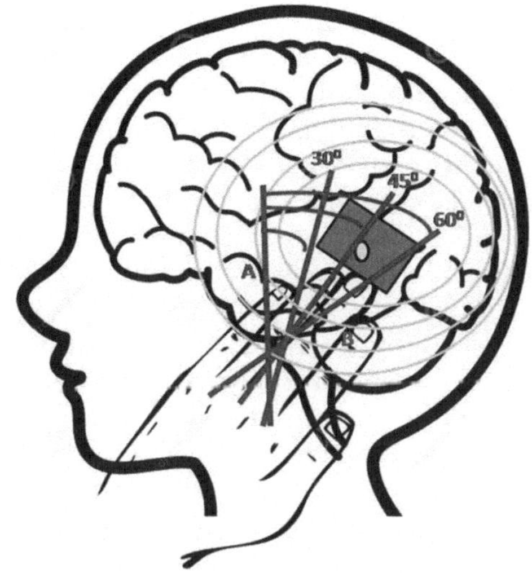

FIGURE 5.3b
Ahead model with telephone in (a) vertical and (b) tilted 30°–45°–60° position.

subsequent absorption is dependent upon several parameters, viz., part body/full body exposure, l/λ (length of the body/wavelength of incident radiation), resonant/nonresonant absorption, deviation and signal type (pulsating sine, triangular, etc.), polarization of the radiation, coupling of the energy to the body, and if the body is grounded or not, besides several others. Some people may also be adversely affected by the environmental impact of mobile phone base stations located near their homes, schools, and several other places. In the phones used, the field emissions may extend over a wide range, which may have different mode of interaction. Also at any instance of time differentiation between thermal and nonthermal effect or their combination is difficult to distinguish (Zhao et al. 2007). Obviously, several of these parameters are uncontrollable and hence the computation of the amount of energy actually deposited on the biological body remains uncertain. This further makes the estimation of the bioeffects and safe exposure criteria from such exposures open to question.

5.2 Mobile and Wireless Communication Technology

The mechanism of cell phones functioning is such that the wave produced from the speaker goes through a transmitter that converts the sound into electrical sine wave. This sine wave then travels to the antenna, which then projects the wave out into space. Average power usage of the transmitter is about 0.75 to 1 W, with a maximum of 2W. The propagation of the electric sine wave through the transmitter circuit also yields an electromagnetic field. As the electric current oscillates back and forth, these electromagnetic fields continue to build up and collapse, resulting in electromagnetic radiation (How cell-phone radiation works 2007).

Since the development of analogue cellular radio systems, the development of cellular mobile communication technology has developed very fast. In the first generation of mobile telephones was the analogue system operating at 800/900 MHz adopting frequency modulation. This service has either been abandoned or is not much used. In 2G carrier frequencies, the frequency bandwidth of each frequency is around 200 kHz, and a 9.6 kbits/s data rate for encoded speech. In Europe and India, GSM (217 Hz with duty ratio of 1/8) is used. Hence, it is a burst type transmission, apart from the access frequency of 217 Hz and its harmonics, there are various control and system signals giving rise to power variations at the frequency of 2 and 8 Hz and are more bioactive producing biological effects by a mechanism different from a single frequency. This provides greater probability of interaction by generating heat energy (thermal interaction) from handsets being held against the head while a call is made.

The mobile phone network consists of a system of adjoining zones called cells (Figure 5.4). Each cell has its own base station that sends and receives radio signals throughout its specified zone. Microcells provide the main structure for the network and the base stations have power outputs of tens of watts and communicate with phones upto a few tens of kilometers distance (35 km in case of GSM). Microcells are used to infill and improve the main network, especially when the volume of calls is high. The microcell base stations emit less power (a few watts) and have an effective range of a few hundred meters. Picocell base station has a lower power gain (fraction of a watt) and provides short-range communication, may be inside buildings.

The modulated wave (RF wave intermixed with an extremely low frequency wave) carries the desired information. The change from analogue to digital technology is to meet the demand for more data and faster transmission. To show the variation in power density, measurements were performed in the vicinity of 20 randomly selected GSM microcells and picocells (Cooper et al. 2006). The antenna heights ranged between 2.5 and 9 m and the total radiated power was in the range 1–5 W. The average power density at a distance of 1m was about $2 \times 10^{-2} Wm^{-2}$, which decreased to about 2×10^{-6} Wm^{-2} at 100 m, well within the limits of safe exposure.

Hand Holding a Handset

Generally, the hand holding the handset is made up of a metal covered with a thin lossless dielectric. This decreases the radiated power due to the

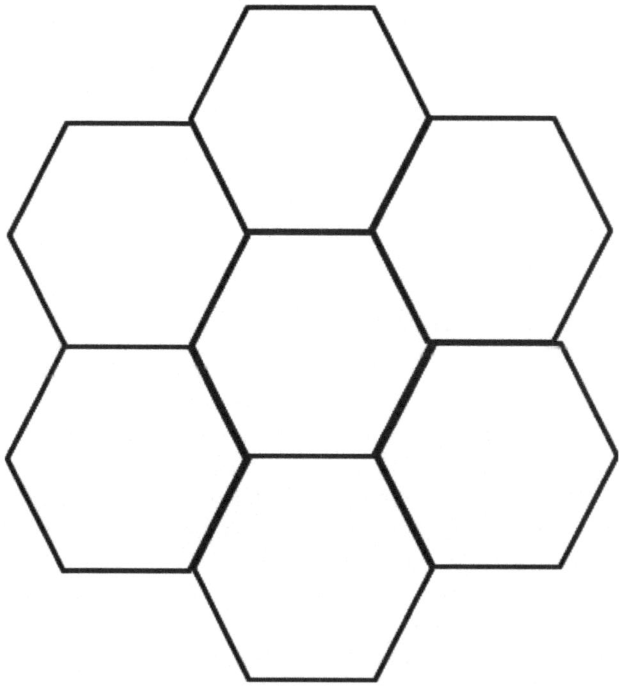

FIGURE 5.4
The mobile phone network and adjoining zones. While normally the base stations are placed at the center of the cells, it is also possible to use edge excited cells where base stations are placed at the vertices.

power absorption in the hand. A simple unoptimized choke that provides an apparent open circuit on the upper surface of the antenna box improves the antenna efficiency from 61 to 70% compared to 77% without the hand (separation of 3 cm between the antenna and the head). Correspondingly, the peak SAR in the head decreases to 5.8 W/kg from 14 W/kg. Handling of a mobile phone is shown in Figure 5.3b. The maximum local SAR decreases as the separation between head and the mobile phone increases. Changes occur in the antenna efficiency, power deposited, and SARs with separation between the antenna and various positions of the head. Since the handheld portable mobile radios are operated at 900MHz or at 1500–1800 MHz, or even above, and as such the wavelength of the EMFs which they produce are much shorter than the whole human body. It is assumed in all the computation that the radio is located in the vicinity of the head.

There are reports indicating adverse health effects of cell phones which emit electromagnetic radiation, with maximum value of 50% of their energy being deposited when held close to the head. Also there is a likelihood that fields emanating from base stations (though very weak) would create a health hazard, though the issue is still being debated. It is therefore suggestive to better understand the mechanism of electromagnetic field effects over a wide frequency band at the existing level of radiofrequency/microwave exposure from various devices and in the environment.

5.3 Antenna Head Separation

The computed values suggest that when the mobile is located within the vicinity of the head, the lower portion of the body does not affect the distribution of SAR within the head. Watanabe et al. (1995) examined the validity of the SAR distribution in an isolated head model and compared with that in a whole body model when both models were exposed to the near field of a short electric dipole at 300 MHz. Subsequently, Watanabe et al. (1996) have also carried out SAR distribution in 1 × 1 × 1 cm cubical cells. The calculations were carried out using finite time difference technique (FTDT). These authors reported that the distribution on the surface of the isolated head model agreed well with that of the whole body model: The difference of the maximum local SARs on the surface was within 2%. The difference between the local SARs calculated with these models were as much as 37% in the deep region of the head, the absorption in the deep region is much smaller (not significant) than the surface absorption. The handheld portable radio was assumed to be a 135 × 42.5 × 25 mm conducting box with either 1/2-wavelength dipole antenna or a 1/4-wavelenth monopole antenna on its upper plane (Figure 5.2). It was located on the left side of the head. These authors rotated the hand and a radio by 60°so that the radio was positioned between the operator's mouth and ear. They reported that the radiation pattern of the antenna is significantly modified with the user's hand.

It was concluded that:

1. The maximum local SAR decreases as the distance between head and antenna increases, and is independent of whether the antenna is a $(1/2)\lambda$ dipole or a $(1/4)\lambda$ monopole. This proportion to $d^{-3/2}$ also does not depend on the frequency (900 MHz or 1.5 GHz).
2. When the auricle is located in the vicinity of the head, the maximum local SARs in the homogenous head model agree well with those in the heterogeneous model.
3. The maximum local SARs in the head do not depend on the position of the head holding the radio as long as the antenna is not obstructed by the hand or by other parts of the body.

TABLE 5.1

Effects of the change in the separation between the antenna and the head model; 915 MHz, 1 W (Partially adopted from Okoniewski & Stuchly 1996)

Model	Separation (cm)	Efficiency (%)	P_{abs} (W)	SAR in the head (W/kg)		
				Peak	1 g	10 g
Homogeneous box	1.5	16	0.84	18.1	14.1	9.25
	3.0	51	0.49	3.2	2.6	1.9
Homogeneous sphere	1.5	46	0.54	13.4	10.9	7.0

SARs obtained experimentally were significantly less than those calculated numerically. This may be because of missing links in the computational modeling.

Effects of the changes in the separation between the antenna and the head model (915 MHz, 1 W) are shown in Table 5.1. Changes in the antenna efficiency, power deposited, and SARs with separation between the antenna and various locations of the head suggest that the box head model is not adequate even for larger separations. The similarities, in terms of the result obtained between the spherical model and the simpler head model without an ear, remain even for larger separation. A comparison between the Gent and Yale heads suggests that the 3.0 and 1.5 cm are equivalent. This observation is further supported by an approximate separation due to the ear thickness. These results are in good agreement with those reported by other workers (Douglas et al. 1995; Jansen & Rahmat-Samii 1995).

5.4 Dosimetry over the Electromagnetic Spectrum

Low frequency has been a source of signal generation and transmission in the biological media to control the physiological events. While estimating the biological implications, it is therefore imperative that their role may also be assessed.

Personal digital assistant (PDA) cell phone units produce extremely low frequency electromagnetic field emissions (Sage et al. 2007). At frequencies below 100 kHz, many biological effects are quantified in terms of the current density in tissue and this parameter is most often used as a dosimetric quantity. At higher frequencies, many (but not all) interactions are due to the rate of energy deposition per unit mass. This is why SAR is used as the dosimetric measure. It is expressed in watts per kilogram (W/kg) and is based on absorption only. This raises questions about using this parameter for evaluating effects that may be of another nature than absorption. In this connection, the possibility of having only the SAR for evaluating all the biological effects is open to further investigations.

In the expression for that of temperature rise (Equation (4.1)), it is assumed that measurements are made where no heat loss occurs by thermal diffusion, heat radiation, or thermoregulation (blood flow, sweating, etc.) With this definition, one measures SAR due to mobile phone emissions in brain and also estimates its value by using complex computation formalism.

It is said that Poynting's theorem expresses equality between the space variation of EM power and the time variation of EM energy. However, temperature is not an EM parameter: It is an absorption loss and there is a temperature elevation when the SAR is positive. Using EM theory, only thermal effects can be evaluated and in principle, possibility of nonthermal effects cannot be investigated.

From Equations (4.2), it is obvious that the basic understanding of the implications of mobile phones is the knowledge of SAR and so of the induced fields, where σ is dependent on the spatial location of the site in question, and hence SAR varies from point to point. A reduction in the output of the mobile phone is a suggestive parameter for immunity from adverse effects. However, a lower power output would require the need to have many more closely spaced base stations, which may not go well with the environmentalists. Moving antennas to a larger distance from the user's head would require a larger handset size, again contrary to the requirement of user. The computation of the induced fields in head is complicated and depends upon a number of parameters, viz., (i) operational frequency and the antenna input power, (ii) position of the device with respect to the head, (iii) design of the device vis-à-vis the outer shape of the head, and (iv) the dielectric properties of the tissue and the shape of head. Out of these (iii) and (iv) are the subject of the technical details and that of the individual. Subsequent to the above computation of SAR in the human head, various approaches using anatomically derived structure, based on magnetic resonance imaging (MRI), were adopted for homogenous and heterogeneous head-shaped volume (Dimbylow & Mann 1994; Gandhi 1995; Jansen & Rahmat-Samii 1995; Martens et al. 1995; Gandhi et al. 1996). Most of these authors have used finite difference time domain technique (FDTD) for the analysis because of the flexibility and efficiency in solving complex heterogeneous geometries.

Okoniewski and Stuchly (1996) used Yee cell rectangular grid (Yee 1996) and the total field formulation (Taflove 1995). The computational space was truncated by a perfectly matched layer (Berenger 1994) of seven-cell thickness with a parabolic profile to ensure reflections below at least 40 dB. Two mesh sizes used were either 5 or 3.4 mm. In case where the metal surfaces did not coincide with the mesh, an algorithm was used that allows for accurate treatment of fields near these surfaces (Anderson et al. 1996). These authors obtained far-field antenna pattern from the computed near-field electric and magnetic field vectors on a box enclosing the modeled structures using the field equivalence principle. The antenna efficiency (η) turns out to be as follows:

$$\eta = P_{\mathrm{rad}}/(P_{\mathrm{rad}} + P_{\mathrm{abs}}). \tag{5.1}$$

where P_{rad} is the power radiated by the antenna and P_{abs} the power absorbed by the head. These authors used distance d between the monopole and the closest head surface. The following formulation applies: (1) the steady-state radiated power from the antenna is 1 W (i.e., the power radiated in the far field plus the power dissipated in the head and hand) and (2) the antenna patterns are normalized in respect to those obtained for the Yale head model and for 3 cm separation between the handset and the head using 5 mm FDTD mesh.

The box model of the head at close distance to the phone gives lower antenna efficiency and higher absorbed power in the head and as such higher SARs in comparison to other models. Spherical models provide estimates of the antenna efficiency and total absorbed power that are in reasonably good agreement with relatively low-resolution head models. These authors have further concluded that spherical (and box) models of the head give overestimated values of the decrease in antenna efficiency as well as of the total power absorbed and various local and limited volume averaged SARs. The box representing the head nearly entirely blocks the radiation in the head direction. In the case of sphere, there is a significant reduction in power radiated toward the half space where the head is located.

Okoniewski and Stuchly (1996) have described three types of models, viz., dielectric covered metal box for a three-layered tissue box, sphere, and an anatomically correct (Yale) head model. The computations were carried out at 915 MHz. They concluded that the effect of the anatomically correct head is well stimulated (±3 dB) by a three-layered sphere. This result further confirms the findings of Jansen and Rahmat-Samii (1995) who used a less anatomically correct model of the head and a different antenna. The differences they computed were somewhat bigger, which are explained by the different antenna geometry. As the distance increases the antenna pattern is less affected and less power is radiated toward the head direction.

In the model of the mobile phone, the calculated peak local SAR over 10 g is lower than the limit of 2 W/kg given by the International Commission for Non-Ionizing Radiation Protection (ICNIRP). The power absorption budget by tissues indicates that more than half of the power is absorbed by the skin (absorption at 1800 MHz is more superficial than at

900 MHz). As the brain is nearer to the mobile phone in the case of the CS head, one finds that the power absorption in the brain of the CS is slightly more significant than that for the adult, while it remains at a weak level of exposure (from one-third to one-half maximum) of the SAR on 10 g in the head.

When EM fields pass from one medium to another (air to biological tissues), they can be reflected, refracted, transmitted, or absorbed, depending on the complex conductivity of the exposed body and the frequency of the source. Absorbed RF energy can be converted to other form of energy and cause interference with the functioning of the living system. Most of this energy is converted into heat (absorption). However, not all EM field effects can be explained in terms of energy absorption and conversion by this process.

5.5 Functioning of Cellular Phone Towers

The location of the cell phone base stations may be free standing towers or can also be mounted on existing structures, for example, trees, water tanks, or tall buildings. The antennas need to be high enough to adequately cover the area and as such the base stations are usually kept 50–200 feet high. At very high power levels, RF waves can heat up body tissues (i.e., how the microwave ovens work). But the levels of energy used by cell phones and towers are much lower.

When a person makes a cell phone call, a signal is sent from the phone's antenna to the nearest base station antenna. The base station responds to this signal by assigning it an available radiofrequency channel. RF waves transfer the voice information to the base station. The voice signals are then sent to a switching center, which transfers the call to its destination. Voice signals are then relayed back and forth during the call. The accidental exposure of these radiations produced at the base station is given off and forms a part of the environment, where they interact with human populations. To assess the total exposure scenario, it often happens that exposure from mobile phones is clubbed with those from base stations. However, the difference between the two lies in that in one case (mobile phone)it is the local exposure and that from towers is the total body exposure. Also, the exposure from mobile towers is over a period of a longer duration (with less intensity) and from mobile phones are of comparatively shorter duration (controllable) but comparatively of higher intensity. The exposures from mobile towers are of several orders of magnitude less than that of INCIRP guidelines.

The energy from a cellular phone tower antenna, like that of other telecommunication antennas, is directed toward the horizon (parallel to the ground), with some downward scatter. Base station antennas use higher power levels than other types of land-mobile antennas, but much lower levels than those from radio and television broadcast stations. The amount of energy decreases rapidly as the distance from the antenna increases. As a result, the level of exposure to radio waves at ground level is very low compared to the level close to the antenna. The RF waves produced at the base stations escape into the environment. However, the public exposure to radio waves from cell phone tower antennas is marginal for several reasons. The power levels are relatively low, the antennas are mounted high above ground level, and the signals are transmitted intermittently, rather than continuously. The GSM cellular phone tower radiation is the dominating HF source in residential areas.

5.6 Health Hazards due to Cellular Phone Frequencies

Christoph and Hacker (2009) found that people who lived within 100 m of cell phone towers had greater salivary alpha-amylase levels. Keeping this in view (and may be many others), special attention has been drawn to the biological effects of EMFs(more due to mobile frequencies)on human body in general, and particularly on nervous and reproductive system. This is because the positioning of the cellular phone may have proximity to one of these organs at a given instance. It can be visualized that cells from higher metabolic rate will be more susceptible to EMF. This is so because more hydrogen peroxide is generated by mitochondria to excite the reaction. The proximity of EMF to interact with iron particles provides a greater clue for higher vulnerability of cell having higher content of intracellular free ions. There are reports confirming biological hazards due to these exposures coming in, while contradictions are also available in literature, the issue appears to be far from resolved. This probably emanates because of different protocols, the type of input signals, the relative orientation and distance between the body and the electronic system devise, and the inherent variability involved in the biological systems.

Scientists are generally in agreement that an exposure to cell phone radiation can possibly cause cancer in humans, thereby putting mobiles in the same risk category as lead, pesticides such as DDT, engine exhaust, and chloroform. The International Agency for Research on Cancer (IARC) also noted that exposure of the brain to RF fields from cell phone base stations (mounted on roofs or towers) is less than 1/100th the exposure of the brain to mobile phones, and yet some adverse effects are reported. Within this the issue of a possible link between cell phone radiation and brain cancer is now a matter of increasing concern and hence has become a subject of renewed investigation.

Whole Body Exposure and Mobile Phone Radiation

When the microwave power from mobile phone falls on the human head, it is nonuniformly distributed over the exposed volume. Inside and outside body geometries also influence the amount of microwave absorption by the human body. It may be mentioned that the maximum absorption in the animal brain exceeds by a factor of two than in the human brain. At 2450 MHz exposure, there is maximum absorption in the anterior (front portion) of the simulated human brain, while there is maximum absorption in the center portion of the simulated animal brain. The animal brain receives a maximum absorption four times that of the human brain. The peak absorption is related to the occurrence of "hot spots" or maxima in the internal absorption. The occurrence of peak is dependent upon the frequency of exposure. With the increase of the exposure frequency ($1/\lambda$) beyond the peak absorption value, the maximum absorption shifts toward the surface with the disappearance of the "hot spots." This is caused by the decreasing depth of the penetration with the increase in the frequency (reducing wavelength) of exposure.

Based on modeling it has been estimated that SAR to head from a 900 MHz cellular telephone vary from 0.16 to 0.69W/kg and for the brain 0.06–0.41 W/kg (Gandhi 1995). However, a similar examination by Dimbylow and Mann (1994) with a vertical or a lateral antenna suggests a 3–4 W/kg averaged over 1 g. The calculations by Excell (1988), based on MRI and FDTD techniques, suggest higher SAR values upto 4.2 W/kg rising to 8.2 W/kg at 1800 MHz. A level of 1 W/kg is expected to increase raise the temperature by <0.5 °C. Even though the power deposited in the head is lower than that prescribed by safety considerations (Gandhi et al. 1996), there are still biological effects (at times called hazards) of nonthermal origin. These effects are caused by low-intensity or ultralow-intensity fields.

Correspondingly, nonthermal effects have also been reported ranging from changes in permeability of the blood–brain barrier and ocular symptoms to biochemical changes (Fritze et al. 1997; Balik et al. 2005; Curcio et al. 2005; Belyaev et al. 2006; Behari 2009; Kumar et al. 2010). Calculation of the maximum temperature rise in the head from RF exposure during mobile phone use suggests the increase in temperature of no more than about 0.1 °C (Tahvanainen et al. 2007). Thus, if there are health effects from RF exposure, they are unlikely to be due to any temperature rise. As further indication to this DNA strand break and generation of micronuclei, there has been a clear indication of genotoxic effects (Zmyslony et al. 2000;Lai & Singh 2004; Belyaev et al. 2006; Kumar et al. 2010). Nittby et al. (2008a) reported cognitive alterations in GSM-exposed animals as compared to sham-exposed ones.

Long-Term Exposure

Long-term exposure of mouse (Repacholi et al. 1997) showed an elevated risk of developing lymphoma in a transgenic strain. Use of phone in driving stimulator leads to negative reaction time. Evidence for a direct memory effect on brain slices from the hippocampus of rat showed changes in long-term potentiation when exposed to 915 MHz (Scott et al. 1998). Mild et al. (1998) looking for a subjective response, suggested increased headache or sensation of warmth when using mobile phones. Braune et al. (1998) reported blood pressure increase (5–10 mm Hg) induced by exposure to the right side of the head. However, Barker et al. (2007) in a double blind study reported no effect of GSM and TETRA signals on blood pressure and related physiological parameters. They also did not report any significant differences between the mean concentration of adrenaline and noradrenaline. Röschke and Mann (1997) did not notice any difference in the awake electroencephalograms (EEG) of subjects exposed to radiation emitted by cellular phones.

A ten year long study carried out by World Health Organization on cell phone and cancer (INTERPHONE Study 2010) confirms that regular use of cell phone by adults can significantly increase the risk of glioma by 40% with 1640 h or more of use. Tumors were more likely to occur on the side of the head most used for calling. The risk is likely to increase to 96% for adults with ipsilateral cell phone use. This study further revealed that the group who ever used mobile phones to those who never used yielded an odd ratio (OR) of 0.81. Association between glioma and cumulative specific energy absorbed at the tumor location was examined in a subset of 553 cases. The OR for glioma increased with increasing RF dose for exposures 7 years or more before diagnosis, whereas there was no association with estimated dose for exposures less than 7years before diagnosis (Baan et al. 2011).

5.7 Biological Implications

The biological implications due to cell phone use have started appearing (Frei et al. 2009), when it was demonstrated to cause dose-dependent difficulty in concentration, fatigue, and headache (Oftedal et al. 2007) and an increase in reaction time (Preece et al. 1999). The emitted microwaves from communication gadgets devises are shown to alter cognitive functions (Keetly et al. 2006; Nittby et al. 2008a), decrease in cholinergic activity (Lai et al. 1989), gene expression alteration in cerebellum (Belyaev et al. 2006), cortex, and hippocampus (Nittby et al. 2008b). Thomas et al. (2008) reported an increase in adult complaints of headaches and concentration difficulties with short-term cell phone use at 0.005–0.04 $\mu W/cm^2$ exposure levels. Heinrich et al. (2010) reported that children and adolescents (8–17 years old) with short-term exposure to base station level RFR (0.003–0.02 $\mu W/cm^2$) experienced headache, irritation, and concentration difficulties in school. Mohler et al. (2010) reported that adults exposed to 0.005 $\mu W/cm^2$ cell phone radiation (basestation exposure levels) had sleep disturbances with chronic exposure, but this effect was not significantly increased over the entire population. Visual symptoms such as flashes, memory loss, and sleep disturbance have been investigated in relations to mobile phone use (Chia et al. 2000; Oftedel et al. 2000; Sandstrom et al. 2001).

Partial or whole body exposure of human and animals to RF radiation due to mobile phone use may lead to a variety of changes in tissues. Communication between brain cells is mediated by a host of chemical substances that both excite and inhibit transaction and transmission of information between them. These substances act by binding to their specific receptors on cell surfaces. Changes in the different tissues may occur depending on the exposure conditions, species, and histological parameters examined. Several authors (Penafiel et al. 1997) have shown that the radiation from TDMA digital cellular phones can cause significant changes in ornithine decarboxylase activity (ODC), which is essential for DNA synthesis. In particular, low level 2.45 GHz exposure affects protein kinase c activity in rat brain (Paulraj & Behari 2004). Kolomytkin et al. (1994) studied specific receptor binding of three neurotransmitters: gamma-aminobutyric acid (GABA), an inhibitory transmitter and acetyl choline and glutamate, both excitatory to rat brain synaptosomes. Microwave exposures used 880 or 915 MHz fields at varying power densities. With incident field intensities of 1.5 mW/cm^2, binding to GABA receptors decreased 30% at 16 Hz, but differences were not significant at 3, 5, 7, or 30 Hz. Conversely, 16 Hz modulation induced a significant increase in glutamate receptor binding. For acetyl choline receptors, binding decreased 25% at 16Hz with similar trends at higher and lower frequencies. As a function of field intensity, sensitivities of GABA and glutamate receptors persisted for field densities as low as 50 $\mu W/cm^2$ at 16 Hz with 915 MHz continuous wave fields.

Results of Zhao et al. (2007) suggest that specific CNS cells may activate different genes in response to cell phone emissions, and there is a variable threshold sensitivity depending on cell type. The variations in culture conditions that could contribute to the observed differences were minimized, since both cells were grown in an attached manner in the same size culture dish and in the same volume of medium. Still, some technical differences are impossible to avoid and disparities may arise because of the amount of total radiation received by the two cell types. For example, the culture media for astrocytes and neurons is slightly different. Astrocytes which are highly proliferative were also plated at a lower density compared to neurons to allow for expansion of the cell population between plating and RF/MW radiation exposure. Inherent differences in cell size and shape, composition of cell membranes, organelle distribution, junctional coupling between adjacent cells, stages of the cell cycle, and other parameters that cannot be controlled will also contribute to different amounts of energy absorption by the cells. Its role in Alzheimer's disease is also reported (Zhang et al. 2016). Since mobile phones are used near to the head and often kept in trousers pockets, we shall discuss the effect of mobile phones on brain and reproductive systems.

(A) Blood–Brain Barrier (BBB)

In order to assess the possible effect on brain, it is suggestive to first look at BBB. Nonthermal effects due to mobile phone exposures are identified by the leakage of albumin through the BBB (Salford et al. 2007, 2008). For this reason, BBB has been a favorable subject of investigation due to electromagnetic field exposure (Nittby et al. 2008), for even a slight variation in its permeability can lead to tissue damage (Sokrab et al. 1988; Lin 2001).

The tight junctions, which seal the endothelial cells together, limit paracellular leakage of molecules. A bilayered basal membrane supports the ablumenal side of the endothelial cells. The glial astrocytes, surrounding the surface of the basal membrane cells, are important for the maintenance, functional regulation, and repair of the BBB. The protrusions of the astrocytes, called end feet, cover the basal membrane on the outer endothelial surface and thus form a second barrier to hydrophilic molecules and connect the endothelium to the neurons. About 25% ablumenal membrane of the capillary surface is covered by pericytes (Frank et al. 1987), which are a type of macrophages. Seemingly, they are in the position to significantly contribute to the central nervous system (CNS) and immune mechanisms (Thomas 1999). Also, perivascular structures such as astrocytes and pericytes as well as a bilayered basal membrane help maintain the BBB (Salford et al. 2007).

Frey et al. (1975) found increase in the BBB permeability of rats to fluorescein after 30 min of exposure to both pulsed and continuous waves at 1.2 GHz with average power densities of 0.2 mW/cm^2. Williams et al. (1984) reported that intensity of sodium fluorescein in brain tissue exposed to EMF for 30 min was larger than that without such exposure. In a study on the transport of D-mannitol across BBB, it was observed that a higher power (larger SAR) generally yielded larger permeability and pulse wave was more effective in the permeability enhancement than continuous wave (Oscar & Hawkins 1977). Further for the higher electromagnetic frequency, the conductivity is larger and correspondingly a higher SAR (Equation (4.2)), and hence producing a greater permeability. Further, a larger modulation induces greater permeability. Also, the conductivity at depth of 50% was larger than that of 0% for AM wave with modulation of 16 Hz (Albert et al. 1987). Twofold increase in BBB permeability of sucrose was obtained after exposure to EMF of 1.8 GHz over 4 days (Schirmacher et al. 2000).

Furthermore, the effects of microwave fields on the BBB have been investigated by exposing male and female Fisher 344 rats in a TEM line chamber to 915 MHz CW microwave as well as pulse-modulated waves with repetition rates of 8, 16, 50, and 200 per second. The SAR varied between 0.016 and 5 W/kg. The rats were not anaesthetized during the 2 h exposure. The results show that both continuous and pulsed microwaves have the potential to open up the BBB for albumin passage, with no significant difference between the two (Salford et al. 1994).

It has been suggested that due to microwave exposure BBB leakage is the major reason for nerve cell injury, such as dark neurons in stroke-prone spontaneously hypertensive rats (Fredriksson et al. 1988). Albumin leaks into the brain and neuronal degeneration is observed in areas with BBB disruption in several circumstances: after intracartoid infusion of hyperosmolar solutions in rats (Salahuddin et al. 1988); in the stroke-prone hypertensive rat (Hassel et al. 1994); in acute hypertension by aortic compression in rats (Sokrab et al. 1988). The linkage between album extravasation over the BBB and neural damage may be a potentiating effect of albumin upon the glutamate-mediated neurotoxicity (Eimerl & Scramm 1991). Indeed, both albumin and glumate-induced lesions have the same histopathological appearance with invasion of macrophages and absence of neuronal cell bodies and axons in the lesion areas. The glumate itself can also increase the BBB opening (Dietrich et al. 1992). Two hours of exposure to radiation from a GSM phone at 915 MHz, at nonthermal SAR values of 12 and 120mW/kg, leads to further albumin extravasation after 14 days of exposure (Nittby et al. 2008b). However, significant neuronal damage occurs after 28 and 50 days (Salford et al. 2003;Eberhardt et al. 2008). These SARs are well below the maximal permissive level for cellular telephone, for instance, 1.6 W kg^{-1}, including extremely low levels (0.016 W kg^{-1}). It is suggested that albumin extravasation into the brain parenchyma is the first observable effect of the mobile phone exposure. The albumin leakage precedes and possibly could be the cause of the damage to the neurons seen as the dark neurons later. In this connection, it is suggested that transient openings of the BBB can result in permanent tissue damage. A higher cellular damage is anticipated in EMF-exposed animals. A plausible question arises that, if by repeated exposure of the human brain to microwave from cellular mobile telephones, it is possible that albumin and other toxic molecules leak into and accumulate in the brain cell (Li et al. 2001).

Shivers et al. (1987) observed that the EMF exposure of the type emitted during a MRI procedure resulted in a temporarily increased BBB permeability in the brain of rats. Through transendothelial channels, a vesicle-mediated transport of horseradish peroxidase (HRP) took place, which was replicated by Garber et al. (1989). The work of Shivers et al. (1987) later got quantitative support from the findings of Prato et al. (1990, 1994). In rats exposed to MRI (an inadvertent exposure), the BBB permeability to diethylenetriameninepentaacetic acid (DTPA) is increased. It is suggested that the increased permeability may be a stimulation of endocytosis, made possible through the time-varying magnetic fields. These findings support the observations (Salford et al. 1992) that BBB permeability to albumin is increased after exposure to MRI radiations.

In another study, Neubauer et al. (2007) reported an increased BBB activity at exposure levels of 2 W/kg and duration of 30–120 min. When the rats were pretreated with colchicines, the EMF-induced rhodamine-ferritin uptake was however blocked. Colchicine is well known for its inhibition of microtubular function, which seems to play an important role for the BBB opening.

Nittby et al. (2009) reported an increased permeability after mobile phone exposures which has also been earlier reported (Fritze et al. 1997). These authors exposed for 4 h at GSM-900 MHz in brain, at power densities ranging from 0.3 to 7.5 W/kg resulting in significantly increasing albumin extravasation not only at the SAR value of 7.5 W/kg, which is a thermal effect, but also at nonthermal levels of 0.3 and 1.3 W/kg. Albumin extravasation was also seen in rats exposed for 2h to GSM-900 MHz at nonthermal SAR values of 0.12, 0.5, and 2 W/kg using fluorescein-labeled proteins (Tore et al. 2002). At SAR of 2 W/kg, a marked BBB permealization was observed at lower SAR value of 0.5 W/kg. However, the extravasation at 0.5 W/kg was seen at a lesser extent as compared to that seen at 2 W/kg. Fritze et al. (1997) and Tore et al. (2002) also concluded that an already disrupted BBB is more sensitive to the RF fields than an intact BBB. Kuribayashi et al. (2005) concluded no BBB alterations after 90 min of daily EMF exposure for 1–2 weeks at SAR values of 2 or 6 W/kg.

Volkow et al. (2011) performed PET scan, both with and without EMF exposure (50 min of GSM with maximum SAR of 0.901 W/kg), and the participants were blinded to the exposure scenario. A 7% increase in metabolism in the exposure situation compared to controls was identified regionally on the same side of the head where the mobile phone was placed, in the right orbitio frontal cortex and in the lower part of the right superior temporal gyrus. The strength of the E-field from the phones correlated positively with the brain activation, which the authors suggested was from an increase in brain neuron excitability. Kwon et al. (2011) carried out another study where he demonstrated that ^{18}FDG uptake decreased after GSM-900 exposure—this time in the temporoparietal junction. Tissue pathophysiology based phenomena could influence the measurable metabolism and perfusion abnormalities via mechanisms such as excitotoxicity, cell stress response, construction of capillary lumen by activated astrocytes, volume effects of vascular extravasation, subtle alterations in blood viscosity due to immune or oxidative stress associated blood chemical changes, with other possibilities.

However, in other experiment no albumin extravasation was seen after 2 or 4 weeks of 1h of daily exposure (average whole body exposure at 0.25 W/kg) (Tsurita et al. 2000). Also in another study, Finnie et al. (2002)

exposed mice for 104 weeks at SAR values of 0.25–4 W/kg, with no alteration in BBB permeability in either case.

It is estimated that the studies showing increased BBB permeability in experimental animals are equal in number with those that do not report BBB disruption at high as well as at low SARs. Some of the apparent discrepancies undoubtedly stem from the complexity of the BBB and from differences in microwave exposure conditions, such as frequency power level and SAR distribution, and from differences in the use of a variety of assays and procedures for detecting changes in BBB permeability. The physical and biological phenomena are highly complex to explain, may be needing more experimental data. From the presently available results, it is apparent that:

Exposed animals are at risk for opening of the BBB ($p = 0.0004$).

The response is independent of pulse repetition rate, and the response is the same for CW as compared with pulse modulation. The response is independent of SAR in the interval 0.016–2.5 W kg^{-1} (odd ratio 3.3) but increases rises for SAR > 2.5 W kg^{-1}.

From all these observations, it is apparent that permeability enhancement is not because of temperature increase, as it was within the variation of 1 °C as happens in daily rhythm.

(B) Tumor Promotion

EM Radiation and Melatonin

The melatonin/serotonin cycle is a primary physiological driver of the daily metabolic, awake/sleep cycle. Melatonin is a vital part of many of the body's biochemical systems, including sleep and learning and is a free radical scavenger in all cells and hence is a potent antioxidant with antiaging and anticancer properties. It helps to protect embryonic fetuses through regulation of the cyclic AMP (cAMP) pathway, hence controlling the serotonin/melatonin transformation. A key element of the cAMP pathway is calcium ion. Calcium ion efflux from the pinealocytes has the effect of reducing melatonin through reducing the cAMP.

Prolonged use of GSM mobile phones may lead to reduced melatonin production (Lai et al. 1992; Burch et al. 2002; Jarupat et al. 2003; Sukhotina et al. 2006), and its possible blockade (Lai & Singh 1997). Melatonin exerts an antigonadotrophic effect mainly at the level of the hypothalamic and pituitary (Jackson et al. 1984; Bittman et al. 1985) and decreases the testosterone secretion in Leydig cells (Valladares et al. 1990; Kus et al. 2002).

Other authors (Vollrath et al. 1997; de Seze et al. 1999; Sukhotina et al. 2006) have not reported any significant variation in the melatonin levels due to continuous RF-EMF exposure. Radon et al. (2001) showed that pulsed RF electromagnetic fields (900 MHz carrier frequency pulsed with 217 Hz) similar to those emitted from mobile radio telephones had no short-term or medium-term effects on salivary melatonin, cortisol, neopterin, and sIgA concentrations. These authors also confirmed the observation that nocturnal melatonin levels are not affected by exposure to RF electromagnetic fields (Mann et al. 1998). The findings are in confirmation with the data showing that daytime melatonin levels are unaffected by exposure to RF electromagnetic fields of 900 and 1800 MHz (de Seze et al. 1999).

Regarding tumor, since the energy of a microwave quantum is too small to effect bonding in a biological system, promotion (not initiation) of tumor is a distinct probability. Neubauer et al. (2007) have recommended focusing initially on short-term effects.

Szmigielski et al. (1982a, 1982b) reported that chronic exposure of mice to RF (2.45 GHz, 2–3 or 6–8 W/kg, 2 h/day, 6 days/week for upto 12 months; 40 or 100 animals or 100 animals/group) resulted in accelerating the development of sarcoma colonies in the lung after subcutaneous injection of sarcoma cells—mammary tumors in mice having a normally high incidence of these tumors by painting the skin with a known chemical carcinogen. Sugimachi et al. (1988) reported that exposure to RF fields (2.45 GHz CW, 4–5 W/kg, 2 h/day, 5–6 days/week for a few months; 40 animals/group) increased the number of chemically induced hepatomas and sarcomas and increased the number of skin tumors in mice with a subcarcinogenic dose of benzo[a]pyrene. The authors suggested that the acceleration of tumor development may have resulted from a direct role of immune competent cells. Repacholi et al. (1997) reported a 2.4-fold increase in the incidence of lymphomas in transgenic mice exposed up to 900 MHz fields pulsed at 217 Hz with pulse widths of 0.6 s. The time to lymphoma development was also shorter in the RF-exposed animals.

These results are however not without contradictions. Salford et al. (1997) reported no effect on the progression of tumor cells injected into rat brain after exposure to continuous or pulsed 915 MHz RF fields (CW exposure, 1 W/pulse, 1.67 W/kg, 0.41 W/kg for 217 Hz modulation, pulse width 0.52 ms, 2 W/pulse, 62 animal/group). Santini et al. (1988) found that the progression of subcutaneously implanted melanoma cells in mice was unaffected by daily exposure to pulsed or CW exposure to RF fields (2.45 GHz CW and pulsed, 10 W/m^2, 1.2 W/kg, 2.5 h/day, 6 days/week for the lifetime of the animal). Wu et al. (1994) reported no effect of RF exposure (2.45 GHz exposed 3 h/day, 6 days/week for 5 months; average SAR 10–12 W/kg) on chemical-induced colon cancer in mice. Rotkvoska et al. (1993) found that the exposure of mice to low level RF fields from police radar (34 GHZ) did not affect biological parameters that could initiate any pathologic reaction.

However, substantial evidence now indicates that the current controversy regarding the carcinogenesis of RF-EMFs might be caused by the lack of accurate information regarding the magnitude of exposure to

RF-EMFs which possibly plays a basic role in RF-induced carcinogenesis (Sri 2015).

Brain Function and Mobile Phone Frequency Exposure

The exposure of brain to mobile phones is maximum; hence, investigating the possibility of EMF-induced genetic damage in brain cells is of utmost concern. These cells have high level of iron and have low capacity of DNA repair and hence such damages could accumulate. The presence of magnetic particles could enhance free radical activity in cell. Thus, the effect of EMF on DNA is more significant on nerve cells than on other type of cells in the body. Since nerve cells do not repair, they may undergo apoptosis or accelerate the process of neurodegeneration. Double-strand breaks if not properly repaired are known to lead to cell death (Phillips et al. 2009). However, another type of brain cells (glial cells) can become cancerous as a result of DNA damage.

The animal research that has followed provides possible importance of localized exposures resulting in development of brain cancer (Kesari & Behari 2010). Development of brain cancer takes years or may be decades to develop, and in view of the difficulty in controlling the exposure parameters over a long period of time, it is difficult to arrive at any definite conclusion. Exposing rats to pulse modulated 837 MHz RF energy similar to that emitted by some digital cell phones does not cause any promotion of brain cancer (Adey et al. 1999). These authors have reported the same finding for continuous wave RF, such as those emitted by analog cell phones. Most studies performed so far have reported conflicting findings, varying from no major effect to severe health risk.

Some studies have already suggested that mobile phones affect brain functioning and behavior (Hamblin et al. 2004; Sievert et al. 2005; Ferreri et al. 2006; Khiat et al. 2006; Krause et al. 2007; Kumlin et al. 2007), though there may be variability in their outcome in varying range. Arai et al. (2003) have shown no short-term adverse effects of 30 min of mobile phone exposure on auditory brain stem responses (ABRs), middle latency responses (MLRs), or somatosensory evoked potentials (SEPs) (Yuasa et al. 2006). Other groups have employed visual evoked potentials (VEPs) to investigate possible bioeffects of mobile phone exposure (Urban et al. 1998) and observed no significant effects. The reaction times were not affected by the mobile phone exposure (Hamblin et al. 2006). Even though transcranial magnetic stimulation (TMS) is very useful in investigating motor cortex physiology in humans, more data on effects of mobile phones on human motor cortex using TMS are needed. Barker et al. (2007) in a double blind study reported no effect of GSM and TETRA signals on blood pressure and related physiological parameters. These authors also did not report any significant differences between the mean concentration of adrenaline nor adrenaline concentrations as a result of exposure.

Several researchers have showed nonthermal bioeffects of mobile phones (Huber et al. 2000; Hamblin et al. 2004; Moby et al. 2005). Some of these authors have used evoked potentials as one kind of objective analysis of human brain exposure. Exposure due to mobile phone frequencies has been found to have an impact on brain EEG activity (Vecchio et al. 2007). This also affects the synchronization of cerebral rhythms. These findings suggest that prolonged exposure to mobile phone emissions affects cortical activity and the speed of neural synchronization by inter-hemispherical functional coupling of EEG rhythms.

Preece et al. (1999) studied the effect of a 915 MHz simulated mobile phone signal on cognitive function in man. They reported an increase in responsiveness (reaction time), strongly in the analogue and less in the digital simulation. They further concluded that this could be associated with mild localized heating, or possibly a nonthermal response. Several workers (Ray & Behari 1987; Lai et al. 1989) have reported that different areas of the brain have different sensitivities to radiofrequency radiations. Chou et al. (1985), measuring energy absorption (SARs), have shown that brain regions less than 1 mm apart can have more than twofold difference in SAR. The situation is more complicated if the animal was moving. Use of phone in driving stimulator leads to negative reaction time. Evidence for a direct memory effect on brain slices from the hippocampus of rat showed changes in long-term potentiation when exposed to 915 MHz (Scott et al. 1998). Mild et al. (1998) looking for a subjective response suggested increased headache or sensation of warmth when using mobile phones. Exposure due to mobile phone frequencies has been found to have an impact on brain EEG activity (Vecchio et al. 2007). This also affects the synchronization of cerebral rhythms. These findings suggest that prolonged exposure to mobile phone emissions affects cortical activity and the speed of neural synchronization by inter-hemispherical functional coupling of EEG rhythms. Use of phone in driving stimulator leads to negative reaction time. This may also point to the possibility of desynchronizing the rhythms between two halves of the brain by deregulating the normal alpha wave 2 (8–10 Hz) and alpha 3 (10–12 Hz) bands. This may affect the brain–immune system. Also human brain EEG beta rhythms energies are reported to be increased by exposure to 450 MHz modulated at different low wave frequencies (Hinrikus et al. 2009). Frequency and intensity windows of Ca^{2+} have been observed in the presence of weak fields below 100 Hz, similar to the ELF-modulated RF fields (Adey 1990; Somossy et al. 1991). However, Röschke and Mann (1997) did not notice any difference in the awake EEG of subjects exposed to radiation emitted by cellular phones.

These findings suggest that there are interactions, resulting in specific EEG changes that are affected by modulated RF fields. Further, different effects of modulated and CW microwave exposure were found on morphology and cell surface negative charges. Static experimental models (i.e., biochemical models) do not give information about the transient effects and functional changes induced by EMF exposure, especially in the nervous system. An electrophysiological approach is more appropriate to explain the phenomena in the CNS.

A study undertaken on transgenic mice due to exposure of 918 MHz (repeated at 217 Hz) for 30 min a day for 18 months showed incidences of lymphomas length in exposed (53%) than in sham exposed (22%). In these experiments, pulse width was 0.6 ms. The average incident power density and SAR were 2.6 to 13W/m^2 and 0.13 to 1.4W/kg, respectively. However, in this study since the transgenic mice were free to move around, a wide venation in SAR value has been possible. It is possible that the incidence of lymphomas might have occurred due to the high value of SAR. The study is however ridden with several dosimetric and experimental problems (Lin 2008).

Evidence of brain tumor promotion from exposure to TDMA fields has been sought in rats exposed to a single dose of the short-lived carcinogen ethyl nitrosourea (ENU) in utero, and thereafter, intermittently exposed to digital phone fields for 243 months (Adey et al. 1996). The mean life span of rats used in this study was 26 months. At a low dose of ENU (4mg/kg) on the day of promotion, animals were exposed by mobile phone fields over the life time of the animals. Far-field irradiation with an 836 MHz circular polarized field began on day 19 and continued after parturition until weaning of offspring at 23 days of age. Near-field exposure of offspring began at 35 days and continued for the next 22 months (4 days/week). Exposures were for 2 h daily, field on and off for 7.5 min. Modeled far-field time averaged SAR were: pregnant dam (uterus) 0.3 W/kg; fetus (brain) 0.29 W/kg isolated pup (brain) 0.035 W/kg; young rat (brain) 0.13 W/kg. Time-averaged near-field thermographic SARs were: larger males 0.75 W/kg (localized maximum 1.0 W/kg); smaller females 0.58 W/kg (localized maximum 0.75 W/kg).

A double blind study (Utteridge et al. 2002) was carried out on mice for two years to an exposure of GSM mobile phone radiation, where the animals were exposed for 1 hour a day. These authors reported no significant effects when compared to sham-irradiated animals. Oberto et al. (2007) carried out investigations on 500 transgenic mice (250 female/250 male) and SAR levels varied between 0.5 and 4.0 W/kg. The exposure was performed 1 h/day 7 days a week for a period of 18 months. The authors reported that the incidence in female being two to three times higher than males. These authors have reported that there was no significant difference in the number of animals with incidence of tumors, regardless of malignancy. However, the incidence was reduced by 34% at 4.0 W/kg for females. Further in female, there was reduction in the time of death at 0.5 W/kg.

Mortazavi et al. (2017) have addressed the shortcoming of some of the papers claiming lack of association between exposure to RF-EMF and cancer. They have provided evidence showing that exposure to RF-EMFs at high levels and long durations can increase the risk of cancer.

However, substantial evidence now indicates that the current controversy regarding the carcinogenesis of RF-EMFs might be caused by the lack of accurate information of the magnitude of exposure to RF-EMFs which possibly plays a basic role in RF-induced carcinogenesis. The carcinogenesis relating to nonionizing RF-EMF may have a nonlinear relationship.

Cancer and Cellular Phone Towers

There is a general concern about the well-being of people living in the region close to cell phone towers (Kundi & Hutter 2009). There are regular reports in media of an unusually high incidence of cancer in the vicinity of mobile phone base stations. Because there are several hundred thousand base stations operating all over the world, it is likely that some coincide with a high local cancer incidence area. Regionally, cancer incidence has a distribution due to variations in the age and gender. Therefore, a much higher number of cases than expected from average incidences can occur.

Lerchl et al. (2015) undertook a study using larger number of animals in each group and used two exposure levels: Sham and SAR values (0.04, 0.4, and 2 W/kg). They reported that number of tumors of the lungs and livers in exposed animals were significantly higher than in sham-exposed controls. In addition, lymphomas were also found to be significantly increased due to exposure. Many tumor-promoting effects were also observed at moderate level of exposure (0.04 and 0.4 W/kg SAR), that is, well below exposure level for users of mobile phones. Long-term exposure of mobile phone frequencies to the mouse (Repacholi et al. 1997) showed an elevated risk of developing lymphoma in a transgenic strain.

Another study by Wyde et al. (2017), which are only a partial finding from a series of RFR cancer studies in rats, contains ten neoplastic and hyperplastic findings only in the brain and heart of HSD. In this study, Sprague Dawley SD (HSD) rats are exposed to RFR starting in utero and continuing throughout their lifetimes. These studies found low incidences of 12 malignant gliomas in the brain and schwannomas in the heart of male rats exposed to RFR of the two types: Code Division Multiple Access (CDMA) and Global System for Mobile 14 Communications (GSM). Potentially preneoplastic lesions were also observed in the brain and heart of male rats exposed to RFR.

McCormick (2017) carried out two-year studies to determine if exposure to nonthermal levels of RF increases the incidence of neoplasia in any site. Male rats exposed to RF demonstrated significantly increased incidences of glioma (brain) and schwannoma (heart) though these increases were not seen in female rats or in either sex of mice.

Kim et al. (2017) assessed neuronal effects of RF-EMF on the cerebral cortex of the mouse brain as a proxy for cranial exposure during mobile phone use. These authors exposed mice to 835 MHz RF-EMF at a specific absorption rate of 4.0 W/kg for 5 h a day during 12 weeks. They aimed to examine the activation of autophagy pathway in the cerebral cortex, a brain region that is located externally. Induction of autophagy genes and production of proteins including LC3B-II and Beclin1 were increased and accumulation of autolysosome was observed in neuronal cell bodies in the cerebral cortex during radiofrequency exposure. The observation that neuronal cell bodies remained structurally stable but demyelation was induced in cortical neurons following prolonged RF-EMF exposure suggest a potential cause of neurological or neurobehavioral disorders.

In real scenario, both the environment and telecommunications networks are inherently time varying, and exposure to environmental RF-EMFs at an arbitrary location shows variation with time. Aerts et al. (2017) undertook more than a year of measurement data collected over an urban environment. Though no global trend was discovered over the measuring period, the difference in measured exposure between two instances could reach up to 42dB (a factor 12,000 in power density). It was found that the surrogate model in the area under study was improved by up to 50% compared to models that neglect the daily temporal variability of the RF signals.

Altuntas et al. (2018) investigated the acute effects of the EMWs emitted by mobile phones on attention in emergency physicians.

These authors reported that the EMW emitted by mobile phones has no deleterious effect on the attention and concentration levels of emergency physicians, and even has a positive impact on selective attention levels.

It is apparent that there are conflicting reports Beghi (2017) also concludes that there is lack of robust evidence of association between use of cell phones and brain tumors. None of the cohort studies found an increased risk of brain tumors in people exposed to cell phones. However, the absence of cohort-proven findings does not necessarily mean that there is no detrimental effect. The confirmed evidences of the free radical formation after exposure to RF-EMF in many studies are suggestive that these exposures should be limited, even without confirmed reports from cohort studies. Secondly, the increased risk of brain tumors in case–control studies, if proven, is at best modest and, as brain tumors are rare diseases, the total number of tumors appears only slightly increased. The author also claims that dose–response effect has never been confirmed. It may be concluded that long-term studies on animals exposed to RF found in wireless networks (Wi-Fi) have, so far, found health effects, while contradictory data have also been reported (Bioinitiative Report 2012).

Mobile Phone Frequency Exposure and DNA Damage: The Nucleus

DNA damage caused by any endogenous and exogenous factors is under a constant repair process. Any imbalance or mistakes in damage and repair result in accumulation of former, causing apoptosis, ageing, or promotion of cancer. While damage to DNA strand has been confirmed by several workers (as detailed next), it is argued that its repair is an ongoing process and the damaged chromosomes can be reconstituted. However, this proposition is not without risk. There is no guarantee that these will replicate in the manner they were originally present. Pieces may be left out (deletions), joined in the backward (inversions), swapped between different parts of the chromosomes (translocations), or even attached to the wrong chromosome. The effect may also be frequency dependent in cases, the new arrangement can work for a while if most of the genes are still present and any metabolic deficiencies can often be made good by the surrounding cells. However, things may be different if it comes to meiosis. During meiosis, the chromosomes line up in pairs (one from each original parent) along their entire length so that corresponding parts are adjacent and can be exchanged. Malformed pairs are torn apart in the later stages of meiosis so that eggs or sperms have an incomplete or unbalanced set of genes, may not function properly, and so reduce fertility and other physiological functioning. There is a possibility that this may lead to permanent genetic damage, which though may not be visible in the first generation but may be seen thereafter.

One of the markers of this is the strand break mostly caused by endogenous process causing free radical generation by mitochondrial respiration and metabolism. This may also be caused by exogenous agents, for example, UV radiation, ionizing and nonionizing radiation, and chemicals (Phillips et al. 2009). Phillips et al. (1998) were the first to study the effects of two forms of cellular phones signal known as TDMA and integrated digital enhanced network (IDEN) on DNA damage in Molt-4 human lymphoblastoid cells using the comet assay, using low-intensity field (2.4–2.6 µW/kg). Diem et al. (2005) exposed human fibroblast and rat granulosa cells to cell phones signal (1800 MHz, SAR 1.2 or 2 W/kg; different modulation for 4, 6, and 24 h; intermittent 5 min on/10 min off or continuous). Intermittent exposure caused a significant stronger effect than continuous exposure. Statistically significant increase in micronucleus formation and in chromosomal aberrations was observed in fibroblast as well. These authors concluded that fragmentation of DNA is similar to that due to gamma rays (ionizing radiations).

Gandhi and Anita (2005) reported increase in DNA strand breaks and micro nucleation in lymphocytes obtained from cell phone users. Markova et al.

(2005) reported that GSM signals affected chromatin conformation and Y-H2AX foci that is also co-localized in distinct foci with DNA double strand breaks in mouse embryonic cells after acute exposure to a 1.7 GHz field. Sun et al. (2006) reported that DNA damage caused by the field at 4 W/kg was irreversible. Zhang et al. (2006) also reported that an 1800 MHz field at 3.0 W/kg induced DNA damage. Erogul et al. (2006) reported changes in morphology and decreased motility in isolated sperm cells, exposed to cell phone radiations. A similar conclusion was arrived by other workers too (Fejes et al. 2005; Yan et al. 2007). Several authors (Lai & Singh 1995, p. 996; Paulraj & Behari 2006) showed an increase in DNA breaks at 2.45 and 50 GHz (Kesari & Behari 2009). Some of these *in vivo* effects are caused by hormonal changes (Ozguner et al. 2005; Forgacs et al. 2006).

Nakamura et al. (2003) found that exposure to 915 MHz CW microwave at 3mW/cm^2 power density exposed for 90 min decreased uteroplacental blood flow and estradiol in pregnant rats. There are other reports regarding the effects on DNA damage in cells (C3H10T) exposed to radiofrequency radiations (Li et al. 2001). These results have found support from in vitro studies of Hook et al. (2004).

The genotoxic effect of EM field exposure is studied on DNA and chromatic levels. Cells with limited ability of DNA repair, such as sperm, are particularly susceptible. DNA double strand breaks, if not properly repaired, may lead to cell death (apoptosis) (Lai & Singh 1996). In the event that EM field has different ways of biological interactions with cellular components, a number of theories have been postulated to delineate the EMF-induced electrical currents in opposite directions (Blank & Goodman 1999). These currents form magnetic forces around each strand in opposite directions as well, leading to progressive repelling effect between the two strands. As a result, gradual separation of the two DNA chains and consequently bending and even breaks may occur. The continuous cloud of delocalized electrons along both faces of the "ribbon" formed by the base pairs provides a conducting path for responding to EMF and makes it more vulnerable to damage. The chemical changes that result from electron transfer reactions are associated with molecular damage in DNA. On the other hand, another theory attributes DNA damage to oxidative stress through ROS. ROS have been frequently implicated in oxidative DNA damage and the increased production of 8-OH-deoxyguanosine (a marker of oxidative stress) (De Iuliis et al. 2009).

The TDMA field had no enhancing effect on incidence, type, or location of spontaneous nervous system tumors. On termination of experiments, the TDMA field appeared to reduce incidence of malignant glial cell tumors in rats that received the ENU drug when compared with rats receiving ENU and no field exposure (4 vs. 13). The TDMA field also appeared to reduce the incidence of spontaneous glial tumors occurring in rats not receiving the ENU drug when they were compared with control animals (2 vs. 7). Tumors in exposed rats were smaller in volume. There were no gender differences in tumor incidence. In rats not surviving to experiment termination (n = 54, 22%), the TDMA field appeared to prolong latency of appearance of both spontaneous and ENU-induced glial cell tumors, but did not alter histological criteria of tumor types. Consistent nonsignificant differences in survival rates were noted between the four rat groups, with higher death rates in a progression: sham/field, sham/sham, ENU/field, and ENU/sham.

Papadopoulou et al. (2017) showed that exposing adult *Drosophila melanogaster* to a mobile phone signal for just 6 min a day for 6 days broke the DNA in the cells into fragments which give rise to their eggs and half of the eggs died.

D'Silva et al. (2017)evaluated the possible tissue and DNA damage in developing liver of chick embryo following chronic exposure to radiofrequency radiation emitted from 2G and 3G cell phones. For this purpose, fertilized chick embryos were incubated in four groups: Group A-experimental group exposed to 2G radiation (60 eggs), Group B- experimental group exposed to 3G radiation (60 eggs), Group C-sham-exposed control group (60 eggs), and Group D-control group (48 eggs). On completion of scheduled duration, the embryos were collected and processed for routine histological studies to check structural changes in liver. The nuclear diameter and karyorrhexis changes of hepatocytes were analyzed using oculometer and square reticule, respectively. The liver procured from one batch of eggs from all the four groups was subjected to alkaline comet assay technique to assess DNA damage. The authors reported that the exposure of developing chick embryos to 2G and 3G cell phone radiations caused structural changes in liver in the form of dilated sinusoidal spaces with hemorrhage, increased vacuolations in cytoplasm, increased nuclear diameter and karyorrhexis, and significantly increased DNA damage. Further to this they also concluded that radiations from these sources resulted in various structural changes and DNA damage Lagroye et al 2004). The changes were more pronounced in 3G experimental group. Based on these findings it is necessary to create awareness among public about the possible ill effects of RFR exposure from cell phone.

The genotoxic effects have also been investigated after short-term exposure (Moulder et al. 1999; Vijayalaxmi and Obe 2004). Statistically significant increase in micronucleus formation and in chromosomal aberrations was observed in fibroblast as well. Speit et al. (2007) used continuous intermittent exposure (1800 MHz, SAR 2W/kg) applied using the same cell system and they reported negative results. Nikolova et al. (2005) reported after a 6h (but not after 48h) RF field exposure a low and transient increase of DNA strand breaks in embryonic stem cell derived neural progenitor cells.

When mice were exposed to 2.45 GHz fields at an SAR of 1.18 W/kg for 2 h/day for 120, 150, and 200 days, structural genomic rearrangements were observed in brain and testes cells (Sarkar et al. 1994). Lai and Singh (1995, 1996) reported that rats exposed to pulsed (2 se pulses, 500 pulses per second)or continuous wave 2.45 GHz fields with SARs of 0.6 or 1.2 W/kg for 2 h increased the number of single and double strand breaks in brain cell DNA when assayed 4 h after RF exposure. Lai and Singh (1997) also reported that treatment of rats immediately before or after exposure with either melatonin (1mg/kg) or N-*tert*-butylphenylnitrone (PBN, 100 mg/kg) blocks the formation of DNA breaks by RF fields. These experiments challenge the belief that RF fields are unable to break molecular bonds. Epigenetic events may be involved. Paulraj and Behari (2006) studied the same phenomena at low dose level, confirming DNA strand break and concluded that hippocampus is the targeted site of such interaction.

However, the findings of DNA strand breaks are not without contradictions. Several authors (Chou et al. 1992; Malyapa et al. 1998;Stronati et al. 2006) showed that 24 h of exposure to 935MHz GSM base signal at 1 or 2 W/kg shows no DNA strand break. Similarly, Verschaeve et al. (2006) did not observe significant affect of DNA strand break to long term (2 h/day, 5 days/week for 2 years) to 900 MHz GSM signal. Hook et al. (2004) showed that a 24 h exposure of Molt-4 cells to CDMA, FDMA, IDEN, or TDMA-modulated RFR did not significantly alter the level of DNA damage. Several other authors (e.g., Lagroye et al. 2004) reported no significant change in DNA strand breaks, DNA–protein cross links, and DNA-DNA cross links in cells exposed to 2450 MHz RFR. Stronati et al. (2006) showed that 24 h of exposure to 935 MHz basic signal at 1 or 2 W/kg did not cause DNA strand breaks in human blood cells. In agreement with these results, Vijayalaxmi et al. (2000, 2004) reported no increase in DNA strand breaks in human lymphocytes exposed in vitro to 2450 MHz RFR at 2.135 W/kg for 2 h.

Brain Cancer

For laboratory studies, cancer can be induced in small animals (mice, rats) by the use of chemical carcinogen (Szmigielski et al. 1982a, 1982b) in a short time frame.

Development of brain cancer takes years or may be decades to develop and in view of the difficulty in controlling the exposure parameters over a long period of time is difficult to arrive at any definite conclusion. Exposing rats to pulse modulated 837 MHz RF energy similar to that emitted by some digital cell phones does not cause any promotion of brain cancer (Adey et al. 1999). These authors reported the same finding for continuous wave RF, such as those emitted by analog cell phones.

Evidence of brain tumor promotion from exposure to TDMA fields has been examined in rats exposed to a single dose of the short-lived carcinogen ENU in utero, and thereafter, intermittently exposed to digital phone fields (Adey et al. 1996). The mean life span of rats used in this study was 26 months. At low dose of ENU (4mg/kg) on the day of promotion, animals were exposed by phone fields over the lifetime of the animals. Far-field irradiation with an 836 MHz circular polarized field began on day 19 and continued after parturition until weaning of offspring at 23 days of age. Near-field exposure of offspring began at 35 days and continued for the next 22 months, 4 consecutive days weekly. Exposures were for 2 h daily, field on and off for 7.5 min. Modeled far-field time averaged SAR were: pregnant dam (uterus) 0.3 W/kg; fetus (brain) 0.29 W/kg, isolated pup (brain) 0.035 W/kg; young rat (brain) 0.13 W/kg. Time-averaged near-field thermographic SARs were: larger males 0.75 W/kg (localized maximum 1.0 W/kg); smaller females 0.58 W/kg (localized maximum 0.75 W/kg). Of the 236 original rats, 182 (77%) survived to the termination of the whole experiment. The 54 rats (23%) that died during the study ("preterm rats") formed a separate group. There was no evidence of tumorigenic effects in the CNS from exposure to the TDMA field. However, some evidence of tumor-inhibiting effects of TDMA exposure was apparent. Overall, the TDMA field-exposed animals exhibited trends toward a reduced incidence of spontaneous CNS tumors ($P < 0.16$, two-tailed) and ENU-induced CNS tumors ($P < 0.16$, two-tailed). In preterm rats, where primary neural tumors were determined to be the cause of death, fields decreased the incidence of ENU-induced tumors ($P < 0.03$).

Children and Cell Phones

Given the rapid introduction of mobile phones and other portable wireless devices into society, and the increased possibility of young children using or being exposed to EMF, the severity of the issue is now increasingly recognized realized. It is possible that there are currently unrecognized health effects from the use of mobile phones. Children have thinner skulls and smaller ears than adults, and so the radiation has a deeper penetration and higher SAR from the phone to the brain. Hence, the brain of a child absorbs a much greater amount of radiation from a cell phone than does the brain of an adult. Children are hence more vulnerable because of their developing nervous system, greater absorption of energy, and a longer lifetime of exposure. As such, unnecessary use of mobile phones by children should be avoided. Other users should use the device with the instructions as supplied by the manufacturers and as sparingly as possible. The hands-free devices that move the handset away from the user's body tend to reduce exposure, though these may cause exposure to other body organs and consequently there is likelihood of other problems.

Study due to Mortazavi et al. (2017) found that a larger proportion of children used cordless phones compared to mobile phones. They found limited evidence to show that change in the use of mobile phones or cordless phones in primary school children was associated with change in cognitive function.

In an attempt to evaluate the exposure of children to electromagnetic fields, realistic head models, which consider the age-specific anatomical structure and age-dependent tissues dielectric properties, are developed (Jin et al. 2002). During postnatal development of human tissues, the number and size of cells increase while the proportion of water content decreases. Such changes generally result in significant changes in the dielectric properties of tissues. The results show that the maximum SAR levels in brain tissues of young children (3 months) are higher by up to 61% and 78% than adults at the lowest (700 MHz) and highest (2600 MHz) frequencies, respectively. The percentage absorption power in the heads of young children (3 months) is higher by up to 40.6% and 24% than the values for adults at 700 MHz and 2600 MHz, respectively. Investigations shows that previous studies, which used scaled head models without considering the age-dependent variations in the head anatomy and/or age-dependent tissues' dielectric properties, underestimated SAR levels in the children's heads. The obtained results using the developed realistic head models indicate that for young children, a lower limit on radiated power is required to meet the acceptable dosimetry levels.

Reproduction Pattern: Animal Study

Male Reproduction

Effects of radio frequency effects on prenatal development in mice have been a constant subject of investigation, particularly on male reproductive system, and results obtained have often been at variance. Male reproductive system is highly compartmentalized sensitive that requires the integration of intrinsic and extrinsic factor to properly function. Because the testis is a superficial organ, it may absorb more EM energy than other organs. Human testis need physiological temperature 2 °C lower than body temperature for optimal spermatogenesis and an elevation of testicular temperature may be a detrimental factor to sperm production (Jung & Schill 2000).

Animal studies indicated that EMWs may exert a wide range of damaging effects on the testicular function and male germ lines (Dasdag et al. 1999). Adverse effects due to microwave radiations in animals showed a decrease in diameter of seminiferous tubule (Dasdag et al. 1999, 2008; Yan et al. 2007; Otitoloju et al. 2010), decreased weight of testicular organs (i.e., caput, cauda, corpus), decreased sperm count (Behari & Kesari 2006), and destruction in Leydig cells. Saunders and Kowalczuk (1981) also showed that microwave radiation of 50 mW cm^2 and frequency 2.45 GHz for 30–40 min resulted in significant degeneration of seminiferous epithelium in mice. Wistar albino rats were exposed through pregnancy (6 h/day) to 915 MHz radiation at a power density level of $10 mW/cm^2$

(Jensh et al. 1982; Jensh 1997). Teratologic evaluation included the following parameters: mean litter size size, maternal organ weight and organ weight/body weight ratios of various organs (brain, liver, kidneys, and ovaries), number of resorptions and absorption rate, number of abnormalities rate, and mean term fetal weight. Mothers were rebred, and the second unexposed litters were evaluated for teratogenic effects. Animals exposed did not exhibit any constant significant alterations in any of the above mentioned parameters.

Sperms lack the capability to repair DNA damage. Human sperms are damaged by cell phone radiation at very low intensities (0.00034–0.07 $\mu W/cm^2$). There is a flood of new studies reporting sperm damage in human and animals, causing substantial concern for fertility, reproduction, and health of the offspring (unrepaired by mutation in sperm). Waist pockets are the sites usually adopted by people to keep their mobile phones. Exposure levels are similar to those resulting from wearing a cell phone on the belt or in the pant pocket (Bioinitiative Report 2012).

Dasdag et al. (1999) experimenting on Wistar albino rats exposed animals to mobile phone for 2 h/day for one month in standby position, where the SAR was 0.141 W/kg. The decrease of epididymal sperm counts in the exposed group was not found to be significant. Histological changes were observed in the testes. Seminiferous tubular diameter of rat testes in experimental group was lower than those of controls. Rectal temperature of rats in the experimental group was found to be higher than in the sham-exposed group. However, the same group of workers could not replicate the same results in Sprague-Dawley rats, exposed to 890–915 MHz pulsed wave (PW) daily for 20 min/day for one month (250mW radiated power, SAR = 0.52 W/kg).

Dasdag et al. (2000) examined the effect of microwaves emitted by cellular phones on males and females (915 MHz, SAR 0.155 W/kg). These authors observed no difference in the rectal temperature between the experimental and control group. The birth weight of offspring in the experimental group was significantly lower than in the sham-exposed group. However, in the next generation of rats the parameters under investigation showed no difference. In another study, Dasdag et al. (2003) reported the decrease in seminiferous tubule diameter in male rat testes after exposure, where they used commercially available 890–915 MHz GSM with 0.141 W/kg whole body SAR. Cobb et al. (2000) exposed pregnant rats to ultra wide band (UWB) 0.1–1 GHz radiation. In order to determine if teratological changes occur in rat pups as a result of (i) daily UWB exposures during gestation days 3±1.8, or (ii) as a result of both prenatal and postnatal (10 days) exposures, dams were exposed either to (a) UWB irradiation with average whole body specific absorption rate 45 mW/kg, (b) sham irradiation, or (c) a positive control. Offsprings were examined regarding litter size, sex ratios, weights, coat appearance, and tooth eruption. The pups postnatally exposed were examined for hippocampal morphology. Generally, no significant differences were found between the exposed and sham group. The medial-to-lateral length of the hippocampus was significantly longer in the UWB-exposed pups than in the sham-exposed animals but could not be correlated with neurological dysfunction. The male offspring exposed in utero to UWB mated significantly less frequently than sham-exposed males, but when they did mate there was no difference in fertilization and offspring numbers from the sham group.

Aitken et al. (2005) assessed the testis of mice irradiated with 900 MHz in a wave guide for 7 days (12 h/day, SAR = 90mW/kg) and reported no abnormalities in sperm count, morphology, and vitality. However, they reported significant damage to the mitochondrial genome as well as to the nuclear globin locus. Also Ozguner et al. (2005) have not reported any adverse affect on rats due to 900 MHz CW microwave exposure (1±0.4 mW/cm^2). The parameters they considered were weight of testis, testicular biopsy score count, and the percentage of interstitial tissue. However, the exposed group showed a decrease in height of germinal epithelium.

Forgacs et al. (2006) have reported that repeated whole body exposure to1800 MHz GSM-like microwave exposure (0.018–0.23 W/kg) below the maximum permissible exposure level recommended by ICNIRP is able to increase the serum testosterone level, RBC, and VPRC volume packed red cells in male mice, though within the physiological limit. These authors further reported that the unaltered in vitro steroidogenic capacity of Leydig cells obtained from microwave exposed mice suggests that Leydig cells were not the primary targets of the applied microwave exposure or the direct action was transient only and it was confined to the period of exposure. It is suggestive that the main target of action is probably located at the higher regulation level of the hypothalamic–pituitary–gonadal axis.

Ribeiro et al. (2007) exposed male rats to RF emitted from a conventional cell phone on their testicular function (1835–1850 MHz, 0.04–1.4 mW/cm^2). These authors have reported that total body weight and absolute and relative testicular and epididymal weight did not change significantly, and so the epididymal sperm count. Yan et al. (2007) exposed 800 MHz digital and 800 MHz analog cell phones to rats for a period of 3h to 30 min for 18 weeks (SAR of 0.9 to 1.8 W/kg). The authors analyzed the morphology of the sperm cells from epididymis of rats and found no significant difference in the deformities among the experimental and control group of animals. They also studied the effects of cellular phone emissions on sperm motility in rats. Rats were exposed to two 3h periods of daily cellular phone emissions for 18 weeks, whereby the sperm samples were then collected for evaluation. These authors concluded that exposed group of rats exhibited a significantly higher incidence of sperm cell death than control group. In addition, abnormal clumping of sperm cells was present in rats exposed to cellular phone emissions and absent from control group rats. Yilmaz et al. (2008) reported that rats exposed to 900 MHz radiation

(SAR 0.87 W/kg) 20 min/day for a period of one month did not alter the antiapoptotic protein in the testes of rats. Dasdag et al. (2008)also reported that 2h/day (7 days a week) exposure to rats for a period of 10 months did not affect the active caspase-3 level in testes of rats.

A related issue is the corresponding effect on male infertility. A study carried out in Poland (Wdowiak et al. 2007) on the population using mobile phone (GSM equipment) spread over a period of 1–2 years has found their sperm quality affected. They reported a decrease in the percentage of sperm cells in vital progressing motility in the semen as well as their structure is correlated with the frequency of using mobile phones. These two findings seem to be mutually consistent.

Batellier et al. (2008) exposed fertilized fertilized chicken eggs to a mobile phone over the entire period of incubation. The cell phone in call position was placed at a distance of <25 cm from the eggs, where in the sham position the cell phone in the off position was kept at a distance of 1.5 m away from the exposed group. A significantly higher percentage of embryo mortality was observed in the experimental group compared to the sham-exposed group.

Sommer et al. (2009) undertook a vey exhaustive study whereby they subjected male and female mice chronically exposed (life-long, 24 h/day) to mobile phone communication electromagnetic fields at 1966 MHz (universal mobile telecommunication service, UMTS). They studied their development and fertility pattern over four generations by investigating histological, physiological, behavioral, and reproductive functions. They considered SAR variation from the time of mating was 0 (sham), and increased to 0.08, 0.4, and 1.3 W/kg. Power densities were kept constant for each group (0, 1.35, 6.8, and 22 W/m^2), resulting in varying SARs due to different number of pups during the course of blind experimentation. The results show no harmful effects of exposure on the fertility and development of the animals. The number and the development of the pups were not affected by the exposure. These authors concluded no harmful effects of long-term exposure of mice to UMTS over several generations.

As a follow-up of the above, Otitoloju et al. (2010) exposed male mice to radiofrequency radiations from mobile phone (GSM) base stations at a workplace complex and residential quarters caused 39.78 and 46.03%, respectively, in sperm head abnormalities compared to 2.13% in control group, which corresponds to P <0.005. The major abnormalities observed were knobbed hook, pin head, and banana-shaped sperm head. The abnormalities were also found to be dose dependent. The results are important as this may have severe consequences on the offsprings.

Salma et al. (2010) examined the accumulating effects of exposure to electromagnetic radiation emitted by a conventional mobile phone (800 MHz, standby position, kept opposite to the testis) on the testicular function and structure. The animals were exposed 8 h daily for a period of

12 weeks in a specially designed cage. The data obtained were semen analysis and sperm function tests conducted weekly. Other parameters evaluated were histological testicular sections and serum total testosterone level. When compared with other two groups (stress control and ordinary), phone group showed a drop in sperm concentration at week 6 which became significant at week 8. Mobile sperm population showed similarity among the three study groups until week 10 when it declined significantly, and thereafter in phone and stress control groups, with more significant decline in the phone group (50, 61, and 72.4%, respectively). Histological examination also showed a significant decrease in the diameter of seminiferous tubules in the phone group versus the stress and ordinary controls (191 μm vs. 206 and 226 μm, respectively). These authors concluded that the pulsed radio frequency emitted by a conventional mobile phone kept in the standby position could affect the testicular function and structure in the adult rabbit.

Gao et al. (2016) investigated the influence of cellphone electromagnetic radiation (CER, 2 h exposure) on the testicular ultrastructure and the apoptosis of spermatogenic cells in male rats. Compared with the normal controls, the exposed group showed swollen basement membrane of seminiferous tubules, separated tight junction of Sertoli cells, increased cell intervals, apparent vacuoles, and medullization in some mitochondria, and increased apoptosis of spermatogenic cells, mainly the apoptosis of primary spermatocytes ($P < 0.05$). Compared to the 2 h CER group, the animals of the 4 h CER group exhibited swollen basement membrane of seminiferous tubules, more separated tight junction of Sertoli cells, wider cell intervals, incomplete membrane of spermatogonial cells, and fragments of cytoplasm. They also observed nuclear pyknosis and notch, slight dilation of perinuclear space, abnormalities of intracellular mitochondria with vacuoles, fuzzy structure, and fusion or disappearance of some cristae, and increased damage of mitochondria and apoptosis of spermatogenic cells, including the apoptosis of spermatogonial cells, primary spermatocytes, and secondary spermatocytes ($P < 0.05$). The authors concluded that CER can damage the testicular ultrastructure and increase the apoptosis of spermatogenic cells of the male rat in a time-dependent manner, and the apoptosis of spermatogenic cells may be associated with the damage to mitochondria.

Kamali et al. (2017) studied the effects of 3G+wi-fi modems on human sperm quality. A total of 40 semen specimens were gathered between March and September 2015 from healthy adult men. It was concluded that electromagnetic waves emitted from 3G+wi-fi modems cause a significant decrease in sperm motility and velocity, especially in nonprogressive motile sperms. Other parameters of semen analysis did not change significantly. EMWs, which are used in communications worldwide, are a suspected cause of male infertility. These studies revealed a significant decrease in the quality of human semen after exposure to EMWs emitted from 3G+wi-fi modems.

It is now generally accepted that human sperm are damaged by cell phone radiation at very low intensities. There is flood of new studies reporting sperm damage in human and animals, causing substantial concern for fertility, reproduction, and health of the offspring (unrepaired by mutation in sperm). Exposure levels are similar to those resulting from wearing a cell phone on the belt or in the trouser pocket. As discussed before, sperms lack the capability to repair DNA damage (Blank & Goodman 2011). Several other international studies have replicated studies showing adverse effects on sperm quality, motility, and pathology in men who in particular keep mobile phone in their pocket or tie with belt (Fejes et al. 2005; Agarwal et al. 2008, 2009; Kumar et al. 2012). Some other studies also support a similar conclusion, that is, exposure to cell phone radiation or keeping of mobile phone close to the testes of human males (and animals) affects sperm counts, motility, viability, and structure (Aitken et al. 2005; Behari & Kesari 2006; Erogul et al. 2006).

To understand the mechanism of EMF biointeraction, Kesari et al. (2011) investigated the role of free radical generation due to mobile phone frequency exposure on 70 days old male rats. The exposure was limited to 2 h/day for a period of 35 days. The mentioned SAR of mobile phone was 0.9 W/kg. Antioxidant enzymes: glutathione peroxidase (P <0.001) and superoxide dismutase (P <0.007) showed a significant decline, while an increase in catalase (P <0.005) was observed. Malondialdehyde (P <0.003) showed an increase, while histone kinase (P <0.003) and micronuclei showed a significant decrease (P <0.002) in the exposed group. A significant change in sperm cell cycle (G(0) – G(1)) (P <0.042) and G(2)/M (P <0.022) was recorded. They have shown a significant increase (P < 0.002) in micro nucleated polychromatic erythrocyte (PCE) of mobile phone exposed group (0.67 ± 0.15) as compared with control group (1.36 ± 0.07) and a decrease in the ratio of PCE to NCE (normochromatic erythrocyte) in blood cells. Poor DNA integrity and chromosomal breaking may ultimately negatively affect jeopardize the male reproductive function. Sperm DNA damage correlates with poor sperm count and abnormal morphology. Nuclear damage in Leydig cells is associated with apoptosis and decreased testosterone production. Free radical generation was significantly increased (P <0.035). An overproduction of reactive oxygen species acting on spermatozoa is an indication of infertility (Figure 5.5a). Animal studies have further demonstrated that oxidative and DNA damage, pathological changes in testes of animals, decreased sperm motility and viability, and other measures of deleterious damage to the male germ line (Salma et al. 2010; Kumar et al. 2012). A summary of animal results of low level exposure of EMF on cell is summarized in Figure 5.5b.

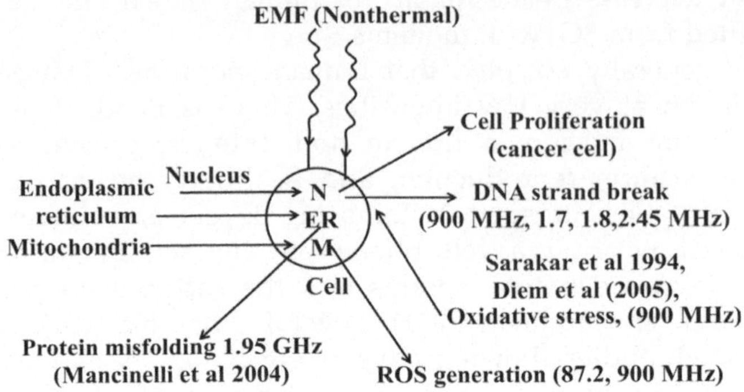

FIGURE 5.5a
Nonthermal EMF effects at cellular level.

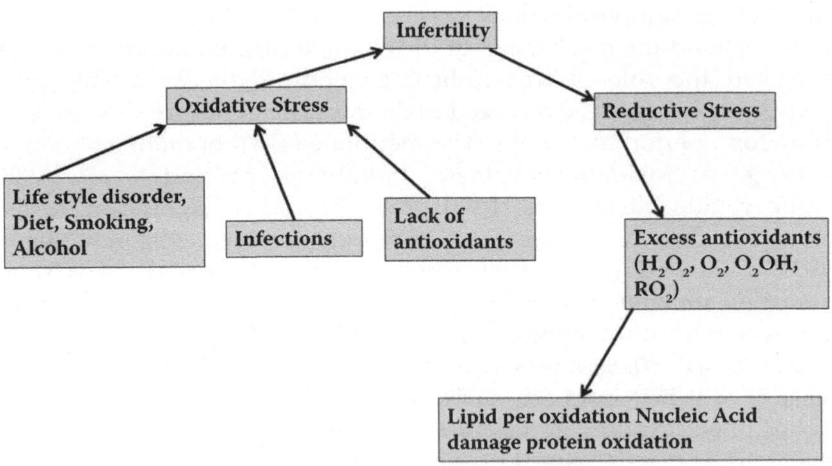

FIGURE 5.5b
Infertility and the oxidative stress.

Female Reproduction

There are comparatively lesser number of animal studies carried out on effects of cell phone radiation on female fertility parameters. Some are described next.

A study as below Magras and Xenos (1997) consisted of in vivo experiments around an "antenna park" where the frequency emission ranged from 88.5 to 950 MHz. At these locations RF power densities were ranging between 168 and 1053 nW/cm^2. The prenatal development of the newborn, evaluated by the crown-rump length, the body weight, and the number of lumbar, sacral, and coccygeal vertebrae, was improved. These authors reported irreversible infertility (progressive decrease in the number of newborn per dam) in mice after five generations of exposure to RFR at cell phone tower exposure levels of less than 1 $\mu W/cm^2$.

Wistar rats were continuously exposed (Bornhausen & Scheingraber 2000) during pregnancy to a low level of 0.1 mW/cm^2 (900 MHz, 217 Hz pulse modulated EMF). Whole body average SAR values for the freely roaming, pregnant animals were measured in models (17.5 and 75 mW/kg). No differences between exposed and sham-exposed dams or offspring were recorded in terms of litter size, evolution of body mass, and developmental landmarks of litter mates. Nakamura et al. (2003) found that exposure to 2.45 GHz CW microwave on female at 2 mW/cm^2 power density for 90 min decreased uteroplacental blood flow, increased progesterone, and $PGF_2\alpha$ in pregnant rats.

Oral et al. (2006) exposed 16 weeks female rats to 900 MHz radiation (30 min/day for 30 days). The animals were exposed at 1 ± 0.4 mW/cm^2 (SAR 0.016–4 W/kg) and experimental group fed vitamin C and E. They found endometrium apoptosis in exposed group. Guney et al. (2007) repeating the same set of experiments (with the inclusion of control group) reported histological changes in endometrium, diffuse and severe apoptosis in the endometrial surface, epithelial and glandular cells in the group exposed to EMF. These authors also reported eosinophilic, leucocytes, and lymphocyte infiltration in the endometrial stroma.

Gul et al. (2009) reported that rats exposed to standby level RFR (phones on but not transmitting calls) caused decrease in the number of ovarian follicles in pups born to these exposed dams.

In utero development and over born were studied by Grigoriev et al. (2010). The animals were divided into three groups: control (1), sham (2), and experimental (microwave irradiated) (3). On 15thday of pregnancy, 5–6 pregnant rats from each group were sacrificed to evaluate embryo mortality. Also, the number of implants, corpora lutea of pregnancy, live embryos, resorbed embryos, as well as the mass of the embryos and placentas were recorded in each group of rats. Embryo development and placental formation was assessed by weight. On day 20 of pregnancy, four female rats from groups 2 and3 were sacrificed to evaluate total in utero mortality and the fertility index; the number of implants and live embryos were also recorded for these rats. In each group, 11–12 pregnant rats were kept alive until delivery to send offspring development and survival. At delivery, the number of newborn in a litter, body mass of newborns, number of stillborns, and apparent birth defects were registered. Study was also carried on the effects on postnatal development of the offspring. This was studied for the first 30 postnatal days using generally accepted integral and specific parameters. Changes in body mass were determined over the first postnatal month by weekly measurements. The specific parameters were appearance of hair cover, detachment of auricles, opening of eyes, eruption of incisors, and onset of independent eating.

On day 15 of pregnancy, that is, 5 days after the injection of blood serum, the number of live embryos per animal did not differ significantly among the studied groups and was equal to 7.5±0.4, 8.3±0.2, and 7.4±0.4 in groups 1, 2, and 3, respectively. The average mass of the embryos of rats from groups 2 and 3 was similar (190.4±5.4 and 185.4±4.7 mg, respectively) and was higher than in the control group (151.1±1.6 mg). The ratios of placenta-to-embryo mass (placental coefficient) were 1.14±0.16, 0.96±0.03, and 0.95±0.04 in groups 1, 2, and 3, respectively, and did not differ significantly between each other. Data on embryo mortality evaluated on day 15 of pregnancy showed that embryo mortality was higher in rats from group 3; however, this was not significantly different compared to the other groups.

On day 20 of pregnancy, that is, 10 days after injection of blood serum, the number of live fetuses per animal did not differ significantly between groups 2 and 3 and was equal to 8.3±0.7 and 7.5±0.8, respectively. The average fetal mass in rats also did not differ significantly between these groups and was equal to 3.8±0.1 and 3.7±0.1, respectively. In utero fetal mortality on day 20 of pregnancy increased compared to that on day 15 and did not differ significantly between the rats from groups 2 and 3, being 19.5±6.3% and 23.1±6.8, respectively.

Of the total number of pregnant rats left for the delivery, offsprings were delivered in 100% of rats in the control group (11 rats from 11 animals), 90% of rats from group 2 (9 rats from 10 animals), and 33.3% of rats from group 3 (4 rats from12 animals). From the group of rats injected with blood serum from the sham-exposed animals (group2), two rats that did not deliver offspring were sacrificed, one was found not to be pregnant and another had all embryos resorbed. Eight rats from the group injected with blood serum from RF-exposed animals (group3) that did not deliver offspring were also sacrificed and all were found to have their embryos resorbed. Because the body mass of rats was not measured during pregnancy, it was not known when the resorption of embryos occurred. It is concluded that in utero mortality among rats from group 3 was significantly higher compared to rats from groups 1 and 2 (55.6±4%, 4.3 ±3.0%, and 11.7±3.3%, respectively).

Panagopoulos (2012) reported that as a result of microwave exposure, there is a decreased ovarian development size of ovaries, and premature cell death of ovarian follicles and nurse cells in *Drosophila melanogaster*.

A summary of biological effects of mobile phone exposure is summarized (Figure 5.6).

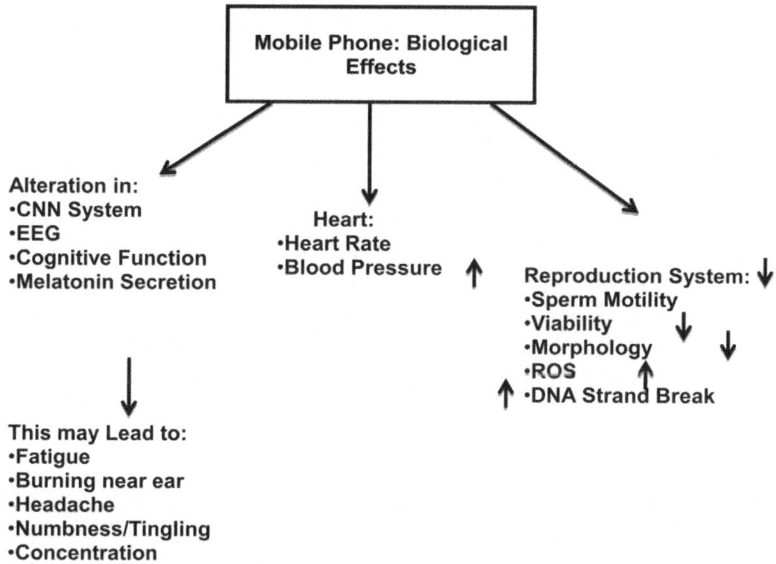

FIGURE 5.6
Mobile phone frequency biointeraction: bioeffects.

5.8 Epidemiological Studies

Presently, it is almost impossible to select control (unexposed groups) because the whole population in many countries is exposed to wide range of microwave frequencies from various sources such as mobile phones, base stations, wireless local area network (WLAN), wireless personal area network (WPAN), and digital enhanced cordless communication (DECT) wireless phones and given that duration of exposure (at least 10 years latency period) is also important for the effects of nonthermal microwaves along power density/SAR. Exposure from downlink sources (base stations, etc.) may contribute up to 90% of total outdoor-urban exposure to DECT phone and is comparable to exposure from mobile phones (Frei et al. 2009; Joseph et al. 2010). Another point of uncertainty is that, because the signals are completely replaced by other signals faster than once per 10 years, a duration comparable with latent period, epidemiologic studies cannot provide basement for assessment of upcoming new signals. Among the initial reports was one from the multicenter Interphone study which focused on acoustic neuroma and was negative though the number of long-term users was small (Christensen et al. 2004). The first case-control study of brain tumors was conducted in Sweden (Hardell et al. 2001, 2002, 2003). This included adult cases diagnosed in two regions in Sweden between 1994 and 1996 and still alive, with two controls per case matched for region of residence. Details of intensity and duration of mobile phone use, preferred side (ear) of use, and whether phones were analogue or digital, and handheld or hands-free, were gathered by postal questionnaire followed by telephone interview (Hardell et al. 1999). 209 cases (only about a third of the malignant cases occurring in the study geographical area in the period) (Ahlbom & Feychting 1999; Ahlbom et al. 2004, 2009) took part along with 425 controls (a reported 91% response rate extraordinarily high for a contemporary population-based study). There was no association of phone use with brain tumors (Hardell et al. 1999), though later reanalysis of side of use in relation to tumor site suggested a possible relationship (Hardell et al. 2001). A second larger study a few years later by the same authors Hardell et al. (2002,2003) was similar in design to the first. It involved 1303 living cases (51% of all brain tumors diagnosed in 1997–2000) and their controls. Cumulative phone use for over 85 h, 10 years before case diagnosis, gave ORs for brain tumors of 1.9 (1.1–3.2) and 3.0 (0.6–14.9), respectively, for analogue and cordless phones, but not raised for digital. There was no adjustment for confounding variables. Ipsilateral use of analogue phones was related to temporal tumors, OR = 2.5 (1.3–4.9), and general analogue phone use was associated with acoustic neuroma, OR = 3.5 (1.8–6.8) (Hardell et al. 2002, 2003). Muscat et al. (2000) conducted two hospital-based case-control studies in the United Stated, one of malignant brain tumors and the other of acoustic neuroma, using the same ascertainment and data collection procedures. The first study included 469 cases of brain cancer (70% response rate) and 422 matched controls from the same hospitals (90% response rate) with a variety of malignant and benign conditions. Information about mobile phone use was obtained by standard interview (of proxies for 9% of cases and 1% of controls). No higher risks were seen relating to frequency or duration of use, or for site or histologic subtype brain cancer. An excess of brain cancer was found on the same side of the head as reported phone use among 41 cases with assessable data ($p = 0.06$), compared with a deficit on the side of mobile phone use for tumors specifically located in the temporal lobe ($p = 0.33$).

In another U.S. hospital-based case-control study (Inskip et al. 2001), interview data obtained from 782 cases with brain tumors (92% response rate via proxies for 16% and 3% of glioma and acoustic neuroma patients, respectively) and 799 matched hospital controls with nonmalignant conditions (88% response; 3% by proxy). Results adjusted for potential confounders showed no association between cumulative use of mobile phones (mainly analogue) and brain tumor overall or by histological subtype or anatomical location.

Subscription records of national network providers were used to identify mobile phone users in a Finnish case-control study (Auvinen et al. 2002). All people (398) diagnosed with brain tumors in 1996, ascertained from the National cancer Registry, were matched with five controls per case drawn from the national population register. The OR for brain tumors with ever subscription to phones was 2.1 (1.3–3.4) for analogue phones and 1.0 for digital, and the OR for glioma was 1.5 (1.0–2.4) (null for other brain tumor histologies) for any phone subscription. The average duration of subscription was 2–3 years for analogue phones and less for digital. Adjusting for potential confounders did not alter results. No information was available about the frequency or duration of calls or about corporate subscriptions.

Of two cohort studies, an early U.S. study (Rothman et al. 1996;Dreyer et al. 1999) analyzed one year of follow-up of mortality in a cohort of 285,561 noncorporate users of mobile phones with at least two billing cycles from two U.S. carriers. No relation was found between mortality from brain cancer (based on six cases ascertained from the National Death Index) and the use of handheld versus non-handheld phones. The overall mortality of the cohort was less than that in the general population. The second cohort study was in Denmark (Johansen et al. 2001) and comprised 420,095 private cellular network subscribers (80% of all subscribers), with average follow-up for analogue and digital subscribers of 3.5 and 1.9 years, respectively. Standardized incidence ratios comparing cancer rates in phone users with national rates allowing for sex, age, and period showed no relation to risk of brain and nervous system cancers (standardized infection ratio, SIR = 0.95, 0.81–1.21) and reduced risk of smoking-related cancers. Risks did not vary by age at, or time since, first subscription, phone type, or tumor location. Again no information was available about the frequency or duration of cells or about corporate subscriptions.

Regarding head and neck cancers, no association with parotid gland tumors (34 cases) was seen in the Finnish case-control study (Auvinen et al. 2002), or in the Danish cohort study (Johansen et al. 2001). A mixed population and hospital-based case-control study of uveal melanoma (Stang et al. 2001) included 118 cases and 475 controls. Occupational exposure to mobile phones for several hours a day for 6 months or more assessed by interview gave a raised OR (4.2, 1.2–14.5), reflecting result in the hospital-based participants (OR = 10.1), although there was no raised risk of uveal melanoma is the Danish mobile phone user cohort (Johansen et al. 2001). Finally, leukemia was assessed in both cohort studies, but no relation with phone use was found.

Studies in a single community, one in Bavaria (Eger et al. 2004) and one in Israel (Wolf & Wolf 2004), have a significantly increased incidence in an area of 400 and 350 m around a base station, respectively. Although incidence in proximity to the base station strongly exceeded the expected values and was significant even considering over dispersion in the case of the Neila study in Bavaria, though no far-reaching conclusions can be drawn due to the ecological nature of the studies. However, both studies underline the urgent need to investigate this problem with an appropriate design. Neubauer et al. (2007) have recommended focusing initially on short-term effects and "soft" outcomes given the problems of exposure assessment. Such a case control design within areas around a sufficiently large sample of base stations would provide answers to the questions raised by the studies of Eger et al. (2004) and Wolf and Wolf (2004). A similar approach chosen in the study of leukemia around nuclear power plants (Kaatsch et al. 2008) may also be applied for studying cancer in relation to base station exposure.

Agarwal et al. (2008) in an epidemiological study have concluded that the use of mobile phone adversely affected the quality of semen by decreasing the sperm count, motility, viability, and morphology. These parameters were found to be lower in mobile user group. In another study conducted on 37 men, the duration of possession and daily transmission time of cell phones correlated negatively with the proportion of rapidly progressive mobile spermatozoa, suggesting that the prolonged use of cell phone has negative result on sperm motility (Fejes et al. 2005). Davoudi et al. (2002) involving 13 men with normal semen analysis also concluded that using GSM phones for 6 h a day for 5 days decreased the motility of spermatozoa. Similarly, Erogul et al. (2006) found a decrease in sperm motility in semen samples of 27 men exposed to 900 MHz cell phone for 5 min. Kilgallon and Simon (2005) found a decrease in sperm concentration in subjects using mobile phone. In spite of consistency in these data, the variability in the lifestyle and possible impact of emitted radiation from other sources are the major instance of uncertainty.

Hutter et al. (2006) reported that short-term exposure to GSM cell phone radiation resulted in complaints of headache, neurological problems, sleep and concentration problem in adults (0.01–0.05 $\mu W/cm^2$ exposure levels). In a study conducted by Buchner and Eger (2011) extending over 18 months, to assess changes in stress hormones in 60 persons exposed before and after a mobile phone base station went into operation in Germany. The study showed that a chronic exposure to whole body exposure (0.006–0.01 $\mu W/cm^2$) had significant impact on stress hormone over time. In the beginning months, adrenaline levels first increased in a dose-dependent manner ($p<0.002$) and then decreased below normal levels ($p<0.005$). Both the average as well as the median adrenaline values increased after the activation of the transmitter and decreased again after one year with exposure levels >0.006 $\mu W/cm^2$. Chronically ill subjects and children showed especially strong responses while healthy subjects showed no effect.

A 6-year study was conducted by Eskander et al. (2012) to assess the role of radiations emitted by mobile phone or base stations and its relations with human hormone profile. The study revealed significant RFR effects on pituitary–adrenal axis, resulting in reduction of ACTH, cortisol, thyroid hormones, prolactin in young females, and testosterone levels in males. These authors however revealed no mention of RFR power density levels.

A study was carried out to evaluate the effect of RFR on the DNA damage and antioxidant status in cultured human peripheral blood lymphocytes (HPBLs) of individuals residing in the vicinity of mobile phone base stations and comparing it with healthy controls. The study groups matched for various demographic data including age, gender, dietary pattern, smoking habit, alcohol consumption, duration of mobile phone use, and average daily mobile phone use. The RF power density of the exposed individuals was significantly higher (p <0.0001) when compared to the control group. The HPBLs were cultured and the DNA damage was assessed by cytokinesis blocked micronucleus (MN) assay in the binucleate lymphocytes. The analyses of data from the exposed group (n = 40), residing within a perimeter of 80 m of mobile base stations, showed significantly ($p < 0.0001$) higher number of micronuclei when compared to the control group, residing 300 m away from the mobile base station(s). The analysis of various antioxidants in the plasma of exposed individuals revealed a significant attrition in glutathione (GSH) concentration ($p < 0.01$), activities of catalase (CAT) ($p < 0.001$) and superoxide dismutase (SOD) ($p < 0.001$), and rise in lipid peroxidation (LPO) when compared to controls. Multiple linear regression analyses revealed a significant association among reduced GSH concentration ($p < 0.05$), CAT ($p < 0.001$), and SOD ($p < 0.001$) activities and elevated MN level ($p < 0.001$) and LPO (p< 0.001) with increasing RF power density. Qureshi et al. (2018) considered human body exposure to radiofrequency electromagnetic waves emitted from smart meters using various exposure configurations. Specific energy absorption rate distributions were determined using three anatomically realistic human models. Each model was assigned with age- and frequency-dependent dielectric properties representing a collection of age groups. Generalized Exposure conditions involving standing and sleeping postures were assessed for a home area network operating at 868 and 2,450 MHz. The smart meter antenna was fed with 1 W power input which is an overestimation of what real devices typically emit (15 mW max limit). The highest observed whole body specific energy absorption rate value was 1.87 mW kg^{-1} within the child model at a distance of 15 cm from a 2,450 MHz device. The higher values were attributed to differences in dimension and dielectric properties within the model. SAR values were also estimated based on power density levels derived from electric field strength measurements made at various distances from smart meter devices. All the calculated SAR values were found to be very small in comparison to International Commission on Non-Ionizing Radiation Protection limits for public exposure.

Papadopoulou et al. (2017) investigated the association between maternal cell phone use in pregnancy and child's language, communication, and motor skills at 3 and 5 years. The study included 45,389 mother–child pairs, recruited at mid-pregnancy from 1999 to 2008. These authors reported no cell phone use in early pregnancy as reported by 9.8% of women, while 39%, 46.9%, and 4.3% of the women were categorized as low, medium, and high cell phone users. Children of cell phone user mothers had 17% lower adjusted risk of having low sentence complexity at three years, compared to children of nonusers. The risk was 13%, 22%, and 29% lower by low, medium, and high maternal cell phone use. Additionally, children of cell phone users had lower risk of low motor skills score at 3 years, compared to children of nonusers, but this association was not found at 5 years. They found no association between maternal cell phone use and low communication skills.

Also they reported a decreased risk of low language and motor skills at three years in relation to prenatal cell phone use, which might be explained by enhanced maternal–child interaction among cell phone users. No evidence of adverse neurodevelopmental effects of prenatal cell phone use was reported.

Röschke and Mann (1997) did not notice any difference in the awake EEG of subjects exposed to radiation emitted by cellular phones.

The TDMA field had no enhancing effect on incidence, type, or location of spontaneous nervous system tumors. On termination of experiments, the TDMA field appeared to reduce incidence of malignant glial cell tumors in rats that received the ENU drug when compared with rats receiving ENU and no field exposure (4 vs. 13). The TDMA field also appeared to reduce the incidence of spontaneous glial tumors occurring in rats not receiving the ENU drug when they were compared with control animals (2 vs. 7). Tumors in exposed rats were smaller in volume. There were no gender differences in tumor incidence. In rats not surviving to experiment termination (n=54, 22%), the TDMA field appeared to prolong latency of appearance of both spontaneous and ENU-induced glial cell tumors, but did not alter histological criteria of tumor types. Consistent nonsignificant differences in survival rates were noted between the four rat groups, with higher death rates in a progression: sham/field, sham/sham, ENU/field, and ENU/sham.

Subjective symptoms, including tinnitus, headache, dizziness, fatigue, sensations of warmth, dysesthesia of the scalp, visual symptoms such as flashes, memory loss, and sleep disturbance have been investigated in relation to mobile phone use (Chia et al. 2000; Oftedel et al. 2000; Sandstrom et al. 2001).

Panagopoulos et al. (2007) showed that exposing adult *Drosophila melanogaster* to a mobile phone signal for just 6 min a day for 6 days broke the DNA into fragments that give rise to their eggs and half of the eggs died. Diem et al. (2005) also found significant fragmentation after exposing cultured rat and human cells for 16 h to a simulated mobile phone signal. It shows that exposing human cells for 24 h to simulated phone signals gave DNA fragmentation similar to that due to the gamma rays emitted from a radioactive isotope.

Human studies are in general open to a lot of uncertainties because of inherent variability in data. On the other hand, animal studies are possible in a comparatively controlled environment. Hence, the index of reliability is higher. These studies are pointer to a trend. Hence, any conclusion of their impact on health needs more data taking with differently designed protocols.

5.9 Free Radical Generation and Oxidative Stress

The present-day controversy regarding the mobile phone biological effect is mostly because of nonthermal effects, causing oxidative stress (Sies et al. 2005). It is unlikely that even a prolong use of mobile phone is capable of producing thermal damage. The theme of argument against its use is that the emitted radiations produce free radicals which damage DNA (Behrend et al. 2003). Another source of damaging the DNA are genotoxic agents (Sun 1990), which are the chemicals that are capable of directly damaging it, which in turn leads to mutation and/or clastogenic changes. A second category of carcinogenic compounds (nongenotoxic) functions through non-DNA or indirect-DNA reaction mechanisms. These compounds modulate cell growth and cell death.

Water chemistry: Mobile phone frequency exposure on humans is considered important from the health point of view because of the fact that biological systems have large water content.

The vast majority of biological molecules are present in an aqueous medium. When water is exposed to radiation, the water absorbs energy, and as a result forms chemically reactive species that can interact with dissolved substances (solutes). Water ionized form a solvated electron and H_2O^+. The H_2O^+ cation can react with water to form a hydrated proton (H_3O+) and a hydroxyl radical (HO). Furthermore, the solvated electron can recombine with the H_2O+ cation to form an excited state of the water. This excited state then discomposes to its species as hydroxyl radicals (HO), hydrogen atoms (H), and oxygen atoms (O). Finally, the solvated electron can react with solutes such as solvated protons or oxygen molecules to form hydrogen atoms and dioxygen radical anions, respectively.

The fact that oxygen changes the radiation chemistry may be one reason why oxygenated tissues are more sensitive to irradiation than the deoxygenated tissue at the center of a tumor. The free radicals such as the hydroxyl radical, and chemically modified biomolecules such as DNA lead to damage such as breaks in the DNA strands. Some substances can protect against radiation-induced damage by reacting with the reactive species generated by the irradiation of water.

While in vitro data are available these are often not confirmative because of the fact that in vivo there is a mechanism of defense built into the system which is not available with the former. Mobile phone exposures are likely to produce mainly nonthermal effects. Blood–brain barrier (Fritze et al. 1997) and ocular effects (Elder 2003) have been reported, but are mainly due to power exposure in the thermal range.

Water is a wide band attenuator of microwaves and hence this property is used utilized for cooking in microwave ovens. The amount of energy deposited inside the body to produce heating is invariably dependent on its frequency, its orientation, with respect to the object and the electrical properties of the tissue. When the intensity increases above the level to maintain homeostats, it starts affecting the biosystems when the temperature exceeds 1 °C. There is a preferential heating near a frequency close to the resonance level. The organs of the body having reduced blood supply are more prone to this leading to cataract formation and reduction in sperm counts (tests) due to acute microwaves exposure.

While in vivo exposure of Wistar albino rats (Yurekli et al. 2006) implies an induction of oxidative stress or an interaction with antioxidant cellular activity, in vitro experiments (Hirose et al. 2006) found no indication of cellular stress in human glioblastoma cells and fibroblasts. One of the major molecular effects of magnetic fields is their interaction on nuclear spins of paramagnetic molecules (Grissom 1995). Results of experimental data in vitro (Grissom 1995; Kula & Drozdz 1996) revealed that intracellular processes occurring under the influence of a power line magnetic field related to free radicals and signal transmission may determine its biological effects. An uncontrolled free oxygen radical release, termed oxidative stress, may cause protein oxidation, enzyme inactivation, and lipid peroxidation within the cellular membranes, resulting in structural and functional abnormalities as well as in oxidative damage to the DNA and RNA leading to increased mutation frequency and correspondingly triggering of carcinogenesis (Sun 1990).

Mitochondrial respiratory chain is the major site for the generation of superoxide radicals (O_2, H_2O_2). It is possible that EMR may affect the mitochondrial membranes to produce large amounts of radicals ROS under experimental conditions. It has been pointed out (De Iuliis et al. 2009) that when SAR is increased (0.4–27.5 W/kg), human spermatozoa motility and vitality significantly reduced after the EMR exposure at 1800 MHz, while the mitochondrial generation of ROS and DNA fragmentation is significantly increased.

Superoxide dismutase (SOD) plays a key role in the system protecting the body from destructive free radical activity (Mc Cord & Fridovich 1969). Its absence or decreased activity may have noxious metabolic outcomes. Hydrogen superoxide, a product of SOD activity, is also a strong inhibitor of this enzyme (Ratilio 1972). That is why the effective detoxication of active oxygen forms takes place with concordant SOD and CAT action.

SOD activity decreases due to the effect of electromagnetic field exposure and CAT activity increases. Glutathione peroxidase (GSH-P_X)

inactivates hydrogen superoxide and organic hydroxides together with glutathione reductase and glucose-6-dehydrogenase with reduced glutathione. The oxidized glutathione generated is then reduced again by NADPH-dependent glutathione reductase, in the process that maintains the peroxidation continuity (Collonce & Hochstein 1981).

A significant decrease in red blood cell GSH-P_X activity indicates a tendency of abnormal function of the antioxidative system caused by the electromagnetic field. Exposure to electromagnetic fields had lower ceruloplasmin activity, which seems to indicate that the free copper plasma concentration increases. However, mechanism of interaction is unclear. In young individuals, cellular defenses against the radical-induced protein oxidation by antioxidant enzymes are likely to be in prime shape and the proteases and protein synthesis machinery are fully functional. Thus, there is no change in the level of protein carbonyl during the first 45 years. However, after attaining the age of 45 years, enzymes including proteases and antioxidant proteins, and smaller antioxidant molecules in the individual become progressively inactivated due to the failure of the antioxidant systems to overcome the constant influx of ROS. Consequently, the accumulation of free radical induced carbonylated proteins accelerates, indicating the age when cells in the individual become increasingly more susceptible to ROS-mediated damage. Cumulated oxidative stress in brain cells can lead to neurodegenerative diseases and an excess of free radicals in cells has been suggested to be the cause of various human diseases (e.g., Parkinson, Alzheimer, amyotrophic lateral sclerosis, etc.).

An enzymatic cascade is initiated within cells when glutamate receptors are activated, leading to the synthesis of nitric oxide (NO). Receptor activation initiates an influx of calcium, triggering the enzyme nitric oxide synthase from the amino acid arginine. It has been identified as a widely distributed neuroregulator and neurotransmitter in many body tissues (Izumi & Zorumski 1993).

Oxidative damage has been reported in brain tissues (Salford et al. 2003; Ilhan et al. 2004). Spermatozoa are known to be susceptible to damage induced by oxidative stress, however, whether RF radiation is capable of inducing oxidative stress is still being explored. Conflicting results have been reported regarding the effect of electromagnetic waves exposure on the secretion of an antioxidant melatonin (de Seze et al. 1999; Gavella & Lipovac 2000; Burch et al. 2002). Studies analyzing the effect of RF radiation on apoptosis have failed to find any significant effect. An exposure of 1800 MHz signal for 12 h failed to induce apoptosis is human mono Mac 6 cells (Lantow et al. 2006). No evidence of apoptosis has been detected after exposing human leukemia cells in vitro to RF waves 25 times higher than the reference levels set by ICNIRP. However, this view has been recently revised by results from this laboratory where RF radiations have been found to increase apoptosis (Kesari & Behari 2010). Seishima et al. (2003) have examined classical contact energy reactions such as chromate allergy. These authors described the clinical characteristics and results of patch tests in eight patients with contact dermatitis possibly caused by handling a cellular phone. The present-day controversy regarding mobile phone is probably because of non-thermal effects.

Extensive research has undergone in investigating a variety of possible effects and includes epidemiologic, in vivo, and in vitro research. The overall epidemiologic evidence suggests that mobile phone use of less than 10 years does not pose any increased risk of brain tumor or acoustic neuroma. For longer duration, data are sparse. The safety standard assumes that EMF exposure causes biological damage only by heating, but several biological effects (including cell damage) have been reported which are caused by exposure below the safety limit (Behari 2009). Cellular stress response occurs where cells produce synthesize stress proteins in response to potentially harmful stimuli in the environment including EMF. The stress response to both radiofrequency and microwaves shows the inadequacy of the thermal SAR standards (macromolecular effects).

It may be concluded that some correlation exists between sperm motility and sperm chromatin structure, which are brought about by distorted epididymal protamination (Giwercman et al. 2003). ROS causes DNA fragmentation in somatic cells reducing protamination (Sun et al. 1997).

5.10 Present Scenario

Exposure to human population is from two man-made sources: handset and base station. There are important differences between the two. The typically very low exposure to microwaves from base stations rarely exceeding 1 mW/cm^2 is unlikely to produce any adverse effect. Assuming energy equivalence of effects to 24 h exposure at 1 mW/cm^2 from a base station would be roughly equivalent to 30 min exposure to a mobile phone operating at a power of 20 mW (average output power in areas of good coverage). Because we do not know whether time dose reciprocity holds for RF-EMF and whether there is a threshold for biological effects, there is an argument that such low exposures in vicinity of homes near base stations could have health effects.

The most important difference between mobile phone use and exposure from base station signals is one of duration of exposure. While mobile phones are used intermittently with normal exposure duration around 1–2 h per day, exposure to base stations is continuous (up to 24 h a day). It may be mentioned that the exposure of mobile phone users is in the near field and localized at the head (or waist) region, while base stations exposure to the whole body is essentially in the far field. Strictly speaking, exposure from mobile phones and their base stations have almost nothing in common except for the almost equal carrier frequency that is likely to be of lesser importance for determining biological effects. However, both the exposure is nonthermal in nature.

There are several field studies of well-being and exposure to base stations signals available to date. Two were in occupational groups working in a building below (Heinrich et al. 2007) as well as opposite a building with a roof-mounted base station antenna (Abdel-Rassoul et al. 2006).

The five studies carried out were in neighbors of base stations: Sanitini et al. (2003), Navarro et al. (2003), Hutter et al. (2006), Blettner et al. (2008), and Thomas et al. (2008). Studies had different methodologics with the least potential for bias.

Despite some methodological limitations of the different studies there are still strong indications that long-term exposure near base stations affects well-being. Symptoms most often associated with exposure were headaches, concentration difficulties, restlessness, and tremor (Huber et al. 2000). Sleeping problems were also related to distance from base station or power density, but it is possible that these results are confounded by concerns about adverse effects of the base station, or more generally, by specific personality traits. While the data are insufficient to delineate a threshold for adverse effects, the lack of observed effects at fractions of an mW/m^2 suggests that exposure around 0.5–1 mW/m^2 is a limit for safe exposure.

5.11 Conclusion

Bioeffects can occur in the first few minutes at levels associated with cell and cordless phone use. Bioeffects can also occur for just minutes after exposure to mobile phone masts (cell towers). Wi-fi and wireless utility smart meters produce whole body exposure. Chronic base station exposures can result in illness. Many of the bioeffects can reasonably be expected to result in adverse health effects if the exposures are prolonged or chronic (Figure 5.6). This may be mentioned that while a lot of data have accumulated on the biological effects of extremely low and mobile phone frequency exposure, many are contradictory and need to be explored further, particularly in relation to human being. There is a need for more independent replications of above findings. Based on these findings it is suggestive that it is necessary to create awareness among public about the possible ill effects of RFR exposure from cell phone, while prudent avoidance is recommended.

References

Abdel-Rassoul G, Abou E, Fatech O, Abou-Salem M, Michael A, Farahat F, El-Batanouny M & Salem E (2006) Neurobehavioral effects among inhabitants around mobile phone base stations. *NeuroToxicology*, *28*: 434.

Adey RW (1990) Electromagnetic fields & the essence of living systems. In *Modern Radio Science* (Andersen JB ed.). Oxford University Press, p. 87.

Adey WR, Byus CV, Cain CD, Higgins RJ, Jones RA, Kean CJ, Kuster N, MacMurray NA, Stagg RB, Zimmerman GJ, Phillips JL & Haggren W (1999) Spontaneous and nitrosourea induced primary tumors of the central nervous system in Fischer 344 rats chronically exposed to 836 MHz modulated microwaves. *Radiat. Res.*, *152*: 293.

Adey WR, Byus CV & Hagggren W (1996) Brain tumor incidence in rats chronically exposed to digital cellular telephone fields in an initiation promotion model, Bioelectromagnetics Society, 18th Annual Meeting, Proceeding, Abstract A-7-3.

Aerts S, Calderson C, Valic B, Maslany J, Addison D, Mee T, Goiceanu C, Verlock L, van Den Bossche M, Gajsek P, Vermenlen R, Roosil M, Cardis L & Joseph W (2017) Measurements of intermediate frequency electric and magnetic fields on households. *Environ. Res.*, *154*: 160.

Agarwal A, Deepinder F, Sharma RK, Ranga G & Li J (2008) Effect of cell phone usage on semen analysis in men attending infertility clinic: An observational study. *Fertil. Steril.*, *89*: 124.

Agarwal A, Desai NR, Makker K, Varghese A, Mouradi R, Sabanegh E & Sharma R (2009) Effects of radiofrequency electromagnetic waves (RF-EMW) from cellular phones on human ejaculated semen: An in vitro pilot study. *Fertil. Steril.*, *92*(4): 1318.

Ahlbom A & Feychting M (1999) Use of cellular phones & the risk of brain tumors. A case control study. *Int. J. Oncol.*, *15*: 1045.

Ahlbom A, Green A, Kheifets LI, Savitz D & Swerdlow A (2004) Epidemiology of health effects of radiofrequency exposure. *Environ. Health Perspect.*, *112*: 1741.

Ahlbom A, Maria F, Green A, Kheifets L, Savitz DA & Swerdlow AJ (2009) Epidemiologic evidence on mobile phones and tumor risk: A review, ICNIRP (International Commission for Non-Ionizing Radiation Protection) Standing Committee on Epidemiology. *Epidemiology*, *20*(5): 639.

Aitken RJ, Bennetts LE, Sawyer D, Wiklendt AM & King BV (2005) Impact of radiofrequency electromagnetic wave radiation on DNA integrity in the male germ line. *Int. J. Androl.*, *28*: 171.

Albert EN, Slaby F & Roche J (1987) Effect of amplitude modulated 147 MHz radiofrequency radiation on calcium efflux from avian brain tissue. *Radiat. Res.*, *109*: 19.

Altuntas G, Sadoglu D, Ardic S, Yilmaz H, Imamoglu M & Turedi S (2018) Acute effects of the electromagnetic waves emitted by mobile phones on attention in emergency physicians. *Am. J. Emerg. Med.*, *36*: 455–460.

Anderson J, Okaniewski M & Stuchly SS (1996) Practical 3-D contour/staircase treatment of metals in FDTD. *IEEE Microwave Guided Wave Lett.*, *6*(3): 146–148.

ANSI/IEEE C95.1 (1992) *American National Standard Safety levels with Respect to Human Exposure to Radio Frequency Electromagnetic Fields, 300 kHz to 100 GHz.* New York: IEEE. 1991.

Arai N, Enomoto H, Kkabe S, Yuasa K, Kamimura Y & Ugawa Y (2003) Thirty minute mobile phone use has no short term adverse effects on central auditory pathways. *Clin. Neurophysiol., 114*: 1390.

Augner C & Hacker GW (2009) Are people living next to mobile phone base stations more strained? Relationship of health concerns, self-estimated distance to base station, & psychological parameters. *Indian J. Occup. Environ. Med., 13*(3): 141.

Auvinen A, Hietanen M, Luukkonen R & Koskela RS (2002) Brain tumors & salivary gland cancers among cellular telephone users. *Epidemiology, 13*: 356.

Azanza MJ, Perez Bruzon RN, Lederer D, Calvo AC, Vander Vorst A & Del Moral A (2002) Reversibility of the effects induced on the spontaneous bioelectric activity of neurons under exposure to 8.3 & 217.0 Hz low intensity magnetic fields, 2nd International Workshop on Biological Effects of EMFs. *Rhodes*, p. 651.

Baan R, Lauby-Secretan B, El Ghissassi F, Bouvard V, Benbhim-Tallaa, Guha N, Islam F, Galiecht L & Straif K (2011) WHO International Agency for Research on Cancer Monograph Working Group, Carcinogenicity of radiofrequency electromagnetic fields. *Lancet Oncol.* DOI: 10.1016/S1470-2045(11)70147-4.

Balik HH, Balik DT, Balikci K & Ozcan IC (2005) Some ocular symptoms & sensations experienced by decrease in central cholinergic activity in therat. *Bioelectromagnetics, 13*: 237.

Barker AT, Jackson PR, Parry H, Coulton LA, Cook GC & Wood SM (2007) The effect of GSM & TETRA mobile handset signals on blood pressure, catechol levels &heart rate variability. *Bioelectromagnetics, 28*: 433.

Barnett J, Timotijevic L, Shepherd R & Senior V (2007) Public responses to precautionary information from the Department of Health (UK) about possible health risks from mobile phones. *Health Policy, 82*: 240.

Batellier F, Couty I, Picard D & Brillard JP (2008) Effects of exposing chicken eggs to a cell phone in "call" position over the entire incubation period. *Theriogenology, 69*: 737.

Beghi E (2017) Use of cell phones & brain tumors: A true association?*J. Neurol. Sci., 1*: 2992.

Behari J (2009) Biological correlates of electromagnetic field exposure. In *Toxicology General & Applied Toxicology* (Ballantyne B, Marrs TC & Syver T eds., 3rd Edition). John Wiley & Sons Ltd., Chapter 106, p. 1.

Behari J & Kesari KK (2006) Effect of microwave radiations on the reproductive system of male rats. *Embryo Talk, 1*(Suppl. 1): 81.

Behrend L, Henderson G & Zwacka RM (2003) Reactive oxygen species in oncogenic transformation. *Biochem. Soc. Trans., 31*: 1441.

Belyaev IY, Koch CB, Terenius O, Roxstrom-Lindquist K, Malmggren LOG, Sommer WH, Salford LG & Persson BR (2006) Exposure of rat brain to 915 MHz GSM microwaves induces changes in gene expression but not double stranded DNA breaks or effects on chromatin conformation. *Bioelectromagnetics, 27*: 295.

Berenger JP (1994) A perfectly matched layer for the absorption of electromagnetic waves. *J. Comput. Phys., 14*: 185.

Bioinitiative Report (2012) *A Rationale for Biologically based Exposure Standards for Low Intensity Electromagnetic Radiation* (Sage C and Carpenter DO eds.). Bioinitiative Working Group.

Bittman EL, Kaynard AH, Olster DH, Robinson JE, Yellow SM & Karsch FJ (1985) Pineal melatonin mediates photoperiodic control of pulsatile luteinizing hormone secretion in the ewe. *Neuroendocrinology., 40*: 409.

Blank M & Goodman R (1999) Electromagnetic fields may act directly on DNA. *J. Cell Biochem., 75*: 369.

Blank M & Goodman R (2011) DNA is a fractal antenna in electromagnetic fields. *Int. J. Radiat. Biol., 87*: 409–415.

Bornhausen M & Scheingraber H (2000) Prenatal exposure to 900 MHz cell phone electromagnetic fields had no effect on operant-behaviour performances of adult rats. *Bioelectromagnetics, 21*: 566.

Braune S, Wrocklage C, Raczek J, Gailus T & Lucking CH (1998) Resting blood pressure during exposure to a radio frequencyelectromagnetic field. *Lancet, 351*: 1857.

Buchner K & Eger H (2011) Changes of clinically important neurotransmitters under the influence of modulated RF fields: A long-term study under real-life conditions. *Umwelt-Medizin-Gesellschaft, 241*: 44.

Burch JB, Reif JS, Noonan CW, Ichinose T, Bachand AM, Koleber TL & Yost MG (2002) Melatonin metabolite excretion among cellular telephone users. *Int. J. Radiat. Biol., 78*: 1029.

Chia SE, Chia HP & Tan JS (2000) Prevalence of headache among hand held cellular telephoneusers in Singapore: Acommunity study. *Environ. Health Perspect., 108*: 1059.

Chou CK, Guy AW, Kunz LL, Johnson RB, Crowley JJ & Krupp JH (1992) Long-term, low level microwave irradiation of rats. *Bioelectromagnetics, 13*: 469.

Chou CK, Guy AW, McDougall J & Lai H (1985) Specific absorption rate in rats exposed to 2450-MHz microwaves under seven exposure conditions. *Bioelectromagnetics, 6*: 496.

Christensen HC, Schuz K, Kosteljanetz M, Poulson HS, Thomson J & Johansen C (2004) Cellular telephone use & risk of acoustic neuroma. *Am. J. Epidemiol., 159*: 277.

Cobb BL, Jauchem JR, Mason PA, Dooley MP, Miller SA, Ziriax JM & Murphy MR (2000) Neural & behavioral teratological evaluation of rats exposed to ultra-wideband electromagnetic fields. *Bioelectromagnetics, 21*: 524.

Collonce JT & Hochstein KP (1981) Red cells glutathione content & stability in oxidant stress. *J. Lab. Clin. Med., 78*: 736.

Cooper TG, Mann SM, Khalid M & Blackwell RP (2006) Public exposure to radio waves near GSM microcell & picocell base stations. *J. Radiol. Prot., 26*: 199.

Curcio GM, Ferrara M, Moroni F, Inzeo GD, Bertini M & De Gennaro L (2005) Is the brain influenced by a phone call? An EEG study of resting wakefulness. *Neurosci. Res., 53*: 265.

D'Silva MH, Swer RT, Anbalagan J & Rajesh B (2017) Effect of radiofrequency radiation emitted from 2G & 3G cell phone on developing liver of chick embryo: Acomparative study. *J. Clin. Diagn. Res., 11*(7): AC05.

Dasdag S, Akdag MZ, Aksen F, Yilmaz F & Bashan M (2003) Whole body exposure ofrats to microwaves emitted from a cell phone does not affect the testes. *Bioelectromagnetics, 24*(3): 182.

Dasdag S, Akdag MZ, Ayyildiz O, Demirtas OC, Yayla M & Sert C (2000) Do cellular phones alter blood parameters & birth weight of rats? *Electromagn. Biol. Med., 19*: 107.

Dasdag S, Akdag MZ, Ulukaya AK & Yegin D (2008) Mobile phone exposure does not induce apoptosis on spermatogenesis in rats. *Arch. Med. Res., 39*: 40.

Dasdag S, Ketani MA, Akdag Z, Ersay AR, Sari I, Demirtas OC & Celik MS (1999) Whole body microwave exposure emitted by cellular phones & testicular function of rats. *Urol. Res.*, *27*: 219.

Davoudi M, Brossner C & Kuber W (2002) The influence of electromagnetic waves on sperm motility. *J. Fururol. Urogynakol.*, *19*: 18.

De Iuliis GN, Newey RJ, King BV & Aitken RJ (2009) Mobile phone radiation induces reactive oxygen species production & DNA damage in human spermatozoa in vitro. *PLoS One*, *4*(7): e6446.

de Seze R, Ayoub J, Peray P, Miro L & Touitou Y (1999) Evolutions in humans of the effects of radiocellular telephones on the circadian patterns of melatonin secretion, a chronobiological rhythm marker. *J. Pineal Res.*, *27*: 237.

Diem E, Schwarz C, Adlkofer F, Jahn O & Rüdiger HW (2005) Non-thermal DNA breakage by mobile phone radiation (1,800 MHz) in human fibroblasts & in transformed GFSH-R17 rat granulosa cells in vitro. *Mutat. Res.*, *583*: 178.

Dietrich WD, Alonsi O, Halley M, Busto R & Globus MYT (1992) Intravesticular infusion of N-methyl-D-aspartate, I: Acute blood-brain barrier consequences. *Acta Neuropathol.*, *84*(1992): 621.

Dimbylow PJ & Mann SM (1994) SAR calculations in an anatomically realistic model of the head for the mobile communication transreceivers at 900 MHz & 1.8 GHz. *Phys. Med. Biol.*, *39*: 1537.

Douglas MA, Okoniewski M & Stuchly MA (1995) Modeling of wireless personal communication transmitters in the presence of the user's body. Wireless'95–7th Int. Conf. Wireless Communication, Calgary, Alberta, p. 77.

Dreyer NA, Loughlin JE & Rothman KJ (1999) Cause-specific mortality in cellular telephone users. *JAMA*, *282*: 1814.

Eberhardt JL, Persson BR, Brun AE, Salford LG & Malmgren LO (2008) Blood-brain barrier permeability & nerve cell damage in rat brain 14 & 28 days after exposure to microwaves from GSM mobile phones. *Electromagn. Biol. Med.*, *27*: 215.

Eger H, Hagen KU, Lucas B, Vogel P & Voit H (2004) Einfluss der raumlichen Nahe von Mobilfunksendeanlagen auf die Krebsinzidenz. *Umwelt-Med.-Ges.*, *17*: 273.

Eimerl S & Scramm M (1991) Acute glutamate toxicity in cultured cerebellar granule cells: Agonist potency, effects of pH, Zn^{2+}& the potentiation by serum albumin. *Brain Res.*, *560*: 282.

Elder JA (2003) Ocular effects of electromagnetic energy. *Bioelectromagnetics* (Suppl 6): 148.

Erogul O, Oztas E, Yildirim I, Kir T, Aydur E, Komesli G, Irkilata HC, Irmak MK & Peker AF (2006) Effects of electromagnetic radiation from a cellular phone on human sperm motility an in vitro study. *Arch. Med. Res.*, *37*: 840.

Eskander EF, Estefan SF & Abd-Rabou AA (2012) How does long term exposure to base stations & mobile phones affect human hormone profiles? *Clin. Biochem.*, *45* (1–2): 157.

Excell P (1988) Computer modeling of high frequency electromagnetic field penetration into the human head. *Meas. Control*, *31*: 170.

Fejes I, Zavaczki Z, Szollosi J, Koloszar S, Daru J, Kovacs L & Pal A (2005) Is there a relationship between cell phone use & semen quality?*Arch. Androl.*, *51*: 385.

Ferreri FG, Curico P, Pasqualetti L, de Gennaro L, Fini R & Rossini PM (2006) Mobile phone emissions & human brain excitability. *Ann. Neurol.*, *60*: 188.

Finnie JW, Blumbergs PC, Manavis J, Utteridge TD, Gebski V, Davies RA, Vermon-Roberts B & Kuchel TR (2002) Effect of long-term mobile communication microwave exposure on vascular permeability in mouse brain. *Pathology, 38*: 63.

Forgacs Z, Somosy Z, Kubinyl G, Bakos J, Hudak A, Surjan A & Thuroczy G (2006) Effects of whole body 1800 MHz GSM-like microwave exposure on testicular steridogenesis & histology in mice. *Reprod. Toxicol., 22*: 111.

Frank RN, Dutta S & Mancini MA (1987) Pericycle coverage is greater in the retinal than in the cerebral capillaries of the rat. *Invest. Opthalmol. Vis. Sci., 28*: 086.

Fredriksson K, Kalimo H, Norberg C, Johansson BB & Olsson Y (1988) Nerve cell injury in the brain of stroke prone spontaneously hypertensive rats. *Acta Neuropathol. (Berlin), 76*: 227.

Frei P, Mohler E, Neubauer G, Theis G, Burgi A, Frohlich J, Braun-Fatrilander C, Bolte J, Egger M & Roosli M (2009) Temporal & spatial variability of personal exposure to radiofrequency electromagnetic fields. *Environ. Res., 109*(6): 779.

Frey AH (1998) Headaches from cellular telephones: Are they real & what are the implications?*Environ. Health Prospect., 106*: 101.

Frey AH, Feld SR & Frey AB (1975) Neural function &behavior: Defining the relationship. In: *Biologic Effects of Non Ionizing Radiation. Ann. NY Acad. Sci., 247*: 433.

Fritze K, Sommer C, Schmitz B, Mies G, Hossman K, Kiessling M & Wiessner C (1997) Effect of global system for mobile communication (GSM) microwave exposure on blood brain barrier permeability in rat. *Acta Neuropathol., 94*: 465.

Gandhi G & Anita (2005) Genetic damage in mobile phone users: Some preliminary findings. *Ind. J. Hum. Genet., 11*: 99.

Gandhi OP (1995) Some numerical methods for dosimetry: Extremely low frequencies to microwave frequencies. *Radio Sci., 30*: 161.

Gandhi OP, Lazzi G & Furse CM (1996) Electromagnetic absorption in the human head & neck for mobile telephones at 850 & 1900 MHz. *IEEE Trans. Microwave Theory Tech., 44*: 1884.

Gao XH, Hu HR, Ma X, Chen J & Zhang GH (2016) Cellphone electromagnetic radiation damages the testicular ultrastructure of male rats [Article in Chinese]. *Zhonghua Nan Ke Xue, 22*(6): 491.

Garber HJ, Oldendorf WH, Braun LD & Lufkin RB (1989) MRI gradient fields increase brain mannitol space. *Magn. Reson. Imaging, 7*: 605.

Gavella M & Lipovac V (2000) Antioxidative effect of melatonin on human spermatozoa. *Arch. Androl., 44*: 23.

Giwercman A, Richthoff J, Hjollund H, Bonde JP, Jepson K, Frohm B & Spano M (2003) Correlation between sperm motility & sperm chromatin structure assay parameters. *Fertil. Steril., 80*: 1404.

Grigoriev YG, Grigoriev OA, Ivanov AI, Ivanov AA, Lyagrinskaya AM, Merkulov AV, Shagina NB, Maltsev VN, Leveque P, Ulanova AM, Osipov V & Shafirkin AV (2010) Confirmation studies of Soviet research on immunological effects of microwaves: Russian immunology results. *Bioelectromagnetics, 31*: 589.

Grissom CB (1995) Magnetic fields effects in biology: A survey of possible mechanisms with emphasis on radical pair recommendation. *Chem. Res., 3*: 95.

Gul A, Celebi H & Urgas S (2009) The effects of microwaves emitted by cellular phones on ovarian follicles in rats. *Arch. Gynecol. Obstet., 280*(5): 729.

Guney M, Ozguner F, Oral B, Karahan N & Mungan T (2007) 900 MHz radiofrequency induced histopathologic changes & oxidative stress in rat endometrium: Protection by vitamin E & C. *Toxicol. Ind. Health, 23*: 411.

Hamblin DL, Croft RJ, Wood AW, Stough C & Spong J (2006) The sensitivity of human event related potentials & reaction time to mobile phone emitted electromagnetic fields. *Bioelectromagnetics*, *27*: 265.

Hamblin DL, Wood AW, Croft RJ & Stough C (2004) Examining the effects of electromagnetic fields emitted by GSM mobile phones on human event related potentials & performance during an auditory task. *Clin. Neurophysiol.*, *115*: 171.

Hardell L, Hallquist A, Mild KH, Carlberg M, Påhlson A & Lilja A (2002) Cellular & cordless telephones & the risk for brain tumours. *Eur. J. Cancer Prev.*, *11*(4): 377.

Hardell L, Hansson Mild K, Pahlson A & Hallquist A (2001) Ionizing radiation, cellular telephones & the risk for brain tumours. *Eur. J. Cancer Prev.*, *10*: 523.

Hardell L, Mild KH & Johansson B. (2003) Cellular & cordless telephones & basal cell carcinoma: A case report. *Arch. Environ. Health*, *58*: 380.

Hardell L, Näsman A, Påhlson A, Hallquist A & Hansson Mild K (1999) Use of cellular telephones & the risk for brain tumours: A case-control study. *Int. J. Oncol.*, *15*(1): 113.

Hassel B, Iversen EG & Fonnum F (1994) Neurotoxicity of albumin in vivo. *Neurosci. Lett.*, *167*: 29.

Heinrich S, Ossig A, Schlittmeier S & Hellbrück J (2007) Elektromagnetische Felder einer UMTS-Mobilfunkbasisstation und mögliche Auswirkungen auf die Befindlichkeit—Eine experimentelle Felduntersuchung. *Umwelt Med. Forsch. Prax.*, *12*: 171.

Heinrich S, Thomas S, Heumann C, von Kries R & Radon K (2010) Association between exposure to radiofrequency electromagnetic fields assessed by dosimetry & acute symptoms in children & adolescents: Apopulation based cross-sectional study. *Environ. Health*, *9*: 75.

Hinrikus M, Bachmann M, Lass J, Karai D & Tuulik V (2009) Effect of low frequency modulated microwave exposure on human EEG: Individual sensitivity. *Bioelectromagnetics*, *29*: 527.

Hirose H, Sakuma N, Kaji N, Suhara T, Sekijima M, Nojima T & Miyakoshi J (2006) Phosphorylation & gene expression of p53 are not affected in human cells exposed to 2.1425 GHz band CW or W-CDMA modulated radiation allocated to mobile radio base stations. *Bioelectromagnetics*, *27*: 494.

Hook GJ, Zhang P, Lagroye I, Li L, Higashikubo R, Moros EG, Straube WL, Pickard WJ, Baty JD & Roti Roti JL (2004) Measurement of DNA damage & apoptosis in Molt-4 cells in vitro exposure to radiofrequency radiation. *Radiat. Res.*, *161*: 193.

How cell-phone radiation works (2007) *Accessedat electronics*. How.stuffworks.com/cell-phone-radiation.htm/printable.

Huber R, Graf T, Cote KA, Wittmann L, Gallmann E, Matter D, Schuderer J, Kuster N, Borbely AA & Achermann P (2000) Exposure to pulsed high frequency electromagnetic field during waking affects human sleep EEG. *NeuroReport*, *11*: 3321.

Hutter HP, Moshammer H, Wallner P & Kundi M (2006) Subjective symptoms, sleeping problems & cognitive performance in subjects living near mobile phone base stations. *Occup. Environ. Med.*, *63*: 307.

Ilhan A, Gurel A, Armutcu F, Kamisili S, Iraz M, Akyol O & Ozen S (2004) Ginkgo biloba prevents mobile phone induced oxidative stress in brain. *Clin. Chim. Acta*, *340*: 153.

Inskip PD, Tarone RE, Hatch EE, Wilcosky TC, Shapiro WR, Selker RG, Fine HA, Black PM, Loeffler JS & Limet MS (2001) Cellular telephone use & brain tumors. *N. Engl. J. Med., 344*: 79.

INTERPHONE Study Group (2010) Brain tumor risk in relation to mobile telephone use: Resultsof the INTERPHONE International case-control study. *Int. J. Epidemiol., 39*(3): 675.

Ismail NH & Ibrahim AT (2002) Temperature distribution in the human brain during ultrasound hyperthermia. *J. Electromagn. Waves Appl., 16*: 803.

Izumi Y & Zorumski CF (1993) Nitric oxide & long-term synaptic depression in the rat hippocampus. *NeuroReport, 4*: 131.

Jackson FL, Heindel JJ, Preslock JP & Berkowitz AS (1984) Alterations in hypothalamic content of luteinizing hormone—Releasing hormone associated with pineal mediated testicular regression in the golden hamster. *Biol. Reprod., 31*: 436.

Jansen MA & Rahmat-Samii Y (1995) EM interaction of hand set antennas & a human in personal communications. *Proc. IEEE, 83*: 7.

Jarupat S, Kawabatam A, Tokura H & Borkiewicz A (2003) Effects of the 1900 MHz electromagnetic field emitted from cellular phone on nocturnal melatonin secretion. *J. Physiol. Anthropol., 22*: 61.

Jensh RP (1997) Behavioral teratological studies using microwave radiation: Is there an increased risk from exposure to cellular phones & microwave ovens?*Reprod. Toxicol., 11*: 601.

Jensh RP, Vogel WH & Brent RI (1982) Postnatal functional analysis of prenatal exposure of rats to 915 MHz microwave radiation. *Int. J. Toxicol., 1*: 73.

Jin MB, Johansen C, Boice, Jr. J, Laughlin J, McLaughlin JK, Christensen HC & Oslen JH (2002) Mobile phones & malignant melanoma of the eye. *Br. J. Cancer, 86*: 348.

Johansen C, Boice, Jr. J, Laughlin J & Oslen J (2001) Cellular telephone & cancer: A nationwide cohort study in Denmark. *J. Natl. Cancer Int., 93*: 203.

Jokela K, Puranen L & Shivonen, AP (2004) Assessment of the magnetic field exposure due to the battery current of digital mobile phones. *Health Phys., 86*: 56.

Joseph W, Frei P, Roosli M, Thuroczt G, Gajsek P, Trcek T, Bolte J, Vermeeren G, Mohler E, Juhasz P, Finta V & Martens L (2010) Comparison of personal radiofrequency electromagnetic field exposure in different urban areas across Europe. *Environ. Res., 110*: 658.

Jung A & Schill WB (2000) Male infertility: Current life style could be responsible for infertility. *MMW Fortschr. Med., 142*: 31.

Kaatsch P, Spix C, Rath RS, Schmiedel S & Blettner M (2008) Leukaemia in young children living in vicinity of German nuclear power plants. *Int. J. Cancer, 122*(4): 721.

Kamali K, Atarod M, Sarhadi S, Nikbakht J, Emami M, Maghsoudi R, Salimi H, Fallahpour B, Kamali N, Momtazan A & Ameli M (2017) Effects of electromagnetic waves emitted from 3G+wi-fi modems on human semenanalysis. *Urologia, 84*(4): 209.

Kang XK, Li LW, Leong MS & Kooi PS (2001) A method of moments study of SAR inside spheroidal human head & current distribution among handset wireless antennas. *J. Electromagn Waves Appl., 15*: 61.

Keetly V, Wood AW, Spong J & Stough C (2006) Neurophysiological sequelae of digital mobile phone exposure in humans. *Neurophysiologica, 44*: 1843.

Kesari KK & Behari J (2009) Fifty gigahertz microwave exposure effect of radiations on rat brain. *Appl. Biochem. Biotechnol., 158*(1): 126.
Kesari KK & Behari J (2010) Effect of microwave at 2.45 GHz radiations on reproductive system of male rats. *Toxicol. Environ. Chem., 92*: 1135.
Kesari KK, Kumar S & Behari J (2011) Effects of radiofrequency electromagnetic wave exposure from cellular phones on the reproductive pattern in male Wistar rats. *Appl. Biochem. Biotechnol., 164*(4): 546.
Khiat N, Charlinet Y & Agoulmine N (2006) The emerging threat of peer-to-peer worms. In: Proceedings of IEEE/1st workshop on monitoring, attack detection & mitigation, Tubingen, Germany: 18.
Kilgallon SJ & Simon LW (2005) Mage content influences men semen quality. *Biol. Lett., 1*: 253.
Kim JH, Yu D-H, Huh YH, Lee EH, Kim H-G & Kim HR (2017) Long term exposure to 835 MHz RF-EMF induces hyperactivity, autophagy & demyelination in the cortical neurons of mice. *Sci. Rep., 7*: Articlenumber 41129.
Klemn M & Troester G (2006) EM energy absorption in the human body tissues due to UWB antennas. *Prog. Electromagn. Res., 62*: 261.
Kolomytkin O, Yurinska M, Zharikov S, Kuznetsov V & Zharikova A (1994) Response of brain receptor systems to microwave energy exposure. In: *On the Nature ofElectromagnetic Field Interactions with Biological Systems* (Frey AH ed.). Austin: R. G. Landes Company, p. 195.
Krause CM, Pesonen M, Haarala-Bjornberg C & Hamalainen H (2007) Effects of pulsed & continuous wave 902 MHz mobile phone exposure on brain oscillatory activity during cognitive processing. *Bioelectromagnetics, 28*: 296.
Kula B & Drozdz M (1996) A study of magnetic field effects on fibroblasts cultures. Part 2. The evaluation of effects of static & extremely low frequency (ELF) magnetic fields on free radical processes in fibroblasts cultures. *Bioelectrochem. Bioenerg., 39*: 27.
Kumar S, Behari J & Sisodia R (2012) Impact of microwave at X-band in the aetiology of male infertility. *Electromagn. Biol. Med., 31*(3): 223.
Kumar S, Kesari KK & Behari J (2010) Evaluation of genotoxic effects in male Wistar rats following microwave exposure. *Indian J. Exp. Biol., 48*(6): 586.
Kumlin T, Liyonen H, Miettenen P, Iunoven A, van Groen T, Puranen L, Pitkaaho R, Juutilainen R & Tanila H (2007) Mobile phone radiation and the developing brain: Behavioral and morphological effects in juvenile rats. *Radiat. Res., 168*: 471.
Kundi M & Hutter HP (2009) Mobile phone base stations: Effects on wellbeing & health. *Pathophysiology, 16*: 123.
Kuribayashi M, Wang J, Fujiwara O, Doi Y, Nabae K, Tamano S, Ogiso T, Asamoto M & Shirai T (2005) Lack of effects of 1439 MHz electromagnetic near field exposure on the BBB in immature & young rats. *Bioelectromagnetics, 26*: 578.
Kus I, Akpolar N, Ozen OA, Songur A, Kavakli A & Sarsilmaz N (2002) Effects of melatonin on Leydig cells in pineal ectomized rat: An immunohistochemical study. *Acta Histochem., 104*: 93.
Kwon MS, Vorobyev V, Kannala S, Laine M, Rinne JO, Toivonen T, Johansson J, Teres M, Lindholm H, Alanko T & Hammalainen H (2011) GSM mobile phone radiation suppresses brain glucose metabolism. *J. Cereb. Blood Flow Metab., 31*(12): 2293.
Lagroye I, Anane R, Wettring BA, Moros EG, Straube WL, Laregina M, Niehoff M, Pickard WF, Baty J & Roti Roti JL (2004) Measurement of DNA damage after acute comet assay methods. *Int. J Radiat. Biol., 80*: 11.

Lai H, Carino MA & Guy AW (1989) Low-level microwave irradiation & central cholinergic systems. *Pharm. Biochem. Behav., 33*: 131.

Lai H, Carino MA, Horita A & Guy AW (1992) Opioid receptor subtypes that mediate a microwave induced decrease in central cholinergic activity in the rat. *Bioelectromagnetics, 13*(3): 237.

Lai H & Singh N (1997) Melatonin & a spin trap compound block radiofrequency electromagnetic radiation induced DNA strand break in rat brain cells. *Bioelectromagnetics, 18*: 446.

Lai H & Singh NP (1995) Acute low intensity microwave exposure increases DNA single-strand breaks in rats brain cells. *Bioelectromagnetics, 16*: 207.

Lai H & Singh NP (1996) Single- & double-strand DNA breaks in rat brain cells after acute exposure to radiofrequency electromagnetic radiation. *Int. J. Radiat. Biol., 69*: 513.

Lai H & Singh NP (2004) Magnetic field induced DNA strand breaks in brain cells of the rat. *Environ. Health Perspect., 112*: 687.

Lantow M, Verqutz T, Weiss DG & Simko M (2006) Comparative study of cell cycle kinetics & induction of apoptosis or necrosis after exposure of human mono mac 6 cells to radiofrequency radiation. *Radiat. Res., 166*: 539.

Lederer D, Azanza MJ, Calvo AC, Perez Bruzon RN, Del Moral A & Vander Vorst A (2001) Effects associated with the ELF of GSM signals on the spontaneous bioelectricity activity of neurons, Proc. 5th Int. Cong. Eur. BioElectromagnetics Assoc., Helsinki,194.

Lerchl A, Klose M, Grote K, Wihelm AF, Spathmann O, Fiedler T, Streckert J, Hansen V & Ciemens M (2015) Tumor promotion by exposure to radiofrequency electromagnetic fields below exposure limits for humans. *Biochem. Biophys. Res. Commun., 459*(4): 585.

Li L, Bisht KS, LaGroye I, Zhang P, Straube WL, Moros EG, Pickard WE & Roti JL (2001) Measurement of DNA damage in mammalian cells exposed to radiofrequency fields at high SAR of 3-5 W/kg. *Radiat. Res., 156*: 328.

Lin JC (2001) The blood-brain barrier, cancer, cell phones, & microwave radiation. *IEEE Microwave Mag., 2*(4): 26.

Lin JC (2008) Studies on tumor incidence in mice exposed to GSM cell-phone radiation [Health Effects]. *URSI, 2008*: 41.

Magras IN & Xenos TD (1997) RF-radiation-induced changes in the prenatal development of mice. *Bioelectromagnetics, 18*: 455.

Malyapa RS, Ahern EW, Bi C, Straube WL, LaRegina M, Pickard WF & Roti Roti JL (1998) DNA damage in rat brain cells after in vivo exposure to 2450 MHz electromagnetic radiation & various methods of euthanasia. *Radiat. Res., 149*: 637.

Manjhi J, Kumar S, Behari J & Mathur R (2013) Effect of extremely low frequency electromagnetic field in prevention of spinal cord injury induced osteoporosis. *J. Rehabil. Res. Dev., 50*(1): 17.

Mann K, Wagner P, Brunn G, Hassan F, Hiemke C & Roschke J (1998) Effects of pulsed high frequency electromagnetic fields on the neuroendocrine system. *Neuroendocrinology, 67*: 139.

Markova E, Hillert L, Malmgren L, Persson BR & Belyaev IY (2005) Microwaves from GSM mobile telephones affect 53BP1 & gamma-H2AX foci in human lymphocytes from hypersensitive & healthy persons. *Environ. Health Perspect., 113*: 1172.

Martens L, De Moerloose J & De Zutter D (1995) Calculation of the electromagnetic fields induced in the head of an operator of a cordless telephone. *Radio Sci., 30*: 283.

Mc Cord JM & Fridovich I (1969) Superoxide dismutase an enzymic function for erythrocuprein (hemocuprein). *J. Biol. Chem., 244*: 60409.

McCormick D (2017) Two year oncogenicity evaluations of cell phone radiofrequency radiation in Sprague-Dawley rats & B6C3F1 mice. *Toxicol. Lett, 280S*, S31.

Mild KH, Oftedal G, Sandstrom M, Wilen J, Tynes T, Haugsdai B & Hauger E (1998) Comparison of systems experienced by users of analogue & digital mobile phones: A Swedish-Norwegian epidemiological study, Report for the National Institute for Working Life, Sweden.

Moby E, Le Bouquim Jeannes R, Faucon G, Liegeois Chauvel C & De Seze R (2005) Effects of GSM signals on auditory evoked responses. *Bioelectromagnetics, 26*: 341.

Mohler E, Frei P, Braun-Fahrlander C, Frohlich J, Neubauer G & Roosli M (2010) Qualifex Team. Effects of everyday radiofrequency electromagnetic field exposure on sleep quality: Across-sectional study. *Radiat. Res., 74*(3): 347.

Mortazavi SAR, Mortazavi G & Mortazavi SMJ (2017) Letter to the Editor: Use of cell phones & brain tumors: A true association?*Neurol. Sci., 87*: 182.

Moulder JE, Erdreich LS, Malyapa RS, Merritt J, Pickarde WF & Vijayalaxmi (1999) Cell phones &cancer: What is the evidence for a connection?*Radiat. Res., 151*: 513.

Muscat JE, Malkin MG, Thompson S, Shore RE, Stellman SD, McRee D, Neugut AI & Wynder E (2000) Handheld cellular telephone use & risk of brain cancer. *J. Am. Med. Assoc., 284*: 3001.

Nakamura H, Matsuzaki I, Hatta K, Nobukuni Y, Kamabayashi Y & Ogino K (2003) Non thermal effects of mobile-phone frequency microwaves on uteroplacental function in pregnant rats. *Reprod. Toxicol., 17*(3): 321.

Navarro EA, Segura J, Portoles M & Gómez-Perretta de Mateo C (2003) The microwave syndrome: A preliminary study in Spain. *Electromagn. Biol. Med., 22*: 161.

Neubauer G, Fevchting M, Hamnerius Y, Kheifets L, Kuster N, Ruiz I, Schutz J, Uberbacher R, Wiart J & Roosli M (2007) Feasibility of future health effects of mobile phone base stations. *Bioelectromagnetics, 38*(3): 224.

Nikolova T, Czyz J, Rolletschek A, Blyszczuk P, Fuchs J, Jovtchev G, Schuderer J, Kuster N & Wobus AM (2005) Electromagnetic fields affect transcript levels of apoptosis-related genes in embryonic stem cell-derived neural progenitor cells. *FASEB J., 19*(12): 1686.

Nittby H, Brun A, Eberhardt J, Malmgren L, Persson BRR & Salford LG (2009) Increased blood brain barrier permeability in mammalian brain 7 days after exposure to the radiation from a GSM-900 mobile phone. *Pathophysiology, 103–112*: 599.

Nittby H, Grafstrom G, Eberhardt JL, Malmgren L, Brun A, Persson BRR & Salford LG (2008) Radiofrequency & extremely low frequency electromagnetic field effects on the blood brain barrier. *Electromagn. Biol. Med., 27*: 103.

Nittby H, Grafstrom G, Tian D, Brun A, Persson BRR, Salford LG & Eberhardt J (2008a) Cognitive impairment in rats after long term exposure to GSM-900 mobile phones. *Bioelectromagnetics, 29*: 219.

Nittby H, Widegren B, Krogh M, Grafstrom, Rehn G, Berlin H, Eberhardt JL, Malmgren L, Persson BRR & Salford LG (2008b) Exposure to human from global system for mobile communications at 1800 MHz significantly changes gene expression in rat hippocampus & cortex. *Environmentalist, 28*(4): 458.

Oberto G, Rolfo K, Yu P, Carbonatto M, Peano S, Kuster N, Ebert S & Tofani S. (2007) Carcinogenicity study of 217 Hz pulsed 900 MHz electromagnetic fields in Pim1 transgenic mice. *Radiat. Res., 168*: 316.

Oftedal G, Straume A, Johnsson A & Stovner LJ (2007) Mobile phone headache: A double blind, sham-controlled provocation study. *Cephalalgia, 27*: 447.

Oftedel G, Wilen J, Sandstrom M & Mild K (2000) Symptoms experiences in connection with mobile phone use. *Occup. Med., 50*: 237.

Okoniewski M & Stuchly MA (1996) A study of the handset antenna & human body interaction. *IEEE Trans. Microwave Theory Tech., 44*: 1855.

Oral B, Guney M, Ozguner F, Karahan N, Mungan T, Comleksi S & Cesur G (2006) Endometrial apoptosis induced by a 900 MHz mobile phone: Preventive effects of vitamin E & C. *Adv. Ther., 23*: 957.

Oscar KJ & Hawkins TD (1977) Microwave alteration of the blood brain barrier system of rats. *Brain Res., 204*: 220.

Otitoloju AA, Obe IA, Adewale OA, Otubanjo OA & Osunkalu VO (2010) Preliminary Study on the induction of sperm head abnormalities in mice, *Mus musculus*, exposed to radiofrequency radiations from global system for mobile communication base stations. *Bull. Environ. Contam. Toxicol., 84*: 51.

Ozguner M, Koyu A, Cesur G, Ural M, Ozguner F, Gokcimen A & Delibas N (2005) Biological & morphological effects on the reproductive organ of rats after exposure to electromagnetic field. *Saudi Med. J., 26*: 405.

Panagopoulos DJ (2012) Effect of microwave exposure on the ovarian development of *Drosophila melanogaster*. *Cell Biochem. Biophys., 63*: 121.

Panagopoulos DJ, Chavdoula ED, Karabarbounis A & Margaritis LH (2007) Comparison of bioactivity between GSM 900 MHz & DCS 1800 MHz mobile telephony radiation. *Electromagn. Biol. Med., 26*(1): 33.

Papadopoulou E, Haugen M, Schjølberg S, Magnus P, Brunborg G, Vrijheid M & Alexander J (2017) Maternal cell phone use in early pregnancy & child's language, communication & motor skills at 3 & 5 years: The Norwegian mother & child cohort study (MoBa). *BMC Public Health, 17*(1): 685.

Paulraj R & Behari J (2004) Radio frequency radiation effects on protein kinase C activity in rats' brain. *Mutat. Res., 545*: 127.

Paulraj R & Behari J (2006) Single strand DNA breaks in rat brain cells exposed to microwave radiation. *Mutat. Res., 596*: 76.

Penafiel LM, Litovitz T, Krause D, Desta A & Mullins JM (1997) Role of modulation on the effect of microwaves on ornithine decarboxylase activity in L929 cells. *Bioelectromagnetics, 18*: 132.

Phillips JL, Ivaschuk O, Ishoda-Jones T, Jones RA, Campbell-Beachler M & Haggren W (1998) DNA damage in Molt-4-T lymphoblastocid cells exposed to cellular telephone radiofrequency fields in vitro. *Bioelectrochem. Bioenerg., 45*: 103.

Phillips JL, Singh NP & Lai H (2009) Electromagnetic fields & DNA damage. *Pathophysiology, 16*: 79.

Prato FS, Frappier RH, Shivers RR, Kraliers M, Zabel P, Drost D & Lee TY (1990) Magnetic resonance imaging increases the BBB permeability to 153-gadolinium diethylenetriaminepentaacetic acid in rats. *Brain Res., 523*: 301.

Prato FS, Wills JM, Roger J, Frappier H, Drost DJ, Lee TY, Shivers RR & Zabel P (1994) BBB permeability in rats is altered by exposure to magnetic fields associated with magnetic resonance imaging at 1.5 T. *Microsc. Res. Tech., 27*: 528.

Preece AW, Iwi G, Davies-Smith A, Wesnes K, Butler S, Lim E & Varey A (1999) Effect of 915 MHz simulated mobile phone signal on cognitive function in man. *Int. J. Radiat. Biol.*, *75*: 447.

Qureshi MRA, Alfadhl Y, Chen X, Peyman A, Maslanyj M & Mann S. (2018) Assessment of exposure to radio frequency electromagnetic fields from smart utility meters in GB; Part II numerical assessment of induced SAR within the human body. *Bioelectromagnetics, 39(3):200.*

Radon K, Parera D, Rose DM & Vollrath L (2001) No effects of pulsed electromagnetic fields on melatonin, cortisol & selected markers of the immune system in man. *Bioelectromagnetics*, *22*: 280.

Ratilio G (1972) Effects of hydrogen peroxide on dismutase & catalase activity in rat liver. *Biochemistry*, *11*: 21.

Ray S & Behari J (1987) Dielectric dispersion in rat brain tissue. Proceedings of the First Asia-Pacific Microwave Conference, Microwave Technology & Applications, February 24–28, 496.

Repacholi MH, Bosten A, Gebski V, Noonan D, Finnie J & Harris AW (1997) Lymphomas in Em-Pim 1 transgenic mice exposed to pulsed 900 MHz electromagnetic fields. *Radiat. Res.*, *147*: 631.

Ribeiro EP, Rhoden EL, Horn MM, Rhoden C, Lima LP & Toniolo L (2007) Effect of subchronic exposure to radiofrequency from a conventional cellular telephone on testicular function in adult rats. *J. Urol.*, *177*: 395.

Röschke J & Mann K (1997) No short term effects of digital mobile radio telephone on the awake human electroencephalogram. *Bioelectromagnetics*, *18*: 172.

Rothman KJ, Chou CK, Morgan R, Bizano Q, Guy AW, Funch DP, Preston Martin S, Mandel J & Carle G (1996) Assessment of cellular telephone & other radiofrequency exposure for epidemiologic research. *Epidemiology*, *7*: 291.

Rotkvoska D, Moc J, Kaustka J, Bartickova A, Keprtova J & Hofer M (1993) Evaluation of the biological effects of police radar RAMER 7F. *Environ. Health Perspect.*, *101*: 134.

Sage C, Johansson O & Sage SA (2007) Personal digital assistant (PDA) cell phone units produce units elevated extremely low frequency electromagnetic field emissions. *Bioelectromagnetics*, *28*: 386.

Salahuddin TS, Johansson BB, Kalimu H & Olsson Y (1988) Structural changes in the rat brain after carotid infusion of hyperosmolar solutions. *Acta Neuropathol.*, *77*(2): 5.

Salford L, Brun A, Eberhardt J, Malmgren L & Persson B (1992) Electromagnetic fields-induced permeability of the blood–brain barrier shown by immunohistochemical methods. In *Interaction Mechanism of Low-Level Electromagnetic Fields in Living Systems* (Ramel C, Norden B eds.). Oxford, UK: Oxford University Press, p. 251.

Salford LG, Brun AE, Eberhardt JL, Malmgren L & Persson BR (2003) Nerve cell damage in mammalian brain after exposure to microwave from GSM mobile phones. *Environ. Health Perspect.*, *111*: 881.

Salford LG, Brun AE, Sturesson K, Eberhardt JL & Persson B (1994) Permeability of the blood brain barrier induced by 915 MHz electromagnetic continuous wave & modulated at 8,16,50 & 200 Hz. *Microsc. Res. Tech.*, *27*(6): 535.

Salford LG, Nittby H, Brun A, Graftstrom G, Eberhardt JL, Malmgren L & Persson BRR (2007) Non thermal effects of EMF upon the mammalian brain: The Lund experience. *Environmentalist*, *27*: 493.

Salford LG, Nittby H, Brun A, Grafstrom G, Malmgren L, Sommarian M, Eberhardt J, Widegren B & Persson BRR (2008) The mammalian brain in the electromagnetic field designed by manwith special reference to blood brain barrier function, neuronal damage & possible physical mechanisms. *Prog. Theor. Phys. Suppl., 174*: 283.

Salford LG, Persson BRR & Brun A (1997) Brain tumor development in rats exposed to electromagnetic fields used in wireless cellular communication. *Wireless Networks, 3*(6): 463.

Salma N, Kshimoto T & Kaneyama HQ (2010) Effects of exposure to a mobile phone on testicular function & structure in adult rabbit. *Int. J. Androl., 33*(1): 88.

Sandstrom M, Wilen J, Oftedal G & Mild KH (2001) Mobile phone use & subjective symptoms comparison of symptoms experienced by users of analogue & digital mobile phones. *Occup. Med., 51*(1): 25.

Sanitini R, Santini P, Danze JM, Le Ruz P & Seigne M (2003) Enquete sur la sente de riverains de stations relais de telephonie mobile: II/Incidneces de I'ae des sujets, de la duree de leur exposition et de leur postion par rapport aux antennes et autres sources electromagnetiques. *Pathol. Biol. (Paris), 51*: 412.

Santini R, Honsi M, Deschaux P & Pacheco H (1988) B16 melanoma development in black mice exposed to low-level microwave radiation. *Bioelectromagnetics, 9*: 105.

Sarkar S, Ali S & Behari J (1994) Effect of low power microwave on the mouse genome: A direct DNA analysis. *Mutat. Res., 320*: 141.

Saunders RD & Kowalczuk CL (1981) Effect of 2.45 GHz microwave radiation & heat on mouse spermatogenic epithelium. *Int. J. Radiat. Biol. Relat. Stud. Phys. Chem. Med., 40*(6): 623.

Schirmacher A, Winters S, Fischer S, Goeke J, Galla HJ, Kullnick U, Ringelstin EB & Sogbauer F (2000) Electromagnetic fields (1.8 GHz) increase the permeability to sucrose of the blood-brain barrier in vitro. *Bioelectromagnetics, 21*(3): 338.

Scott IR, Wood SJ & Tattersall JEH (1998) Effects of radiofrequency radiation on long term potentiation in rat hippocampus slices, In Proceedings of Bioelectromagnetics Society 20th Annual Meeting, St Petersburg, Florida.

Seishima M, Oyama Z & Oda M (2003) Cellular phone dermatitis with chromate allergy. *Dermatoloty, 207*: 48.

Shivers RP, Kavaliers M, Teskey GC, Prato FS & Pelletier RM (1987) Magnetic resonance imaging alters BBB permeability in the rat. *Neurosci. Lett., 76*: 25.

Sies H, Stahl W & Sevanian A (2005) Nutritional, dietary & postprandial oxidative stress. *J. Nutr., 135*: 969.

Sievert U, Eggert S & Pau HW (2005) Can mobile phone emissions affect auditory functions of cochlea or brain stem?*Otolaryngol. Head Neck Surg., 132*: 451.

Sokrab TEO, Johansson BB, Kalimo H & Olsson Y (1988) A transient hypertensive opening of the blood-brain barrier can lead to brain damage. *Acta Neuropathol., 75*: 557.

Sommer AM, Grote K, Reinhardt T, Streckert J, Hansen V & Lerchl A (2009) Effects of radiofrequency electromagnetic fields (UMTS) on reproduction & development of mice: A multi-generation study. *Radiat. Res., 171*(1): 89.

Somossy Z, Thuroczy G, Kubasova T, Kovacs J & Szabo LD (1991) Effects of modulated & continuous microwave irradiation on the morphology & cell surfaces of 3T3 fibroblasts. *Scan Microsc., 5*: 1145.

Speit G, Schütz P & Hoffmann H (2007) Genotoxic effects of exposure to radio-frequency electromagnetic fields (RF-EMF) in cultured mammalian cells are not independently reproducible. *Mutat. Res.*, *626*(1–2): 42.

Sri KN (2015) Mobile phone radiation: Physiological &pathophysiological considerations. *Indian J. Physiol. Pharmacol.*, *59*(2): 125.

Stang A, Anastassiou G, Ahrens W, Bromen K, Bornfeld N & Jöckel KH (2001) The possible role of radiofrequency radiation in the development of uveal melanoma. *Epidemiology*, *12*(1): 7.

Stronati LA, Testa J, Moquet A, Edwards E, Cordelli P, Villani C, Marino AM, Fresegna M, Appolloni M & Lloyd D (2006) 935 MHz cellular phone radiation. An in vitro study of genotoxicity in human lymphocytes. *Int. J. Radiat. Biol.*, *82*: 39.

Stuchly MA (1994) Wireless communications & the safety of the user. *Int. J. Wireless Inf.*, *1*: 223.

Sugimachi K, Matsuda H, Ohno S, Fukuda A, Matsuoko H, Mori M & Kuwano H (1988) Long term effects of hyperthermia combined with chemotherapy & irradiation for the treatment of patients with carcinoma of esophagus. *Surg. Gynaecol. Obstet.*, *169*: 319.

Sukhotina I, Streeckert JR, Bitz AK, Hansen VW & Lerchl A (2006) 1800 MHz electromagnetic field effects on melatonin release from isolated pineal glands. *J. Pineal Res.*, *40*: 86.

Sun JG, Jurisicova A & Casper RF (1997) Detection of deoxyribonucleic acid fragmentation in human sperm: Correlation with fertilization in vitro. *Biol. Reprod.*, *56*: 602.

Sun LX, Yao K, He JL, Lu DQ, Wang KJ & Li HW (2006) DNA damage & repair induced by acute exposure of microwave from mobile phone on cultured human lens epithelial cells. *Zhonghua Yan Ke Za Zhi*, *42*(2006): 1084.

Sun Y (1990) Free radicals, antioxidant enzymes & carcinogenesis. *Free Rad. Biol. Med.*, *8*: 583.

Szmigielski A, Pietraszek A, Janiak M, Wrembel J, Kalczek M & Szmigielski S (1982a) Acceleration of the development of benzopyrene induced cancer in mice by microwave radiation. *Arch. Dermatol. Res.*, *274*: 303.

Szmigielski S, Szmigielski A, Pietraszek A, Bielee M & Wrembel JK (1982b) Accelerated development of spontaneous & benzopyrene induced cancer in mice exposed to 2450 MHz microwave radiation. *Bioelectromagnetics*, *3*: 179.

Taflove A (1995) *Computational Electrodynamics: The Finite-Difference Time Domain Method*. Artechhouse.

Tahvanainen K, Niño J, Halonen P, Kuusela T, Alanko T, Laitinen T, Länsimies E, Hietanen M & Lindholm H (2007) Effects of cellular phone use on ear canal temperature measured by NTC thermistors. *Clin. Physiol. Funct. Imaging*, *27*(3): 162.

Thomas S, Kuhnlein A, Heinrich S, Praml G, Nowak D, von Kries R & Radon K (2008) Personal exposure to mobile phone frequencies & wellbeing in adults: A cross-sectional study based on dosimetry. *Bioelectromagnetics*, *29*: 463.

Thomas WE (1999) Brain macrophages: On the role of pericytes & perivascular cells. *Brain Res. Rev.*, *31*: 42.

Tore F, Dulou PE, Haro E, Veyret B & Aubineau P (2002) Effect of 2h GSM-900 microwave exposures at 2.0, 0.5 & 0.12 W/kg on plasma protein extravasation in rat brain & dura matter. In: Proceedings of the 24thAnnual Meeting ofthe BEMS, 61.

Tsurita G, Nagawa H, Ueni S, Watanabe S & Taki M (2000) Biological & morphological effects on the brain after of rats on the brain after exposure rats to a 1439 MHz TDMA field. *Bioelectromagnetics, 21*: 364.

Urban P, Lukas E & Roth Z (1998) Does acute exposure to the electromagnetic field emitted by mobile phone influence visual evoked potentials? A pilot study. *Cent. Eur. J. Public Health, 6*(1998): 288.

Utteridge TD, Gebski V, Finnie JW, Vernon-Roberts B & Kuchel TR (2002) Long term exposure of E-Mu-Pim 1 transgenic mice to 898.4 MHz microwaves does not increase lymphoma incidence. *Radiat. Res., 158*: 357.

Valladares L, Moraga P, Ronco AM & Ahumada A (1990) A direct effect of melatonin on testicular steroidogenesis. *J. Steroidogenesis Biochem., 36*(Suppl): 7.

Vecchio F, Babilono C, Ferreri F, Curcio G, Fini R, Del Percio C & Maria Rossin FP (2007) Mobile phone emission modulated interhemispheric functional coupling of EEG alpha rhythms. *Eur. J. Neurosci., 25*: 1908.

Verschaeve L, Heikkinen P, Verheyen G, Van Gorp U, Boonen F, Vander Plaetse F, Maes A, Kumlin T, Mäki-Paakkanen J, Puranen L & Juutilainen J (2006) Investigation of co-genotoxic effects of radiofrequency electromagnetic fields in vivo. *Radiat. Res., 165*: 598.

Vijayalaxmi, Leals BZ, Szilagyi M, Prihoda TJ & Meltz ML (2000) Primary DNA damage in human blood lymphocytes exposed in vitro to 2450 MHz radiofrequency radiation. *Radiat. Res., 153*: 479.

Vijayalaxmi & Obe S (2004) Controversial cytogenetic observations in mammalian somatic cells exposed to radiofrequency radiation. *Radiat. Res., 162*: 481.

Volkow ND, Tomasi D, Wang G, Vaska P, Fowler JS, Telang F, Alexoff D, Logen J & Wong C (2011) Effect of cell phone radiofrequency signal exposure on brain glucose metabolism. *JAMA, 305*(8): 808.

Vollrath L, Spessert R, Kartzsch T, Keiner M & Hollmann H (1997) No short term effects of high frequency electromagnetic fields on the mammalian pineal gland. *Bioelectromagnetics, 18*: 376.

Watanabe S, Taki H, Nojima T & Fujiwara O (1996) Characteristics of the SAR distributions in a head exposed to electromagnetic fields radiated by a hand held portable radio. *IEEE Trans. Microwave Theory Tech., 44*(10): 1874.

Watanabe S, Tanaka T & Taki M (1995). Effects of the body on the SAR distribution in the head of a human model exposed to the near field of a small radiation source & to the far field of the source. In Proc. Convention Rec. IEICE Japan, IEICE: p. B-241.

Wdowiak A, Wdowiak L & Wiktor H (2007) Evaluation of the effect of using mobile phones on male fertility. *Ann. Agric. Environ. Med.: AAEM, 14*(1): 169.

Williams WM, Hoss W, Formaniak M & Michaelson SM (1984) Effect of 2450 MHz energy on the blood brain barrier to hydrophilic molecules. A. Effect on the permeability to sodium fluorescein. *Brain Res. Rev., 7*: 165.

Wolf R & Wolf D (2004) Increased incidence of cancer near a cellphone transmitter station. *Int. J. Cancer Prev., 1*: 123.

Wu RY, Chiang H, Shao BJ, Li NG & Fu YD (1994) Effects of 2.45 GHz microwave Radiation and phorbol ester 12-0 tetradeca noylphorbol-13 acetate on dimethylhydrazine-induced colon cancer in mice. *Bioelectromagnetics, 15*: 31.

Wyde M, Cesta M, Blystone C, Elmore S, Paul Foster P, Hooth M, Kissling G, Malarkey D, Sills R & Stout M (2017) Report of Partial Findings from the National Toxicology Program Carcinogenesis Studies of Cell Phone Radiofrequency Radiation in Hsd: Sprague Dawley® SD rats (Whole Body Exposure).

Yan J, Agresti M, Bruce T, Yan Y, Grnalund A & Matloub H (2007) Effects of cellular phone emissions on sperm motility in rats. *Fertil. Steril., 88*: 957.

Yee KS (1996) Numerical Solution of initial boundary value problems involving Maxwells equations in isotropic media. *IEEE Trans. Antenna Propag., 14*: 302.

Yilmaz F, Dasdag S, Akdag MZ & Killine N (2008) Whole body exposure of radiation emitted from 900 MHz mobile phones emitted does not seem to affect the levels of anti-apoptic bcl-2 protein. *Electromagn. Biol. Med., 27*: 65.

Yuasa K, Arai N, Okabe S, Tarusawa Y, Nojima T, Hanajjma R, Terao Y & Ugawa Y (2006) Effects of thirty minutes mobile phone use on the human sensory cortex. *Clin. Neurophysiol., 117*: 900.

Yurekli AI, Ozkan M, Kalkan T, Saybasili H, Tuncel H, Atukeren P, Pinar K, Gumustas K & Seker S (2006) GSM base station electromagnetic radiation & oxidative stress in rats. *Electromagn. Biol. Med., 25*: 177.

Zhang DY, Xu ZP, Chiang H, Lu DQ & Zeng QL (2006) Effects of GSM 1800 MHz radiofrequency electromagnetic fields on DNA damage in Chinese hamster lung cell. *Zhonghua Yu Fang Yi Xue Za Zhi, 40*: 149.

Zhang X, Huang W-J & Chen W-W (2016) Microwave & Alzheimer's disease (Review). *Exp. Ther. Med., 12*: 1969.

Zhao T-Y, Zou S-P & Knapp PE (2007) Exposure to cell phone radiation up-regulates apoptosis genes in primary cultures of neurons & astrocytes. *Neurosci. Lett., 412*: 34.

Zmyslony M, Palus J, Jajte J, Dziubaltowska E & Rajkowska E (2000) DNA damage in rat lymphocytes treated in vitro with iron cations & exposed to 7 mT magnetic fields (static or 50 Hz). *Mutat. Res., 453*: 89.

6

Safety Guidelines for Electromagnetic Field Exposure and Mobile Towers

6.1 Introduction

There is a growing concern among the population about the effects of environmental exposure (due to "uncontrolled" exposure of non-ionizing radiation) on public health. As discussed in previous chapters, the adverse effects of non-ionizing radiations on biological systems (ranging from cells to organisms) are causing immense concern. There are conflicting reports about the mechanism and the nature of the effects, indicating the possible relationship to human diseases (Frey 1967, 1974). It appears that a thorough application of standardized protocols is the key to reliable data acquisition and subsequent interpretation that could create a clearer picture for scientists and general public at large. Specific tuning of radio-frequency (RF) radiation in a clinical environment may lead to beneficial health effects. However, there is a need to know the level of microwave exposure at various times in different local environment. This necessitates the need to define the limits of electromagnetic fields EMF safe exposure for humans over a wide frequency band. The exposure due to ionizing radiation and the subsequent dosimetry is vastly different than due to non-ionizing radiations. Ionizing radiation can cause stochastic and deterministic effects, while most effects due to exposure from non-ionizing radiation appear to be only deterministic. Stochastic effects have been demonstrated due to exposure to ultraviolet radiation. This bridges the continuity between ionizing and non-ionizing parts of the electromagnetic spectrum. For ionizing radiation, there is a greater emphasis on optimization of protection even at low levels of exposure, whereas correspondingly for non-ionizing radiation there is a greater emphasis on keeping exposures below thresholds. Controlling adverse effects through the marking of safe level is still full of uncertainties.

For non-ionizing radiations, the exposure limits have a direct relation to the dose (maybe there is some proportionality). On the other hand, the relationship between the exposure and the induced fields or between SAR computation and its distribution is significantly dependent on various exposure parameters, e.g., the frequency and field polarization, as well as on the location and surroundings of the exposed biological bodies (Chapter 4). The human body has complex surfaces and internal geometries and is composed of tissues with spatially varying dielectric properties. The mere presence of other body/bodies also alters the field distribution. In the case of near-field exposures, the coupling between the body and the electromagnetic source can even alter the behavior of the source. Consequently, the limits of safe exposure are difficult to define and more so over a broad range of frequency spectrum and in an unknown environment (Vecchia, 2007).

In view of this, it is customary to define exposure limits in worst-case scenario, i.e. when it is assured that the basic limits are satisfied under all conditions. Absorption under various exposure conditions was extensively investigated in numerous studies in the late 1970s. From these studies the current exposure limits for electric and magnetic field strengths have been derived. These field quantities can be easily measured using existing equipment (IEEE, 1992, 2005). It leads us to conclude that the most efficient absorption occurs under plane wave conditions with an upright human body is parallel to the incident E-field. Other, more unusual body postures might also result in enhanced absorption. This occurs when the body or body parts form a part of near field of the radiation source and re-radiating structures. For example, in the closest vicinity of low power transmitters, these exposure limits are easily exceeded, although the actually induced absorption might only be a small fraction of the SAR limits, though in the close vicinity of these handheld devices the SAR values are difficult to estimate.

Alternately it may be mentioned that the exposure limits do not apply for the safety assessment of handheld telephones. Subsequently, the testing of compliance of handheld mobile communication transrecievers with safety limits has lately become the key problem in the area of dosimetry. Keeping in view the importance of this issue, the focus of this chapter confines to discussions of methods and procedures to assess the basic dose for safe exposure standards, i.e., the SAR distribution inside biological tissues with respect to the level of incident power density.

Absorption of RF energy exposed to high field strengths can be thermogenic to man and animals. Under ambient environmental conditions, where the temperature and humidity are already elevated, the same SAR could produce body temperatures that reach well beyond normal levels permitted by the 1°C increment. This could precipitate undesired heat-stress-related responses (adverse thermal effects).

Safety guidelines outline two different categories of restrictions for what concerns electromagnetic exposures, namely: (i) basic restrictions and (ii) reference levels or maximum permissible exposure. The basic restrictions, which also include a proper safety factor, define the threshold values above which specific biological effects can be expected and are reported to occur. Basic restrictions are defined in terms of the appropriate biologically effective quantities and are set below the threshold for the appropriate critical effects. Since the direct measurement of the basic restrictions is technically difficult or often impractical in many daily situations, reference levels are derived from basic restrictions and they are derived and reported in terms of a directly measurable parameter of the external electromagnetic exposures. Such a formulation makes the exposure guidelines more practical and versatile. Indeed, while the basic restrictions are closely related to the biological effect, the reference levels (RL) are directly related to the emission levels of the different electromagnetic sources and are thus easier to be evaluated (Vecchia 2007; Christ et al. 2013).

Different scientific committees from several national and international organizations have developed the safety guidelines for electromagnetic field exposure. The most relevant of these organizations are the International Commission for Non-Ionizing Radiation Protection (ICNIRP 1998, 2010) and the Standards suggested by coordinating Committee 28 (SCC28) of the Institute of Electrical and Electronic Engineers (IEEE 2005). These committees constantly monitor scientific literature and reports in order to tune exposure limits based on the effects that the scientific community has established. These limits are under constant revision and as such the guidelines are also under revision (ICNIRP1998; ICNIRP 2010; IEEE 1992). To protect people from EMF overexposure, ICNIRP and IEEE have defined limits. In the radiofrequencies domain, an exposure to EMF is quantified by the specific absorption rate (SAR) (expressed in watts per kilogram). The basic restrictions (BR) are the fundamental limits expressed in terms of the whole-body averaged SAR (WBSAR) as well as local SAR averaged on 1 or 10 g of tissues.

BR are difficult to check in situ; hence, the ICNIRP has also defined RL derived from the BR (ICNIRP 1998). RL give the maximum permissible EMF strength or power density (in the absence of a person). Compliance to RL is deemed to ensure compliance to BR. The link between RL and BR was established by Gandhi (1980) based on simplified human models and assuming maximum coupling. Numerical dosimetry is intensively used to analyze the SAR distribution in tissues and design exposure setup. Numerical methods, such as the well-known finite difference in time domain (FDTD), enable us to achieve a very good accuracy in the SAR computation. Based on this, several studies have used 3D human body models to analyze the relationship between the WBSAR induced in a human model and the incident field. Recent studies have shown that the WBSAR induced by a plane wave with a vertical electric field strength set to the RL can be non-conservative regarding the BR for some phantoms (Dimbylow 1997; Conil et al. 2008). These studies emphasize the variability of the WBSAR with frequency due to the variation in the morphology. In the European Union (2004), the 1998 ICNIRP Guidelines yield the basis for the national regulators to endorse appropriate legislation. In 2004, the

European Union (2004) gave a directive with the aim to guard workers from possible dangerous effects caused by electromagnetic fields The United States considers parts of both the guidelines of the National Council on Radiation Protection (NCRP 1986) and the 1992 issue of the guidelines of the IEEE C95.1 standard (IEEE 1992). In Switzerland, national regulation uses ICNIRP Guidelines 1998 and was the first country to introduce precautionary limits below the ICNIRP guidelines for fixed installations in sensitive areas (e.g., schools, living areas, hospitals) (SAEFL 1999).

A major consideration of existing guidelines is the prevention of adverse biological effects resulting from either whole body or partial body exposure. This exposure could bring about a rise in temperature of the order of 1°C in humans and laboratory animals. The central theme of the exposure guidelines is to protect exposed subjects against temperature increase, thereby breaching the temperature threshold for induction of adverse thermal effects. The tissue heating due to RF exposure is caused not only by the power absorbed but also by the distribution of power due to the exposure in the surrounding volume.

6.2 Exposure of Body to Cell Phone and Base Station

The widespread use of cell phones has led to the installation of cell phone towers being spread over in many communities. These towers, also called base stations, have electronic equipment and antennas that receive and emit RF signals.

Ever since the adverse biological effects of low-level microwave radiations have been reported, there is an increasing demand to lay down the criteria of safe limits of exposure. Guidelines for limiting EM exposure provide protection against known adverse health effects. Since the criteria for safe exposure of microwave radiation, was first established, emissions from mobile tower and handheld cell phones have greatly increased, which are identified as essentially nonthermal. There is a concern among the people about possible adverse biological effects due to cellular telephone base stations, i.e., the possible effects of low-intensity exposure, and health issues.

The basic to EMF biointeraction lies in the electric field induced inside the tissues. There are nonthermal effects, while there might also be isothermal effects. Thermal effects depend on the SAR distribution. It may be mentioned that microwaves as a whole form a group of frequencies, traditionally from 100 MHz to 1THz, exhibiting essentially the same effects throughout the whole frequency range. From a biological point of view, it is even considered microwaves from 50 MHz up, including TV frequencies.

For mobile telephony, the interaction between a handset antenna and the human body is obviously one of the special interests (Okoniewski &

Stuchly 1996).Absorbed power density is the main cause of reported effects: 1 W/kg may yield an increase of (<1°C) in human body, taking thermal regulation into account (WHO 1993). As mentioned in Chapter 3, the SAR is the ratio of absorbed power to absorbing mass (skin effects taken into account). At 900 MHz, the lowest GSM cellular telephone frequency, the skin depth is approximately the absorbing mass of a human body. For a person weighing 65 kg and 1.70 m high, the SAR is approximately 8.5 W/kg at the above frequency. Pulsed waves produce a detectable effect at power levels smaller than due to CW.

Experiments concerning thermal effects due to GSM exposure from hand-held mobile telephones have been made (Taurisano & Vander Vorst 2000). The temperature rise of different parts of the head has been measured when exposed to microwaves from GSM at 900 MHz. Three different phones have been used from three different manufacturers located in Europe, the United States, and Japan, respectively. An infra red (IR) camera measured the temperature by taking a thermographic image every 20s using a pattern of 10,000 thermocouples located in the lens. Measurements were made during the different phases of the phone operation: stand-by, ringing, talking, and switching off. Total temperature is measured, taking into account microwave heating, temperature rise due to the electronic part of the device, and possible reduction in ventilation because of the presence of the device near the face. The most significant temperature increase has been observed on the ear lobe, at the end of the talking phase, for the highest duration (20 min). This temperature increases from 1.0°C to 2.4°C, depending on the location and phone type. The temperature trend for cheek and neck areas follows a similar trend. The temperature increases in the first 5–7 min of exposure.

Another dimension of uncertainty arises, as some people describe themselves as hypersensitive to EMF. This hypersensitivity is mentioned at levels largely below those of international recommendations. However, the severity of the effect being accepted is related to the field intensity, but the relationship between electric and magnetic fields and associated effects is not convincingly demonstrated. A dose-effect relationship at such low levels remains to be established because the phenomena is largely nonlinear. In this connection, this may be mentioned that the prime issue is the field emission from the towers which need to be measured in the first instance (for assessing the exposure levels).If it is so demanded, these measurements need to be performed over a long period of time under a variety of environmental conditions.

6.3 Field Emission from Tower

Electromagnetic measurement systems are used to measure power densities, or power spectral densities, of electromagnetic fields at a point in space. Power density is defined as the "power per unit area normal to the direction of propagation and is usually expressed in units of Watts per square meter (W/m^2)." Plane-waves, power densities, electric field strengths (E (v/m)), and magnetic field strengths (H(A/m)) are related by free-space impedance, i.e., 377 ohms (Ω). Field strength is therefore defined as:

$$E = (120\pi P_D)^{1/2} \tag{6.1}$$

$$P_D = (E^2/120\pi)$$

Where E = rms value of field strength in volts/meter,

P_D = power density in watt/meter^2,

120π = impedance of free space in ohms.

Power density (P_D) is related to the electric field strength (E) and the magnetic field strength (H) as:

$$P_D = E^2/377\Omega = 377H^2\Omega \text{ (far field)} \tag{6.2}$$

The power transmitted by an antenna is given by the equation:

$$P_D = P_T/4\pi r^2 \tag{6.3}$$

Where

P_T = transmitted power in watts,

r = distance in meters.

Radiated electromagnetic fields (radiated emissions)can be produced from several sources. Sources of electromagnetic energy range from man-made sources such as commercial broadcast stations and automobile ignition systems to natural sources such as galactic noise and lightning. These emissions can drastically differ in frequencies and in their magnitudes.

The power received by the antenna ($\mathbf{P_r}$) is then defined by:

$$P_r = P_D G\lambda^2/4\pi \text{ (Watts)} \tag{6.4}$$

Where

G = antenna (power) gain,

λ = wavelength in meters.

Combining these equations with the field strength equation yields:

$$P_r = E^2 G\lambda^2/480\pi^2 \tag{6.5}$$

Also,

$$Pr = Vr^2/Zo$$

Where

V_r = received voltage,
Z_o = receiver input impedance.
Then,

$$V_r^2/Z_o = E^2G\lambda^2/480\pi^2 \tag{6.6}$$

And:

$$\lambda = \mathbf{C/frequency}.$$

6.4 Power Density and Radiation Level

The power density at any distance from an isotropic antenna is simply the transmitter power divided by the surface area of a sphere at that distance. The surface area of the sphere increases by the square of the radius; therefore, the power density, PD (watts/square meter), decreases by the square of the radius (Figure 6.1a, b).

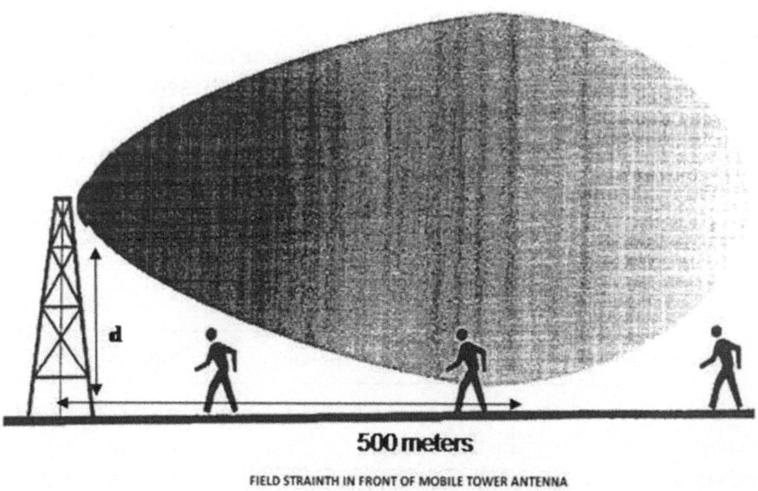

FIGURE 6.1a

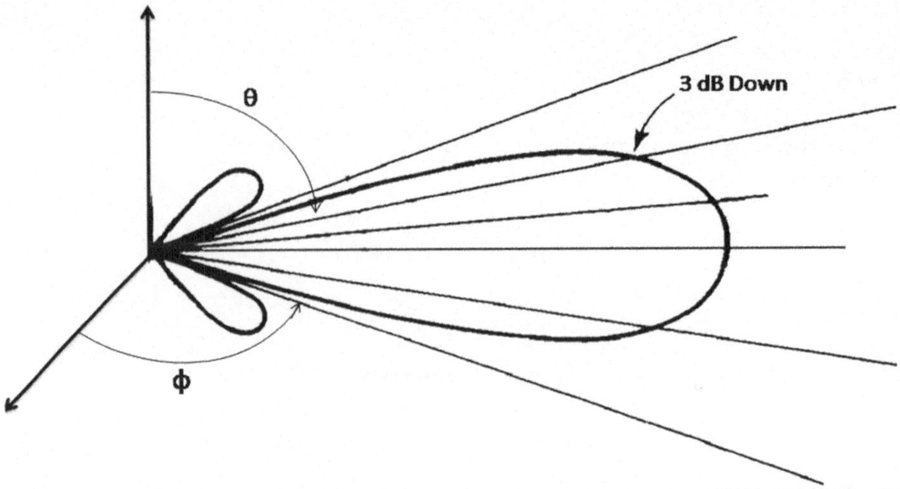

FIGURE 6.1b
Radiation pattern of antenna and beam width and side lobe.

$$S = PG/4\pi R^2 \tag{6.7}$$

Where

S = power density (W/m^2),
P = power input to the antenna (W),
G = power gain of the antenna,
R = distance to the center of radiation of the antenna (m).

Compliance distance recommended by ICNIRP (based on ITU K.70 fact sheet formula) is given in the table below.

Here r is compliance distance (meters), f is the frequency (MHz), and erip is equivalent isotropically radiated power in the direction of maximum antenna gain (watts), and erp is effective power in the direction of maximum antenna gain (watts).

Radio frequency range	General public exposure	General public exposure
1 to 10 MHz	$r = 0.10 \sqrt{eirp \times f}$	$r = 0.129 \sqrt{erp \times f}$
10 to 400 MHz	$r = 0.319 \sqrt{eirp}$	$r = 0.409 \sqrt{erp}$
400 to 2000 MHz	$r = 6.38 \sqrt{eirp/f}$	$r = 8.16 \sqrt{erp/f}$
2000 to 300,000 MHz	$r = 0.143 \sqrt{eirp/f}$	$r = 0.184 \sqrt{erp}$

The field in front of the usual parabolic antenna is divided into two parts:

1. The "near-field," or the region where the radiation is substantially confined within a cylindrical pattern, is called the Fresnel region.
2. The "far-field," or Fraunhofer region, lies beyond the Fresnel region in free space, where the radiation is essentially confined to a conical pattern and the power density along the beam axis falls off inversely with the square of the distance.

The power density in the near-field, assuming a circular "dish" antenna, is given by

$$W = \frac{16P}{\pi D^2} = \frac{4P}{A} \tag{6.8}$$

Where
P = average power output,
D = diameter of antenna,
A = area of antenna.

In the far-field region W_f, the free-space power density on the beam axis can be computed from the relationship:

$$W_f = GP/4\pi r^2 = AP/\lambda^2 r^2 \tag{6.9}$$

Where λ = wavelength.

The power collected by the receiving antenna is

$$(P_r = WA = AP/4\pi)$$

The distance from the antenna to the intersection of the near-field (1) with the far-field (2) is given by

$$r_1 = \frac{\pi D^2}{8\lambda} = \frac{A}{2\lambda} \tag{6.10}$$

These formulas do not include the effect of ground reflection which could cause an increase in the value of power density which is upto four times the free-space value.

For power density falling on the human population, equal to the potentially hazardous level of 10 mW/cm^2, one may calculate the distance to that of the potentially hazardous zone. Base station antennas use higher power levels than other types of land-mobile antennas, but much lower levels than those from radio and television broadcast stations.

6.5 Methods in RF Measurements

In present-day measurements, a spectrum analyzer is used for identification of RF sources and for assessment of the relative magnitude of signals in different frequency ranges, and in fact this is the heart of the entire measuring setup. This instrument is tunable over a vast frequency range, is used to detect the frequency range, and can be used to display the variation of amplitude over the desired portion of the spectrum (Figures 6.2 and 6.3). The use of this instrument with a calibrated antenna will allow a sensitive and accurate precise power measurement across selected frequency ranges or measurement of the strength of an individual broadband signal. This process completely eliminates the problem of inaccuracy in the presence of multiple strong signals. The instrument also permits a determination of the amount of power that is present in different parts of the RF spectrum (ranging from GHz to MHz frequencies).

Measurements can be conducted at different distances and directions, inside and outside of representative public and residential buildings. Frequency-selective spectrum analysis is used to obtain GSM power densities following the current recommendations for GSM cellular phone radiation measurements. In far-field region, the electric (E) and magnetic (H) field distributions are essentially independent of the distance from the source. The field has thus a predominantly plane wave character, i.e., completely uniform distribution of electric field and magnetic field strength

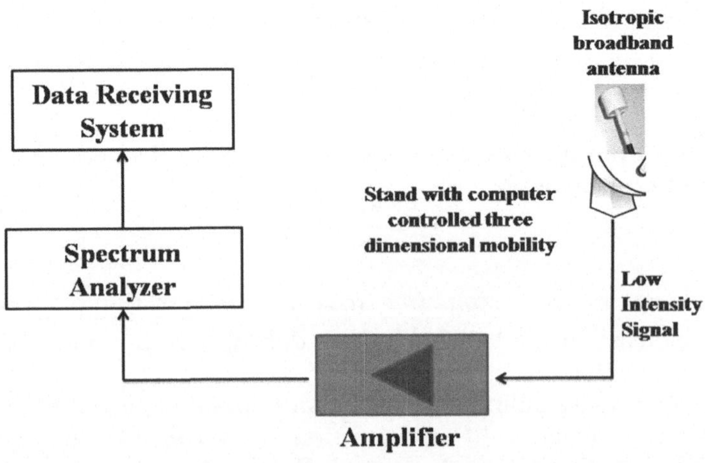

FIGURE 6.2
A schematic representation of a microwave receiving isotropic broadband antenna for field measurements. Measurements made at nominal distances from base station tower (W/m^2).

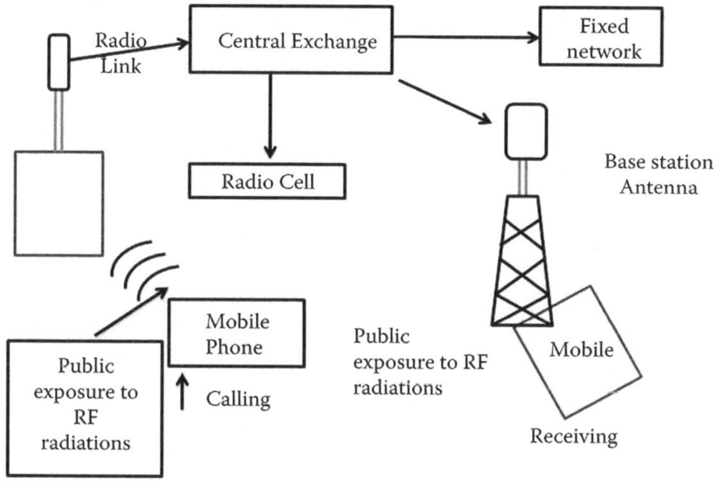

FIGURE 6.3
Public exposure to mobile phone radiations and RF signal propagation with a transmission receiver setup.

in a plane normal to the direction of propagation.The E and H fields are related by the equation:

$$|E|/|H| = 377 \text{ ohms}$$

Where the figure on the right (377 ohms) is the **characteristic impedance** of free space. It is that in this scenario that the electric and magnetic fields are uniquely defined through the intrinsic impedance of the medium. Thus the knowledge of electric and magnetic field behavior is sufficient to characterize the exposure in terms of power density. The spatial distribution of RF energy from an RF antenna is directional and varies with distance from it. At distances greater than the far-field distance (radiation zone), the RF energy changes only with distance (independent of the angle of orientation between antenna and receiving probe). A typical high-frequency spectrum analysis of the signal is shown in Figure 6.4.

Technical Challenges for RF Site Surveys

Measurement of the emissions from cell towers presents particular technical challenges beyond those encountered for broadcast antenna sites. These are twofold: inherent problems in the measurements at site and the instrumentation.

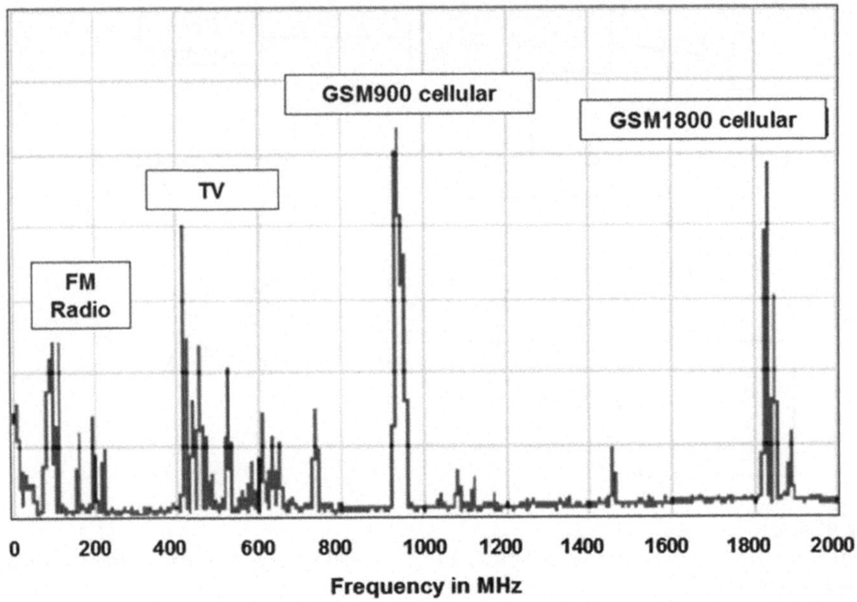

FIGURE 6.4
Aschematic representation of a microwave intercepted by isotropic broadband antenna for free field measurements. Broad based antenna is directed toward the emission tower.

Protocols for the measurement of RF energy for the purpose of human exposure assessment often recommend the use of an "isotropic broadband probe" because this type of sensor responds equally to energy arriving from any direction, and over a broad frequency range, as falling upon the human body. These instruments are commonly used because they permit a quick and simple measurement.

Isotropic Broadband RF Meter

Most types of antennas used in conjunction with spectrum analyzers for narrow band measurements are not isotropic. Measuring antenna is kept on a tripod stand in order to reduce minimize interaction with the operator and the objects around it. The term broadband implies that characteristic of the isotropic meter will measure range of emitted signals across a wide range of frequencies from the source. The instrument is also calibrated to measure the strength of any signal in the range. The reading produced by the instrument will be the combination of all signals present. In a large number of cases, the other signals present near a cell tower will be as strong as the cellular signals that one is trying to measure. Realistically, this composite measurement of all signals may be the most relevant exposure data.To understand the significance of these data requires that one know the frequency of the signal that produced it.

One of the most significant RF measurement problems, and one responsible for some of the greatest inaccuracy, involves an instrument erroneous response that can occur when there are two or more strong signals present at the same time. A very large proportion of antenna sites (cell and broadcast) now have multiple strong signals. Instrument design can minimize this problem and presently broadband meters are available of sufficient accuracy.

Some of the meters used for typical RF compliance surveys are unable to accurately measure the low power densities at some cell sites, demand constant recalibration, and besides being expansive. An additional problem results from the fact that power density levels at a cell tower site are not always constant, as these usually are at a broadcast antenna site. The amount of cell phone use is more during the day, and on some days of the week, than at others. The cellular service providers maintain additional capacity in the form of multiple channels which will become active as needed to meet the fluctuating demand. Each active channel adds to the measured power density at the cell site.

6.6 Exposure of People to the RF Energy from Cellular Phone Towers

The RFspectrum allocated to mobile communication is limited to a narrow bandwidth. To overcome this, constraint, designers have adopted the cellular approach: using multiple antennas (base stations) to cover a geographic area. With each base station covering a geographic area, a base station covers a roughly circular area called a cell (see Figure 5.4 for how a large region can be split into seven smaller cells, approximated by hexagons). This allows different base stations to use the same frequencies as long as they are separated by a sufficient distance. This permits many users just to share a few channels. Another aspect is that with each base station covering a smaller area, the mobile phones need less transmit power to reach any base station (thus remaining connected with the mobile network). In an attempt to adjust its use with growing demand, two methods are found to be useful. The first is the cell splitting; that is, by dividing the cell into several cells, the cellular provider can increase its capacity in high demand areas. The second is sectoring: in this method, instead of a single omnidirectional antenna covering a cell, a cell is sectorized into N_s regions, each being served by an antenna that covers an angular span of $2\pi/N_s$ (N_s=3, a typical value). Note that both approaches increase handoff rates,thus requiring concurrent upgrading of network management.

The mobile phone works by communicating with a nearby base station (also called a "cell site") which connects it to the main phone network (Figure 5.5). When moving, if the mobile phone gets too far away from the cell it is connected to, that cell sends a message to another cell to convey the new cell to take over the call. This is termed a "hand off," and the call continues with the new cell the phone taking over. The taken over is done so well and carefully that the user does not know that the call was transferred to another cell. The level of RF energy inside buildings where a base station signal is available is typically much lower than the level outside, depending on the construction materials of the building. The RF waves transmitted and reflected to and from these base stations and in the process are given off into the environment, where people are exposed to these radiations. Since this is a chronic phenomenon, their biological effects may be important and need to be examined in detail.Their biological effect is now well documented (French et al. 2001; Behari 2009). An estimate of power emission from a tower is shown in Tables 6.2a, b, c, and 6.3).

Cellular phone system covers an area when the signal strength reaches as low of about 0.001 $\mu W/cm^2$. Table 6.2a, b, c gives a measurement of power levels from various technical mobile specifications under various conditions.

6.7 Safety Criteria

Guidelines for Safe Exposure

At very high levels, RF energy can be dangerous, as it produces heating effects. It can heat the body's tissues rapidly. However, such high levels are rare and found only near certain equipment, such as powerful long-distance transmitters, and human exposure to these is a mere chance and does not form a part limits of safe exposure.

Regulations adopted by the Federal Communications Commission (FCC, USA) in 1996, and fully implemented in 2000, limit human exposure to electromagnetic radiation from cell phone, broadcast, and other radio communication systems. Both U.S. and international standards governing exposure to RF fields have long existed, and the FCC regulations were adapted from a pre-existing standard. They establish maximum permissible exposures (MPEs) for the full range of frequencies encountered near transmitting equipment, towers, and antennas.

For cellular antennas on towers, the level of RF energy that one would realistically be exposed to is usually less than 1% of the MPE. For broadcast towers and building mounted cellular antennas, much higher exposures are possible, although the MPEs are still unlikely to be exceeded in areas accessible to the public. However, there are reasons for concern:

1. Since there are several suggestive guidelines for field measurements from mobile tower antenna, people are skeptical about utility agencies to put up a comprehensive data. In fact in many places only self-certifications suffice,validity of which is open to question.
2. Many people equate the adverse health effects of cell phone use, with the presence of cell towers, though the energy that one is exposed to while holding a cell phone is far greater than the one that is exposed to in the vicinity of a cell tower. Main limitations of the present day suggested standards stems from the fact that it is primarily based on RF energy heating the tissue, while nonthermal effects reported suggest a type of phenomena pointing to electromagnetic–cellular interaction. It is then possible to identify a range of numbers below which no adverse effects are expected to occur and above which potentially adverse effects are likely to occur. This range of numbers can form the basis for a guideline,since this number is dependent on a number of parameters, whose uniqueness is difficult to control. The scientific basis for revision of the conceptual basis needs a relook, maybe by including (or adopting) some other parameter, internal to the biological system.

Inadequacies in the Presently Available Guidelines

Sometimes there are questions about precautionary guidelines referenced or developed by various organizations. The frequency at which this occurs has prompted drafting various scientific organizations to come out with some propositions for the entire frequency segment. A large amount of data (due to low-level microwave exposure) that now has gathered suggests that the presently available data of safe exposure are inadequate for public protection. In fact, a long exposure to such fields may cause illness. In one of the earliest observations of threshold response to nonthermal MW was published by Frey (1967, 1974), and the value was 30 $\mu W/cm^2$. This value is approximately four orders of magnitude smaller than the intensities needed to cause an increase in internal body temperature. However, even this low level (or even lower than this)of exposure causes harm to different types: human cells, human sperm, and developing fetus in-utero (Chapters 4 and 5).

Major difficulties in complying with the recommended levels are that measured field data following a standard uniform protocol are not available in many situations. Recommended levels are difficult to achieve in a typical suburban or an urban environment without a shield of the building, or a part of it. Any recommendation which implies that most people in the world today are living in a hazardous environment needs attention, with a long-term measurements over a prolong period of time.

Most of the levels of radio frequencies in the environment are well below the level of producing thermal effects. They can only produce nonthermal effects. This and many other emerging evidences suggest that the SARconcept is insufficient to evaluate the health risks from nonthermal emission of microwaves from mobile communication. Other emerging parameters (e.g., lifestyle disorders) are also important and should be taken into consideration, though their method of inclusion is difficult to decide.

While working the dose dependence, the exposure duration and electric field intensity should be taken into account. Lower intensities, if allowed to impinge for a longer duration, may produce irreversible effects. These exposures can also cause health risks. In view of the mounting evidences underlying the low-level RFradiation exposure causing biological effects, present guidelines, such as IEEE (2005), FCC (1996), and ICNIRP (1998, 2010), are not adequate to protect humans from such exposures. In the first place, it is not possible to evolve a uniform methodology for such measurements. Secondly, many presently available data are taken with uncalibrated instruments. As such, the presently available safety standards data are not very reliable.

There are data about the effects of microwave at super-low intensities and significant role of duration of exposure in these effects. Adverse effects of nonthermal microwave from GSM/UMTS (Universal Mobile Communication Service) mobile phone depend on carrier frequency, and types of microwave signal suggest that microwave from base stations/mast, wireless routers, WI-FI, and other wireless devices and exposures in common use today can also produce adverse effects at prolonged durations of exposure. In many cases,extremely low frequency (ELF) modulation and additional ELF fields created by the microwave sources (e.g., mobile phones) are difficult to distinguish from the effects of exposure to ELF and microwaves.

Therefore, these combined exposures and their possible cancer risks are also pertinent and need consideration. The measurement on animal phantoms has been attempted by Behari and Nirala (2013) by adopting the use of 3G mobile phones. The other type of microwave signals prevalent in the environment (carrier frequency, modulation, polarization, far field and near field, intermittence, coherence, etc.) may produce different effects, may also involve cancer risk, and can be estimated for each microwave signal separately.

Guidelines for Safety Limits:Present Scenario

The question of laying down the criteria for safe exposure is undoubtedly ridden with problems because of various reasons mentioned above and may be some more. Like ionizing radiations, the dose needs to be assessed not just as external field intensity but also due to cumulative exposure. Since in the computation of SAR, conductivity appears, which is a spatially dependent parameter, and hence SAR needs to be computed for different anatomical locations, for various input signals. This further demands the need to have an accurate knowledge of RF exposure. The intensity of incoming radiations invariably assumes a field-free scenario. These radiations (even a low-level exposure) can cause health risks (Behari 2009) and are termed as silent killer. Its impact is not being immediately visible. Also the epidemiological study for an extended period of time (10years or more) is difficult to carry out along with the control subjects. Importantly, the signals of mobile communication are completely replaced at least once in 10 years, making the result of epidemiological studies uncertain, as a new database needs to be undertaken to take care of new signal parameters, in respect of cancer risk assessment. Moreover, the basic restrictions are expressed in quantities that are internal to the body (e.g., SAR). On the other hand, the reference levels are expressed (measured) in the free-space situation, such as electric field. Such data are not easy to measure at any place over an extended period of time. It is also anticipated that some part of the human population, such as children, pregnant women, and groups of hypersensitive person, could be especially sensitive to the nonthermal microwave exposures.

It is generally agreed that behavioral disruption is the potentially adverse effect found in animals at the lowest exposure level. The term "behavioral disruption" refers to the tendency of animals to stop performing a complex learned task when exposed to a sufficient amount of RF energy, without producing any thermal damage to the tissue. This disruption occurs at a threshold level of SAR of about 4W/kg of bodyweight. The standard for partial bodyweight has been set at 8W/kg, though the rational for this is unclear. Nonetheless, the attempts to draw the safety limits and their criteria have been in operation since long. A factor of 1/10 has been introduced to provide a safety margin for people running the risk of having exposed to some sources of unknown exposure. RF exposures are defined by the ICNIRP (1998) and are set to 0.08W/kg for the general public and 0.4 W/kg for occupational exposure. It is possible that because of the large interspecies differences among the small animals (rodents) and primates, the data may not be representative of human responses under identical exposure conditions over the whole body.

The Federal Communication Commission (FCC 1996) has set a limit for the exposure of a user to RF radiation from a wireless handset which is 1.6 W/kg of body tissue averaged over any 1 g of tissue. The limit of 1.6 W/kg is based on thermal effects of total heat load in animals being subjected to whole body exposure; averaging requirements depend upon engineering considerations. The development of public exposure standards for RF/MW fields is based on acute, but not on chronic exposures, and hence fails to take into account intermittent exposures. It also fails to consider special impacts of pulsed RF and ELF-modulated RF and does not take into account bioeffects from long-term, low-intensity exposures that may lead to adverse health impacts. RF exposures are defined by the ICNIRP (1998, 2010) (Table 6.1a, b).

However, the new basic restriction for localized exposure is 2 W/kg for most part of the body (Lin 2006). For the extremities (arms and legs distal from the elbow and knees, respectively, including the fingers, toes, hands, and feet) and for pinnae, the basic restriction expressed in terms of SAR is 4 W/kg. The value of SAR is obtained by averaging over some specified time periods (i.e., 6 to 30 min) and by averaging over any 10 g of tissue. For frequencies between 3 GHz and 100 GHz, the basic restrictions are the same as the derived limits of MPE.

The IEEE standard includes several major differences from the 1991 edition. First and the foremost, the IEEE standard instituted an exclusion for the pinnae or the external ears by relaxation of the abovementioned basic SAR restriction from 2 W/kg to 4 W/kg. Further, the SAR value increases raised from 1.6 W/kg averaged over any 1g of tissue to 2 W/kg over any 10 g of tissue. This effectively means relaxing the criteria, because deposition of energy over 10 g would be inherently low as compared to SAR over 1g. This revised choice (10 g in the shape of a cube) would permit the deposition of RF or microwave energy in different part of the eye that exceeds the basic SAR restriction by a large margin, while keeping the SAR for the entire eye below the prescribed limit (2 W/kg).

TABLE 6.1a

Reference levels for occupational exposure to time-varying electric and magnetic fields (unperturbed rms values)

Frequency range	E-filed strength (V/ m)	H-field strength (A/ m)	B-field (μT)	Equivalent plane wave power density S (Wm)
Up to 1 Hz	—	1.63×10^5	2×10^5	-
1-8 Hz	20,000	$1.63 \times 10^5/f^2$	$2 \times 10^5/f^2$	-
8-25 Hz	20,000	$2 \times 10^4/f$	$2.5 \times 10^4/f$	-
0.025-0.82 kHz	500/f	20/f	25/f	-
0.82-65 kHz	610	24.4	30.7	-
0.065-1 MHz	610	1.6/f	2.0/f	-
1-10 MHz	610/f	1.6/f	2.0/f	-
10-400 MHz	61	0.16	0.2	10
400-2,000 MHz	$3f^{1/2}$	$0.008f^{1/2}$	$0.01/f^{1/2}$	f/40
2-300 GHZ	137	0.36	0.45	50

In terms of average power density (mW/cm^2), exposure limits can be classified as follows: >10 potentially hazardous, 1-10 safe for occasional exposure, and <1 safe for prolonged or permanent exposure.

TABLE 6.1b

Basic restrictions for time-varying electric and magnetic fields for frequencies up to 10 GHz

Exposure characteristics	Frequency range	Current density head and trunk (mA m^{-2})(rms)	Whole-body average SAR (Q kg^{-1})	Localized SAR (head and trunk) (W kg^{-1})	Localized SAR (limbs) (W kg^{1})
Occupational exposure	Up to 1 Hz	40	-	-	-
	1-4 Hz	40/f	-	-	-
	4 Hz-1 kHz	10	-	-	-
	1-100 kHz	f/100	-	-	-
	100 kHz-10 MHz	f/100	0.4	10	20
	10 MHz-10 GHz	-	0.4	10	20
General public exposure	Up to 1 Hz	8	-	-	-
	1-4 Hz	8/f	-	-	-
	4Hz-1 kHz	2	-	-	-
	1-100 kHz	f/500	-	-	-
	100 kHz-10 MHz	f/500	0.08	2	4
	10 MHz-10 GHz	-	0.08	2	4

Exposure characteristics, frequency range,current density for head and trunk (mA/m ^{2}) (rms), whole-body average SAR (W/kg), localized SAR (head and trunk) (W/kg), localized SAR (limbs) (W/kg), general exposure limits are five times less than the occupational exposure limits.

In the 1991 edition, the MPE between 30 and 300 MHz were 10 W/m^2. The new MPE in terms of power density is 2 W/m^2 between 30 and 400 MHz, the region most susceptible for human exposure. It ramps up from 2 to 10 W/m^2, between 400 and 2000 MHz. For frequencies greater than 2000 MHz, the maximum permissible exposure is 10 W/m^2. Also, the designated frequency bands and the MPE are different. The ramp up from 10 to 100 W/m^2 took place between 300 MHz and 3000 MHz. For frequencies greater than 3000 MHz, the MPE was 100 W/m^2 (Figure 6.5).

In general, the new IEEE standards are more restrictive between 30 MHz and 100 MHz, frequency range corresponding to the resonance absorption in the humans (worst-case scenario). The major differences also include the tissue mass and the time period over which the SAR values are to be averaged and the applicable frequency bands for the MPE exposure. Also, the most significant difference is the exclusion of pinnae from the head by IEEE, which made it possible to allow a higher local SAR value for the basic restriction at 4 W/kg. In the ICNIRP guidelines, pinnae are not excluded and are treated as the integral part of the human head.

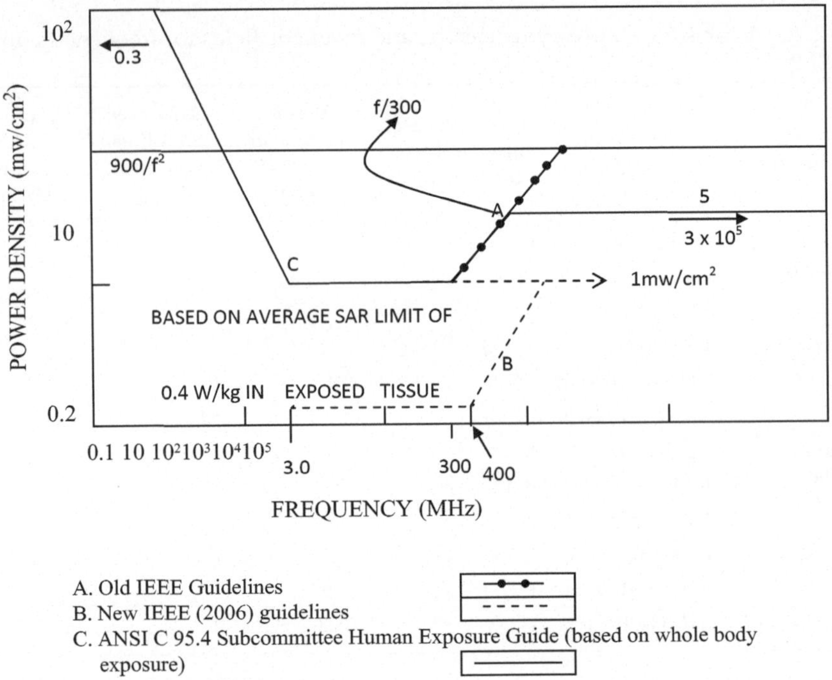

FIGURE 6.5
Exposure guidelines for whole body exposure.

Moreover, localized SAR values in the ICNRP guidelines are to be averaged over any 10-gmass of contiguous tissue. ICNIRP guidelines do not specify a cubic volume of tissue as the averaging mass. In addition, all SAR values are to be averaged over a 6-min period in the ICNIRP guidelines, in contrast to the 2.5 to 30 min stipulated in the new IEEE standard.

The revised IEEE standards are not identical with ICNIRP guidelines (Table 6.1a, b). This may also be true for frequencies used in cellular mobile communications and wireless device and systems. Global harmonization of radiofrequency exposure standards for the general public would be a future goal. Some of the points of contradiction as mentioned above will continue to be a point of investigation and should also include: more accurate assessment of SAR values, more reliable (reproducible) biological results, and an assessment of their impact on health. It may be mentioned that immune system is critical for evaluation of the effect of RF at low intensity and should be taken into consideration for development of standards.

Handsets (Okoniewski & Stuchly 1996)

GSM (Global System for Mobile Communication) and **CDMA** (Code Division Multiple Access) are two dominant technologies for mobile communication. These two technologies differ in the way calls and data travel over the mobile phone networks. On comparing both the technologies, GSM has some limitation when the call quality is concerned but still has more flexibility and an easy implementation relative to the CDMA technology. The major difference between the two lies in terms of security factors, their global reach and the data transfer speeds. While in use, the distance from the antenna to user head is about 2 cm or less. Therefore, the user is in the near-field of the source and simple field calculations are not appropriate for the purpose or even a measurement offers no reliability to assess the actual exposure and any field measurement is not possible, more so to calculate the dose.

(e) RF Radiation from Cellular Towers

A study (internet data) presents data related to GSM cellular phone radiation resulting from antenna sites and towers inside residential areas in Germany. A statistical evaluation of over a large number of study representative high-frequency field measurements is presented here in Table 6.2a, b.

TABLE 6.2a

A GSM cellular tower base station power density levels—percentiles.

	Total	With line of sight	Without line of sight	Outside	Inside
Number of measurements (n)	272	177	95	140	132
Distance in meter (median)	150	100	250	200	100
Power density in $\mu W/m^2$					
Mean	1,800	2,650	130	1,150	2,450
20th percentile	10	70	2	20	10
50th percentile (median)	200	430	20	200	170
70th percentile	640	1,700	70	580	640
90th percentile	3,400	5,200	280	3,260	3,770
95th percentile	6,300	8,500	610	6,490	5,330
99th percentile	23,000	25,000	1,340	12,350	32,000
Maximum	103,000	103,000	2,200	14,400	103,000

(Haumann et al. 2001)

TABLE 6.2b

Comparison of standard values and recommendation

Comparison of standard threshold values and recommendations (electromagnetic fields, non ionizing radiation)	**Total power density**
Standards, e.g., GSM1800/GSM1900/UMTS/DECT	
FCC/ANSI—USA	10,000,000 μW/m^2
Germany, England, Finland, and Japan	10,000,000 μW/m^2
Belgium	1,200,000 μW/m^2
Switzerland and Italy	90,000 μW/m^2
Recommendations	
Ecolog Study, Germany (Ecolog 2000)	10,000 μW/m^2
Cellular tower radiation—significant exposure level, 95th percentile (this study)	6,300 μW/m^2
Salzburg, Austria (Resolution 2000)	1,000 μW/m^2
Cellular tower radiation—median level, 50th percentile (this study)	200 μW/m^2
High exposure, Oeko-Test (OekoTest 2001)	100 μW/m^2
EU Parliament (STOA 2001)	100 μW/m^2
Cellular tower radiation—background level, 20th percentile (this study)	10 μW/m^2
Low exposure, Oeko-Test (Oeko Test 2001)	10 μW/m^2
Nighttime exposure, Baubiology Standard (SBM 2000)	0.1 μW/m^2
Successful communication with GSM mobile phone, system coverage requirements	0.001 μW/m^2
Natural cosmic microwave radiation	0.000001 μW/m^2

Cooper et al. (2006) carried out power density measurements in the vicinity of 20 randomly selected GSM microcells and picocells. The base stations employed a single antenna and between one and four transmitters. The antenna heights ranged between 2.5 m and 9 m and the total radiated power was in the range of 1–5 W. 95% of the data fell within two "tramlines" separated by 21 dB. The average power density at a distance of 1m was about $2{\cdot}10^{-2}Wm^{-2}$ which decreased to about $3{\cdot}10^{-3}Wm^{-2}$ at 10 m and $2{\cdot}10^{-6}Wm^{-2}$ at 100 m. The "tramlines" had a gradient of −10 dB up to a distance of 20 m and a gradient of −40 dB per decade to longer distances.

Statistical Data and Percentiles

The percentiles for the observed power density values are presented in Table 6.2a, b, with the median distance being 150 m. This is in the range of typical residential distances to GSM base stations in larger cities. The 20th

TABLE 6.2c

Radiation power density (P_d) at different distances from the cellphone tower power density.

Distance (m)	P_d (w/m^2)
10	0.398
20	0.0995
50	0.0195
100	0.004
500	0.000159

(Pd = $\frac{P_t\, G_t}{G\Pi R^2}$ watt/m^2); where G_t = gain of the transmitting antenna = 17dB (50)
G_{pt} = 10 w, R is the distance from antenna in meters

percentile value is shown to be 10 μW/m^2 and is considered as residential background. The 50th percentile value is found at 200 μW/m^2 (median). The 95th percentile is observed at 6,300 μW/m^2 and can be considered as a significant exposure radiation level. The maximum value of 103,000 μW/m^2 was found in a residential building in the fourth floor (line-of-sight propagation, and it is in the same height to the antenna site at a horizontal distance of 30 m). In addition, data sets for line of sight, without line of sight, inside and outside locations are also obtained (see Table 6.2a, b and Figures 6.6–6.8). This is apparent that the level of radiation intensity in the line-of-site propagation and otherwise is significantly different, with the former being much higher.

Distance, Line of Sight, and Exposure Parameters

In the Figures (6.6 and 6.7), the power density values are shown in two configurations: in respect to with and without line of sight and the distance to the antenna site. Close to the antenna site (<250 m), the GSM radiation levels are scattered due to various influencing parameters and cannot be easily estimated with knowledge of antenna power and distance only. Table 6.2a shows a significant systematic difference between the percentile data from line of sight and without line-of-sight measurements. Figures 6.6–6.8 display the separated sets of data with trend lines decreasing exponentially to larger distances with lower exposures for without line-of-sight measurements in the range of 90% reduction (−10 dB). In general, the radiation exposure is predominantly determined by the following parameters:

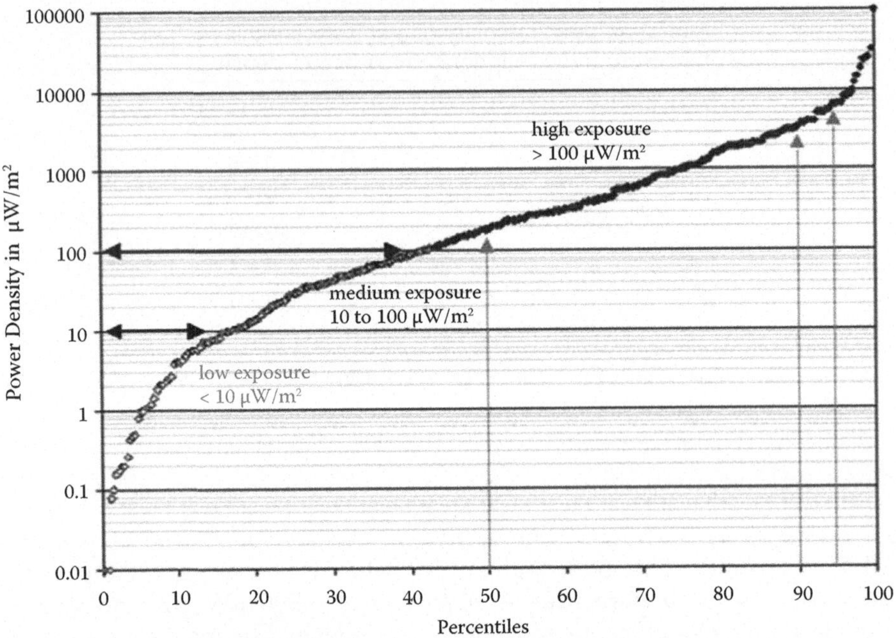

FIGURE 6.6
GSM cellular tower base station power density levels—percentiles.

- Distance (line of sight or not) to the antenna position, type of the antennas (e.g., omnidirectional or directional antennas), and their number, power of each, and their orientation,
- Capacity of the antenna site (number of channels/frequencies),
- Vertical distance(d) between the location and antenna site and the point below (where the measurement is to be performed),
- Type of building construction and that of window glass, and the building material from where the radiations enter the room,
- Physical objects in the environment (e.g., if there are metallic objects, scatters around etc.).

Distance and Phone Tower Positions

The distance profiles were taken for some locations and different antenna heights and positions. For high antenna positions, the power at various positions on the ground is a function of distance (e.g., 50–90 m, pole mount position); the maximum power at ground level is reached in about 300 m and can be considered moderate. As the antenna height is decreased

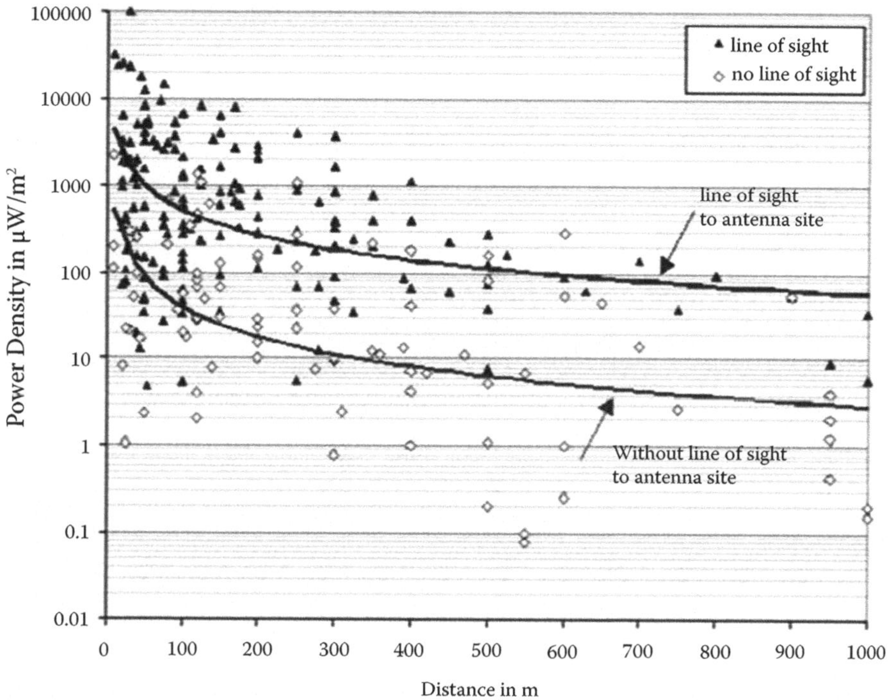

FIGURE 6.7
GSM cellular tower base station power density levels—line of sight and distance.
(Haumann et al. 2001)

(low antenna positions 15–20 m, typical roof top position), the maximum power at ground level will increase and is reached in about 50 m. Figure 6.4 shows the average (mean) density values found in distance ranges. The authors have explained that slight increase in the distance range of 150–200 m (1,480 µW/m^2) is due to the influence of high antenna positions and correspondingly maximum values shifted to larger distances.

Below and Close to Roof Top Positions

Another point of interest is the power levels right below the antenna positions (e.g., schools, preschools, homes) significant exposures in the range of a few 1,000 µW/m^2 are observed due to secondary side lobes and reflections. Highest exposure values in the range of 10,000–100,000 µW/m^2 are observed very close to low antenna/roof top positions at inside and outside locations in line of sight and distance <100 m, a situation which can be avoided in real situation.

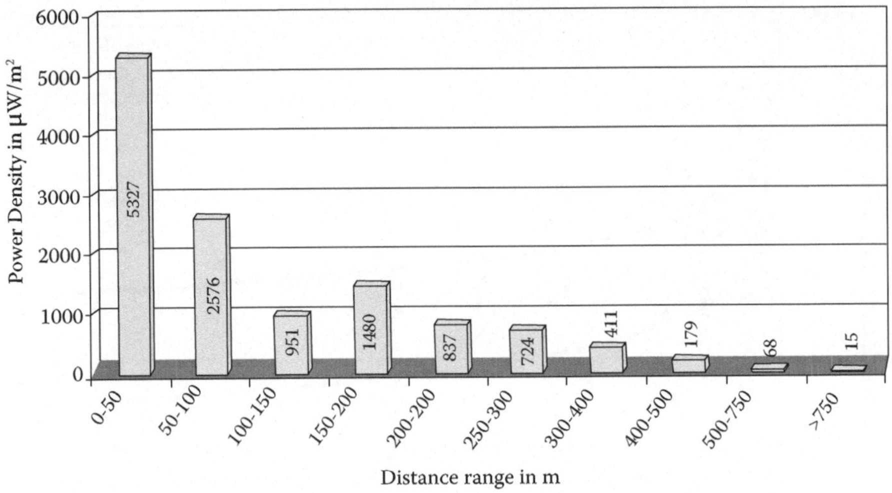

FIGURE 6.8
GSM power density and distance.

DECT, TV,and FM Radio

The data for FM radio, TV, and DECT (Digitally Enhanced Cordless Telecommunication) (cordless phone and other significant HF sources) show that the GSM cellular phone tower radiation is the dominating HF source in residential areas. DECT signals were detected in inside locations. The maximum DECT power density levels were 0.01 $\mu W/m^2$ (20th percentile), 1 $\mu W/m^2$ (50th percentile), and 1,680 $\mu W/m^2$ (95th percentile). High exposure levels > 1,000 $\mu W/m^2$ were only detected when the DECT cordless base station was located in the same room or very close to the testing site.

Summary

The results show that the GSM cellular phone tower radiation is the dominating HF source in residential areas in Germany (and may be in other parts of the world). The median power density is found in the range of 200 $\mu W/m^2$ (50 percentile) with the maximum value exceeding 100,000 $\mu W/m^2$. It may be noted that no location reached or exceeded the official standard values in USA or Germany. For comparison, thermal (official threshold), other nonthermal (recommendations), and cellular tower exposure reference values are listed in the Table 6.2a, b. Average of measured power flux density from various towers at distances (50–500m) is shown in Table 6.3.

TABLE 6.3

Variation of power density with distance

	Measured power flux density levels			
Technology	**50 m**	**200 m**	**500 m**	**Maximum**[1]
CDMA (29 towers)	$2.7 \cdot 10^{-5}$	$3.3 \cdot 10^{-5}$	$5.9 \cdot 10^{-6}$	$8.1 \cdot 10^{-5}$
GSM900 (51 towers)	$3.3 \cdot 10^{-4}$	$2.6 \cdot 10^{-4}$	$2.3 \cdot 10^{-5}$	$7.1 \cdot 10^{-4}$
GSM1800 (12 towers)	$3.1 \cdot 10^{-4}$	$4.1 \cdot 10^{-5}$	$4.7 \cdot 10^{-6}$	$4.3 \cdot 10^{-4}$
3G (35 towers)	$4.1 \cdot 10^{-5}$	$5.6 \cdot 10^{-5}$	$7.6 \cdot 10^{-6}$	$1.4 \cdot 10^{-4}$
All mobile	$3.8 \cdot 10^{-4}$	$2.8 \cdot 10^{-4}$	$2.8 \cdot 10^{-5}$	$8.1 \cdot 10^{-4}$

1 Maximum occurred at distances varying between 50 and 200 m.

Therefore, in respect to recent studies and review of articles regarding nonthermal biological effect of, e.g., digital pulsed GSM radiation, the STOA study concluded with a considerable concern revealing a need for the consideration of RF safety. For example, in 25% of the locations, the long-term exposure levels are very high above 1,000 μW/m², which has been suggested to be the average threshold value for nonthermal biological effects. These levels are reached especially in proximity of the antenna sites (directly below antenna sites) and in line of sight at a distance of <250 m. Two of the most important limiting factors are the distance and the direct line-of-sight to the antenna site. But, in proximity to the antenna sites, the GSM radiation levels are scattered due to various influencing parameters and cannot be calculated easily by using antenna power and distance models only. It has been concluded that, in general, the exposures for without line-of-sight locations are about 90% (−10 dB) lower than those for line of sight.

A criterion for safe exposure is invariably related with the occurrence of biological effects; a threshold of <1,000 μW/m² was marked for nonthermal biological effects. For locations with any long-term exposure, a further safety factor of 10 was recommended for pulsed cellular phone radiation sources as cellular phone base stations. In this case, the power densities should not exceed 100 μW/m². Although, the power density of the radiation used in these experiments is typically found in the head area when using a cellular phone, the information content of the radiation emitted by the latter is the same; accordingly, these results are still relevant to the consideration of potential adverse health effects associated with chronic exposure to cellular or cordless base-station radiation.

Measurements are taken in all distances locations, the median distance being kept as 150 m (450 feet), which is in the range of typical residential distances to GSM base stations in larger cities. The 20th percentile value is 10 μW/m^2 and can be considered as residential background GSM radiation level. The 50th percentile value is found at 200 μW/m^2 (median). The 95th percentile is observed at 6,300 μW/m^2 and can be considered as a significant exposure radiation level. The maximum value of 103,000 μW/m^2 is in a residential building, may be on the fourth floor, falling in the line of sight and lie in the same height to the antenna site at a horizontal distance of 30 m. In addition, data sets for line of sight, without line of sight, and inside and outside locations can be calculated to find out the power distribution in a given area.

In comparison to recommendations for exposure assessment (Test 2001), the statistical data evaluation is done as follows (see Table 6.2a):

a) 20% of data in the range of **low exposure** below 10 μW/m^2 (20th percentile, background level)
b) 25% of data in the range of **medium exposure** between 10 and 100 μW/m^2
c) 55% of data in the range of **high exposure** above 100 μW/m^2.

There is need to perform more data taking in areas where exposure exceeds >10,000 μW/m^2 (Figure 6.6).

Studies on Humans

While the data on human exposure are laden with lot of uncertainties, with corresponding studies focusing on cellular phone towers emissions at various locations and time vis-a-vis the cancer risk needs investigation. This is because of the fact that monitoring human population over a period of time introduces an element of uncertainty which is difficult to estimate.

Buchner and Eger (2011) exposed human fibroblasts to modulated GSM 1800 MHz at 2 W/kg. While acute studies (within 2 hours) did not significantly alter the proteome, an 8-hour exposure caused a significant and reproducible increase in protein synthesis. Most of the proteins are found to cause a significant and reproducible increase in protein synthesis. Most of the proteins found to be induced were chaperones,which are mediators of protein folding. Heat-induced proteome alterations detectable with used proteome methodology would require heating greater than 1°C. GSM-induced heating was less than 0.15°C and hence excluded. These data further supported the notion that the exposure time seems to be a critical factor.

Laboratory studies have looked at whether the types of RF waves used in cell phone communication can cause DNA damage. Some of the studies have supported the idea that the RF waves given off by cell phones and towers donot have enough energy to damage DNA directly. However, the evidences are mounting on to the contrary (e.g.,Lai & Singh 1996; Paulraj & Behari 2006; Behari 2009). While several hypotheses have put forward in support of this, a final picture has yet to emerge.

Several studies in rats and mice have looked at whether RF energy might promote the development of tumors caused by other known carcinogens (cancer-causing agents). These studies did not find evidence of tumor promotion, but this needs confirmation.

A Study by the US Federal Communications Commission (FCC 1996)

A large study by the US National Toxicology Program (NTP) exposed groups of laboratory rats and mice to RF energy over their entire bodies for about 9 hours a day, starting before birth and continuing for up to 2 years. According to the findings of NTP, an increased (although low) risks of brain and heart tumors in male rats exposed to RF radiation, although there was no increased risk among female rats. Some aspects of this study, such as the high doses of RF radiation and the long amount of time the rats were exposed to it, make it hard to know just how well these results might be applied to people. However, the results add evidence to the idea that the signals used in cell phone communication might potentially impact human health.

Recommendations

While a complete blackout of these radiations is not possible, it is probably safe to suggest the principle of prudent avoidance (prevention). This includes implementation of residential exposure minimization and prevention procedures in the frame of the technical feasibility. These will include especially sensitive locations as preschools, schools, hospitals, residential areas, and the workplace.

By official definition, the cellular phone system covers an area when the signal strength of about 0.001 $\mu W/m^2$is reached. We expect that with some technical management, cities, communities, and the service providers will be able to significantly reduce the long-termRF radiation exposures due to cellular phone towers in residential and other areas of choice.

To protect people from EMF overexposure, the International Commission on Non-Ionizing Radiation Protection (ICNIRP 1998; ICNIRP 2010) and the Institute of Electrical and Electronic Engineers (IEEE 2005) have defined limits. In the radiofrequencies domain, exposure to EMF is quantified by the Specific Absorption Rate (SAR, W/kg), whose variability is open to question. The Basic Restrictions (BR) are the fundamental limits expressed in terms of the whole-body averaged SAR as well as local SAR averaged on 1 g or 10 g of tissues.

BR are difficult to check in situ; hence the ICNIRP has also defined Reference Levels (RL) derived from BR (ICNIRP 1998; ICNIRP 2010). RL give the maximum permissible electromagnetic field strength or power density (in the absence of a person). Compliance to RL is deemed to ensure compliance to BR.

HF-Radiation Levels of GSM Cellular Phone Towers in Residential Areas

The GSM technology of wireless communication produces constant pulsed microwave radiation. The cellular base stations are transmitting continuously even when nobody is using the phone. We know from a variety of scientific studies that significant biological effects result from the nonthermal effects of extremely periodic—pulsed—HFradiation as are used in the most common modern digital cellular and cordless phone systems. Official international and national standards and safety guidelines (based on ICNIRP recommendations) take into consideration the risk of thermal effects of high-energy HFradiation. Most of the official HF public exposure measurements are conducted to observe the percentage of the current standard with only broadband—not frequency-selective—measurements. However, it is likely that, in some cases, the guideline value is reached or exceeded close to antenna sites (thermal). Exposure recommendations based on nonthermal effects are lower by many orders of magnitudes. Frequency-selective measurements are necessary to observe the cellular base station downlink frequencies and differentiate from other radiation sources as FM radio or TV transmitters. Therefore, limited information is available on the exposure to cellular base station radiation in residential areas at different distances and directions to antenna sites.

The power density values are displayed in Figure 6.2a, b in respect to line of sight/without line of sight and the distance to the antenna site. The GSM cellular phone tower radiation may be the dominating HF source in residential areas.

The STOA (2001) study concluded: in 25% of the locations, the long-term exposure levels are very high above 1,000 $\mu W/m^2$, which have been suggested to be the average threshold value for nonthermal biological effects. These nonthermal levels of HF radiations could be acute or chronic and may be pulsed or constant HF radiation.

Another concern is that time-averaging of radiofrequency radiations (RFR) to give a single numeric recommendation for a precautionary action guidelines does not address the critical difference with peak power levels. Since biological responses can last over seconds of time or have even longer effects on proteins and enzymes, while the RFR pulses may be in microseconds or millisecond duration, it is entirely possible that what causes bioeffects is the high, intermittent spikes that the body perceives and responds to as one continuous, high power assault. For example in Digital Enhanced Cordless Telecommunication (DECT), the phone peak power is about 100 times larger than what RFR is measured with time-averaging. A person near a cell power station producing an RFR measurement of 0.1 $\mu W/cm^2$ is probably getting RFR power density spikes eight times higher.

These and many other research considerations on the cellular stress response has drawn attention to the inadequacy of EMF safety standards. The synthesis of stress proteins at EMF levels that are currently considered safe indicates that ambient exposure levels can influence the molecular processes involved in protein synthesis needed to provide new molecules and replace damaged ones. The ability of EMF to interfere with normal function and to damage the protein and DNA molecules that are being produced synthesized is a reason to consider this effect for guidance regarding its health implications. It may be emphasized that SAR is the safety standard in the radiofrequency range. A standard based on stress proteins would have several advantages over SAR computation:

1. It is based on cellular protective mechanism that is stimulated by a variety of potentially harmful environmental agents.
2. It is exhibited by a wide range of frequencies in the EM spectrum so there would be no need for different standards in different frequency ranges, as is done presently.

Cancers are believed to arise from mutations in DNA,and changes in DNA induced by interaction with EMF could be a better measure of the biologically effective dose. It may be possible to measure the changes by transcriptional alterations and/or translational changes in specific proteins (Blank 2012).

A study undertaken by Thomas et al. (2008) have shown effects at "lowest observed effect level" (LOEL) of 0.005 μ W/cm^2 on adults exposed to short-term cell phone radiation only (this is not chronic exposure study). Other similar studies are Thomas et al. (2010) with a LOEL of 0.003 $\mu W/cm^2$ and Heinrich et al. (2010) at the same level. Both the studies refer to a mixture of child/adolescent populations of students, but refer to short-term exposure. Buchner and Eger (2011) show a 0.006 μ W/cm^2 "effect level" and tests adult populations, but achieve "chronic" level exposure testing criterion (over 18 months).Applying a tenfold reduction to compensate or the lack of long-term exposure (to provide a safety buffer for chronic exposure) or for children as a sensitive subpopulation yields a 300 to 600 picowatts/cm^2precautionary action level. It may in general be mentioned that the results are available to suggest that a constant exposure may be in the range of micro to nano range to have adverse effects (Kesari & Behari 2009). However, more investigations are needed.

References

Behari J (2009) Biological correlates of electromagnetic field exposure. In: *Toxicology General & Applied Toxicology* (Ballantyne B, Marrs TC & Syver T eds., 3rd Edition). John Wiley & Sons Ltd: Chapter 106, p. 1.

Behari J & Nirala JP (2013) Specific absorption rate variation in brain phantom due to exposure by a 3G mobile phone: problemsin dosimetry. *Indian J. Exptl Biol.*, 51: 1079.

Blank M (2012 supplement) The cellular stress response: EMF-DNA interaction. In: Bioinitiative Working Group, Section 7 p. 14.

Buchner K & Eger H (2011) Changes of clinically important neurotransmitters under the influence of modulated RF fields – A long-term study under real-life conditions. (study reported in German) *Umwelt- Medizin- Gesellsshaft*, 24: 44.

Christ A, Douglas M, Nadakuduti J & Kuster N (2013) Assessing human exposure to electromagnetic fields from wireless power transmission systems. *Proc. IEEE*, 101: 1482.

Conil E, Hadjem A, Lacroux F, Wong MF & Wiart J (2008) Variability analysis of SAR from 20MHz to 2.4GHz for different adult & child models using FDTD. *Phys. Med. Biol.*, 53: 1511.

Cooper TG, Mann SM, Khalid M & Blackwell RP (2006) Public exposure to radio-waves near GSM microcell and picocell base stations. *J. Radiological Protection*, 26(2): 199.

Dimbylow PJ (1997) FDTD calculations of the whole-body averaged SAR in an anatomically realistic voxel model of the human body from 1 MHz to 1 GHz. *Phys. Med. Biol.*, 42: 479.

Ecolog (2000) Hennies K., Neitzke H.-P. &Voigt H., Mobilfunk und Gesund-heit – bewertung des wissenschaftlichenErkenntnisst&esunterdemGesicht-spunkt des vorsorgendenGesundheitsschutzes. ImAuftrag der T-Mobil. Hannover, April 2000. Hannover, Germany: ECOLOG-Institutfürsozial-öko-logischeForschung und Bildung, Nieschlagstr. 26, D-30449.

European Union (2004) Directive 2004/40/EC of the European Parliament & of the Council of 29 April 2004 on the minimum health & safety requirements regarding the exposure of workers to the risks arising from physical agents (electromagnetic fields). 18th Individual Directive Within the Meaning of Article 16 (1) of Directive 89/391/EEC, April 2004.

FCC (1996) Federal Communications Commission, USA.

French PW, Penny R, Laurence JA & McKenzie DR (2001) Mobile phones, heat shock proteins & cancer. *Differentiation*, 67(4–5): 93.

Frey AH (1967) Brain stem evoked responses associated with low intensity pulsed UHF energy. *J Appl. Physiol.*, 23(6): 984.

Frey AH (1974) Pulsed & continuous electromagnetic fields & mechanism of effect. *Annals NY Acad. Sci*, 238: 273.

Gandhi OP (1980) State of the knowledge for electromagnetic absorbed dose in man & animals. *Proc. IEEE*, 68(1): 24.

Haumann T, UWE M, Mares W & Sierck P (2001) HF-Radiation levels of GSM cellular phone towers in residential areas. p. 327. (Internet download).

Heinrich S, Thomas S, Heumann C, Kries R & Radon K (2010) Association between exposure to radiofrequency electromagnetic fields assessed by dosimetry & acute symptoms in children & adolescents: a population based cross- sectional study. *Environ. Health*, 9: 75.

ICNIRP (2010) Guidelines for limiting exposure to time varying electric & magnetic fields (1 Hz to100 kHz). *Health Phys.*, 99: 818.

IEEE (2005) IEEE (95.7) recommended practice for radiofrequency safety programs, 3KHz to 300 GHz.

IEEE Standard for Safety Levels with respect to Human Exposure to Radio Frequency Electromagnetic Fields, 3 kHz to 300 GHz, ANSI/IEEE,C95. 1-1992(2005). (1992). New York: IEEE Press.

International Commission on Non-Ionizing Radiation Protection (ICNIRP) (1998) Guidelines for limiting exposure to time-varying electric, magnetic, & electromagnetic fields (up to 300 GHz). *Health Phys.*, 74(4): 494.

Kesari KK & Behari J (2009) Fifty –gega hertzMicrowave exposure effect of radiations on rat brain. *Appl. Biochem. Biotech.*, 158: 126.

Lai H & Singh NP (1996) Single & double-strand DNA breaks after acute exposure to radiofrequency radiation. *Int. J. Radiation Biol*, 69: 13. See also: Singh N.P. & Lai H. (1996) Use of the microgel electrophoresis assay to study DNA strand breaks after microwave exposure. Proc. Asia Pacific Microwave Conf. (Editor: R.S. Gupta). 1 (B1-4).

Lin JC (2006) Subjective symptoms & mobile phones, (Health aspects of wireless communication). *ACM Mobile Computing & Communication Review*, 10(2): 51.

National Council on Radiation Protection (NCRP) (1986) Biological effects & exposure criteria for radiofrequency electromagnetic fields. Rep. 086.

Oeko Test (2001) Test "Mobilfunk-Sendeanlagen", Öko-Test 4/2001 Germany, April 2001, pp. 32–40. (www.oekotest.de)

Okoniewski M & Stuchly MA (1996) A study of the handset antenna & human body interaction. In: Rosen A & Vander Vorst A (Eds.), Special Issue on Medical Applications & Biological Effects of RF/Microwaves. *IEEE Trans. Microwave Theory Tech*, 44(10): 1855.

Paulraj R & Behari J (2006) Single strand DNA breaksin brain cells exposed to microwave radiation. *Mutation Research*, 596: 76.

SBM 2000 Baubiologic Macs and IBN, Standard der Baubiogischen, Mess technik SBM-2000, Richtwerte fur Schlafbereiche. In "Stress durch Strom und Strahlung", Maes W, 4th Baubiologie und Oekolougie IBN, Neubeuem, Germany.

STOA (2001) The physiological and environmental effects of non-ionizing electromagnetic radiation, STOA-Scientific and Technology options. Assessment, options. Brief and Executive Summary, PE Nr.297.574. March 2001.

Swiss Agency for Environment, Forest & Landscape (SAEFL) (1999) Ordinance regarding protection against non-ionizing radiation (ONIR). December.

Taurisano MD & Vander Vorst A (2000) Experimental thermographic analysis of thermal effects induced on a human head exposed to 900-MHz fields of mobile phones. *IEEE Trans. Microwave Theory Tech*, 48(11): 2022.

Thomas S, Heinrich S & von Kries RK (2010) Exposure to radio-frequency electromagnetic fields & behavioural problems in Bavarian children & adolescents. *Eur. J Epidemiol*, 25(2): 135.

Thomas S, Kuhnlem A, Heinrich S, Prami G, Nowak D, Kries R & Radon K (2008) Personal exposure to mobile phone frequencies & well–being in adults: a cross – sectional study based on dosimetry. *Bioelectromagnetics*, 29: 463.
Vecchia P (2007) Exposure of humans to electromagnetic fields. Standards & regulations. *Ann. Ist. Super*, Sanita, 43: 260.
World Health Organization (1993) *Electromagnetic Fields (300 Hz to 300 GHz)*. Geneva: WHO.

Index